THE
PRIMATE OVARY

SERONO SYMPOSIA, USA

Series Editor: James Posillico

ACROMEGALY: A Century of Scientific and Clinical Progress
Edited by Richard J. Robbins and Shlomo Melmed

THE PRIMATE OVARY
Edited by Richard L. Stouffer

SOMATOSTATIN: Basic and Clinical Status
Edited by Seymour Reichlin

forthcoming

GROWTH HORMONE: Basic and Clinical Status
Edited by Barry B. Bercu

A Continuation Order Plan is available for this series. A continuation order will bring delivery of each new volume immediately upon publication. Volumes are billed only upon actual shipment. For further information please contact the publisher.

THE
PRIMATE OVARY

Edited by
Richard L. Stouffer

Oregon Regional Primate Research Center
Beaverton, Oregon

PLENUM PRESS • NEW YORK AND LONDON

Library of Congress Cataloging in Publication Data

Primate Ovary Symposium (1987: Beaverton, Or.)
   The primary ovary.

   (Publication no. 1546 of the Oregon Regional Primate Research Center)
   ''Proceedings of The Primate Ovary Symposium, sponsored by Serono Symposia, USA, and the
Oregon Regional Primate Research Center, held May 16–17, 1987, in Beaverton, Oregon''—T.p. verso.
   ''Supported in part by Grant RR-00163 from the National Institutes of Health''—T.p. verso.
   Includes bibliographies and indexes.
   1. Ovaries—Physiology—Congresses. 2. Ovulation—Congresses. 3. Primates—Physiology—Congress-
es. I. Stouffer, Richard L. II. Serono Symposia, USA. III. Oregon Regional Primate Research Center. IV.
National Institutes of Health (U.S.) V. Title VI. Series: Publication . . . of the Oregon Regional Primate
Research Center; no. 1546. [DNLM: 1. Corpus Luteum—physiology—congresses. 2. Corpus Luteum
Hormones—physiology—congresses. 3. Graafian Follicle—physiology—congresses. 4. Ovaluation—
congresses. 5. Primates—physiology—congresses. WP 540 P952p 1987]
QP261.P89   1987   599.8'04166   88-2545

ISBN-13: 978-1-4615-9515-1   e-ISBN-13: 978-1-4615-9513-7
DOI: 10.1007/ 978-1-4615-9513-7

Publication No. 1546 of the Oregon Regional Primate Research Center, supported in part by Grant
RR-00163 from the National Institutes of Health

The views expressed in this volume are the responsibility of the named authors. Great care has been
taken to maintain the accuracy of the information contained in the volume. However, neither Plenum
Press, Serono Symposia, USA, nor the editors can be held responsible for errors or any consequences
arising from the use of information contained herein.

Some of the names of products referred to in this book may be registered trademarks or proprietary
names, although specific references to this fact may not be made; however, the use of a name without
designations is not to be construed as a representation by the publisher or editors that it is in the public
domain. In addition, the mention specific companies or of their products or proprietary names does not
imply any endorsement or recomendation on the part of the publisher or editors.

Proceedings of The Primate Ovary Symposium, sponsored by Serono Symposia, USA, and the Oregon
Regional Primate Research Center, held May 16–17, 1987, in Beaverton, Oregon

SCIENTIFIC COMMITTEE

Series Chairmen:
Dr. Robert M. Brenner
Dr. Charles H. Phoenix

Topic Chairman:
Dr. Richard L. Stouffer

Oregon Regional Primate Research Center
Beaverton, Oregon

ORGANIZING SECRETARY

Dr. James T. Posillico
Serono Symposia, USA
Randolph, Massachusetts

ORPRC SYMPOSIA ON PRIMATE REPRODUCTIVE BIOLOGY

Series Editors:
Charles H. Phoenix and Robert M. Brenner
Oregon Regional Primate Research Center
Beaverton, Oregon

1. Fetal Endocrinology, Miles J. Novy and
    John A. Resko, Editors, 1981

2. Neuroendocrine Aspects of Reproduction,
    Reid L. Norman, Editor, 1983

3. The Primate Ovary, Richard L. Stouffer,
    Editor, 1987

FOREWORD

This 1987 ORPRC Symposium on Primate Reproductive Biology, the third in a series, marked the twenty-fifth anniversary of the Oregon Regional Primate Research Center (ORPRC). In organizing these symposia, we have emphasized the dedication of many ORPRC staff members to research with nonhuman primates as models for human reproduction.

The first symposium in this series, organized by William Montagna, was held in May 1981. Appropriately for a beginning series, its topic was fetal endocrinology. The subject of this year's symposium was the primate ovary, and, as in the past, scientists from around the world, including Sweden, Scotland, England, West Germany, and India met in Beaverton, Oregon, to exchange ideas and information on this important aspect of reproduction. The international scope of the symposium reflects our belief that both the problems and their solutions extend beyond national boundaries. Many of the nonhuman primates that we rely on as models are endangered as civilization, through population pressure, encroaches on their natural habitats. Without a deeper understanding of how primate reproduction is regulated, and without the control over human population that such an understanding can bring, the quality of life for all primate species may well become substantially diminished.

Consequently, we dedicate these symposia to the thesis that a deeper understanding of primate reproductive biology will ultimately improve all primate life.

Robert M. Brenner
Charles H. Phoenix

PREFACE

Today there is renewed interest in the processes controlling the gametogenic and endocrine functions of the ovary. Researchers are identifying novel substances within the ovary and attempting to integrate their roles with those of classical hormones. Studies on ovarian function in various species have contributed significantly to the development of methods to control fertility and infertility, including the recent clinical programs on in vitro fertilization and embryo transfer. Nevertheless, the fundamental processes regulating the selection and development of the dominant follicle, the events surrounding ovulation, and the functional life span of the corpus luteum in primates remain obscure. Recognizing the interest in ovarian function in both basic and clinical areas, the editors proposed a gathering to promote scientific exchange on the biology of the primate ovary.

The third ORPRC Symposium on Primate Reproductive Biology, entitled "The Primate Ovary," took place in Beaverton, Oregon on May 16-17, 1987. This event, co-sponsored by Serono Symposia, USA, marked the first scientific meeting dedicated exclusively to the basic biology of the primate ovary and the ovarian processes governing the menstrual cycle and early pregnancy. The symposium (and these published proceedings) were intended to stimulate further research in this field and to promote interest in the biology of nonhuman primates. The format was designed to foster interactions between basic and clinical scientists, as well as primatologists and nonprimatologists. Three sessions (Folliculogenesis, Ovulation and Superovulation, and Corpus Luteum Function) were chaired masterfully by Doctors Stephen Hillier, Gary Hodgen, and Gordon Niswender, respectively. In addition to state-of-the-art topics, submitted abstracts were presented in a poster session. Finally, the task of summarizing the conference and focusing on critical questions was handled superbly by Dr. David Baird. The editors hope that those who read these proceedings will gain a perspective of the meeting and its accomplishments.

Richard L. Stouffer

ACKNOWLEDGMENTS

This year we were fortunate to have assistance from Serono Symposia, USA in organizing the meeting and editing the proceedings for publication. Special thanks go to Dr. James Posillico, Serono Symposia, USA, and Angela Adler, Oregon Regional Primate Research Center.

We also wish to thank the National Institute of Child Health and Human Development (grant No. HD22427), March of Dimes, American Heart Association (Oregon Affiliate), and the Medical Research Foundation of Oregon for their support.

Finally, we wish to thank Dr. Vaughn Critchlow, Director of the Oregon Regional Primate Research Center.

CONTENTS

I. FOLLICULOGENESIS

1. Follicle Maturation and Atresia: Morphological Correlates . .   3
   Marilyn J. Koering, Ph.D.

2. Regulation of Follicle Development by Gonadotropins and
   Growth Factors   25
   David W. Schomberg, Ph.D.

3. Recent Advances in Inhibin Research   35
   Thomas A. Bicsak and Aaron J. W. Hsueh

4. Follicle Regulatory Protein: An Intraovarian Regulator of
   Follicular Response to Gonadotropin Stimulation   49
   Gregor Westhof, Katsuhiko Fujimori, Sharon A. Tonetta,
   Karin Westhof, James Ireland, Jeffrey Fay, Gere S. diZerega

5. Granulosa Cell Differentiation in Primate Ovaries: The Marmo-
   set Monkey (Callithrix jacchus) as a Laboratory Model . .   61
   Stephen G. Hillier, Christopher R. Harlow, Helen J. Shaw,
   E. Jean Wickings, Alan F. Dixson, J. Keith Hodges

II. OVULATION AND SUPEROVULATION

6. Factors Controlling Mammalian Oocyte Maturation   77
   John J. Eppig, Ph.D.

7. Regulation of Ovulatory Processes   91
   William J. LeMaire, M.D., Thomas E. Curry, Jr., Ph.D.,
   Nobuyuki Morioka, M.D., Mats Brannstrom, M.D., Martin R.
   Clark, Ph.D., J. F. Woessner, Ph.D., Robert D. Koos, Ph.D.

8. Angiogenesis in the Ovary   113
   Kenneth J. Ryan, M.D., and Anastasia Makris

9. Oocyte Maturation and In Vitro Fertilization in the
   Rhesus Monkey   119
   Barry D. Bavister

10. Perspectives on Ovarian Stimulation and In Vitro
    Fertilization in Primate Models   139
    Gary D. Hodgen, Ph.D.

III. CORPUS LUTEUM FUNCTION

11. Luteotropic Actions of LH on the Macaque Corpus Luteum 163
    Anthony J. Zeleznik and James Hutchison

12. Luteolysins and Mechanisms of Luteolysis 175
    H. R. Behrman, R. F. Aten, J. J. Ireland, L. K. Soodak,
    J. R. Pepperell, and B. Musicki

13. The Role of Prostaglandins and Catecholamines for Human
    Corpus Luteum Function 191
    Lars Hamberger, Mats Hahlin, and Bo Lindblom

14. Regulation of the Primate Corpus Luteum During Early
    Pregnancy 207
    Richard L. Stouffer, Joseph S. Ottobre, and Catherine A.
    VandeVoort

IV. CORPUS LUTEUM FUNCTION (CONTINUED)

15. The Production and Function of Ovarian Relaxin 223
    Gerson Weiss, M.D.

16. Receptor-Mediated Differences in the Actions of Ovine
    Luteinizing Hormone vs. Human Chorionic Gonadotropin . . 237
    G. D. Niswender, D. A. Roess, and B. G. Barisas

17. The Primate Ovary: Critique and Perspectives 249
    David T. Baird

Keynote Address: Scientific, Legal and Ethical Issues in
    Reproductive Research 261
    Luigi Mastroianni, Jr., M.D.

Speakers and Chairmen 267

Author Index 269

Subject Index 271

I. FOLLICULOGENESIS

FOLLICLE MATURATION AND ATRESIA:

MORPHOLOGICAL CORRELATES

Marilyn J. Koering, Ph.D.

Department of Anatomy, George Washington University
Medical Center, Washington, DC 20037

INTRODUCTION

In most primates studied, the ovary is characterized by its ability to select a single dominant follicle from a pool in which all competing follicles degenerate. This process of follicle maturation and atresia in the adult is cyclic and under control of the hypothalamic-pituitary axis (1). In all primate ovaries, the basic components are similar, consisting of the developing and atretic follicles, corpora lutea, interstitial gland tissue and accessory luteal tissue. It is the numbers and arrangement of these components that vary both during the cycle as well as between the types of primates (Fig. 1-6) (2). The cells composing these structures are responsible for the activity. Therefore, the morphological status of the ovary can reveal important information on ovarian function.

Most information available on primate folliculogenesis and accompanying atresia centers on the selection and growth of the dominant follicle (3) and on ovulation with little understanding of what controls the earlier stages. In addition, the basic structural events that occur from the primordial follicle stage through ovulation are similar in most species with variability existing in the length of time involved. Therefore, studies must now focus on early events of follicle development, both the structural relationships and the hormonal control, which will ultimately expose the mechanisms involved in the early events. Although there are numerous classes of primates, only three genera of old-world monkeys have been studied in detail, and the mechanism closely resembles what is understood about the human. Therefore, most experimental studies have utilized the macaque monkeys, as they have a 28-day cycle and permit a certain amount of manipulation.

The morphological features of follicle maturation and atresia will now be reviewed and correlated with the hormonal events. In addition, the effects of estrogen on follicle maturation will be examined.

BASIC MORPHOLOGICAL FEATURES

Folliculogenesis

In the primate ovary, all primordial follicles are located in the cortex (Fig. 1-6), embedded in dense cellular connective tissue (Fig. 7).

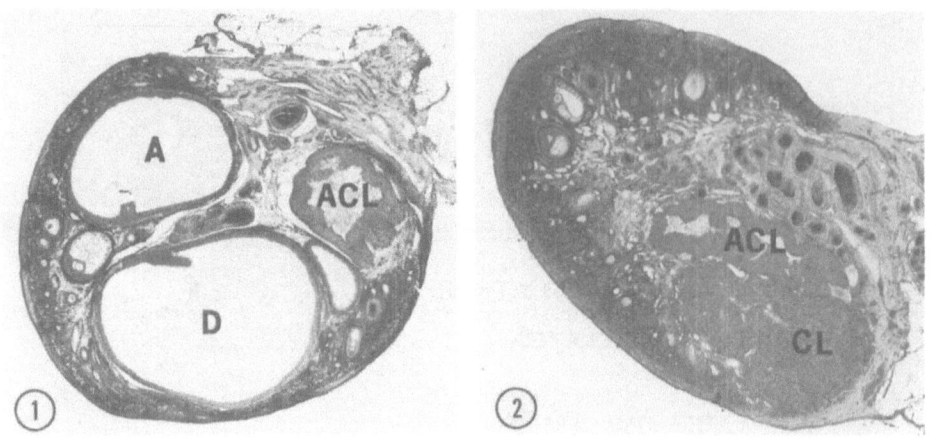

Figures 1 and 2. Sections from a pair of rhesus monkey ovaries
at day 5 of the menstrual cycle. Each section has a definitive
outer cortex in which the primordial and preantral follicles are
located. The left ovary (Fig. 1) contains the dominant follicle
(D), the competing follicle, which is in early atresia (A), and
an aberrant corpus luteum (ACL). The right ovary (Fig. 2) contains the corpus luteum of the last cycle (CL) and an aberrant
corpus luteum. 12x

Although similar numbers occur in the left and right ovaries of a given
individual, major variations occur between individuals (4,5,6). Those
follicles closest to the medulla are the first to be stimulated (Fig. 2,
4, 6). With proper stimulation during subsequent cycles, the follicles
closer to the periphery respond, suggesting that a positive influence is
derived from the microenvironment nearer the medulla. The primordial
follicle in juvenile and adult monkeys is composed of an oocyte surrounded
by a single layer of flattened granulosa cells (Fig. 7). As growth
ensues, the preantral follicle forms. In it, the granulosa cells increase

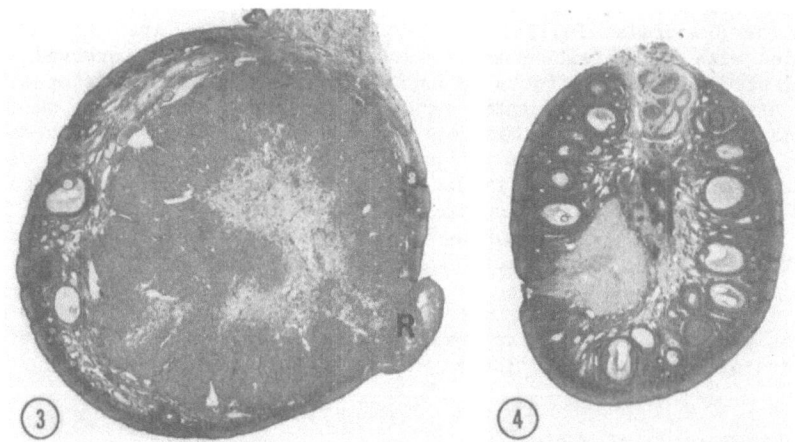

Figures 3 and 4. Sections from a pair of rhesus monkey ovaries
at day 23 of the menstrual cycle. The left ovary (Fig. 3)
contains the active corpus luteum and its rupture point (R).
The right ovary (Fig. 4) contains numerous developing antral
follicles (>1.00 mm in diameter) in the inner cortex. 12x

4

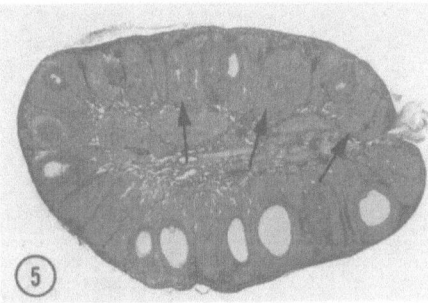

Fig. 5. A section from an adult squirrel monkey ovary. Several developing antral follicles are dispersed between an abundance of interstitial gland tissue (arrows) that formed from atretic follicles. 9x

in size and number with the formation of numerous layers. Simultaneously, the oocyte enlarges (6,2). As growth of the preantral follicle continues, the mean percentages of preantral follicles decrease with increase in size (Fig. 8). Since atresia is minimal during these stages (2), it appears that the rate of growth declines with size. In addition, there is a significant increase in follicles 100-200 μm in diameter during the periovulatory period, suggesting that the hormonal milieu is conducive to stimulation.

Antrum formation begins when a follicle reaches 200-250 μm in diameter, the first sign being the development of fluid-filled spaces between granulosa cells (Fig. 9). Following antrum formation, increase in follicle size is largely a result of accumulation of follicular fluid (Fig. 1), and there is minimal growth of the oocyte (2). As antral follicles develop, all but one will degenerate (Fig. 1). The majority of follicles become atretic when they attain medium size (0.5-1 mm in diameter) (Fig. 11), and it is possibly from this size category that selection of the dominant follicle takes place (7).

When relating this process to the stage of the menstrual cycle, the first sign of an increase in the percentage of developing antral follicles over 1 mm in diameter occurs following the initiation of the demise of the corpus luteum (Fig. 11). Although there are numerous nonatretic follicles

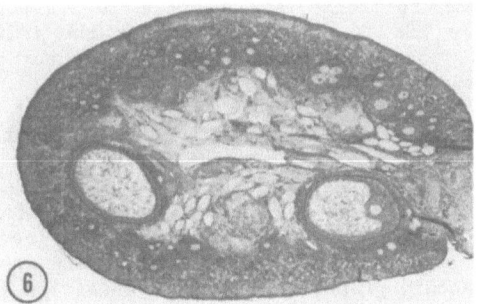

Fig. 6. A section from a juvenile cynomolgus monkey ovary. Primordial and preantral follicles are located in the cortex, while 2 developing antral follicles are more deeply located in the medulla. 22x

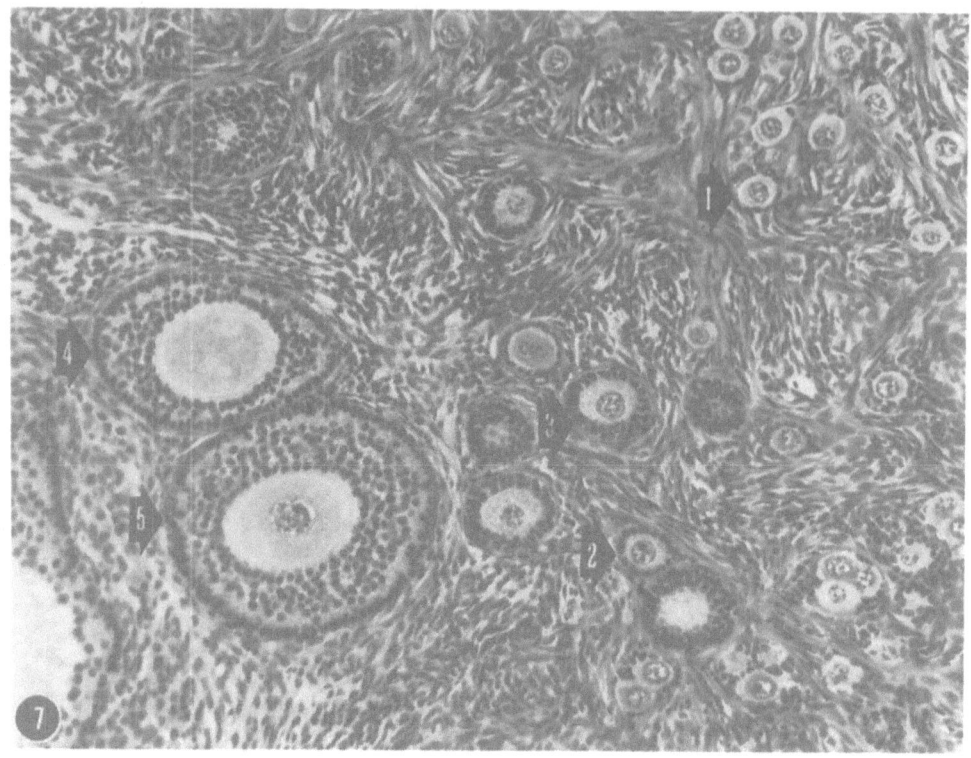

Fig. 7. A portion of the cortex of an ovary from a rhesus
monkey. Primordial follicles (1) are located in the outermost
region. As development occurs, the granulosa cells of the
primordial follicles become cuboidal in shape (2), and the
layers increase in numbers (3, 4, 5). The largest preantral
follicle (5) is 180 μm in diameter, and a thin layer of theca
interna (arrow) can be seen. 196x. (Reprinted with permission
of Alan R. Liss, Inc.)

just under 1 mm during the luteal phase, they have no mitotic activity
(8). However, the progesterone-dominated inhibition of follicle growth
can be overcome by administration of supraphysiological doses of
gonadotropin to monkeys when a corpus luteum is present (9,10). This
suggests that some follicles are capable of responding to hormones.
Although intercycle FSH is not essential for the initiation of follicle
growth (11), it is normally present (12) and may act in a stimulatory or
facilitatory capacity.

During the early follicular phase of the cycle, there is an increase
in the percentages of medium-size antral follicles (7) and large follicles
(Fig. 8). If supraphysiological doses of gonadotropins are given at this
time, more than one dominant follicle will develop (13), suggesting that
more than one follicle can become dominant. In contrast, when normal
levels of FSH are suppressed by the use of inhibin, the larger developing
follicles do not attain proper follicular composition (14). Even though a
follicle ruptures in these monkeys, the resulting corpus luteum is defective and a normal luteal phase is not maintained.

Selection of the dominant follicle occurs prior to day 8 of the
menstrual cycle in most monkeys (3,7). Following selection, there are
elevated levels of estradiol, androstenedione and progesterone in the

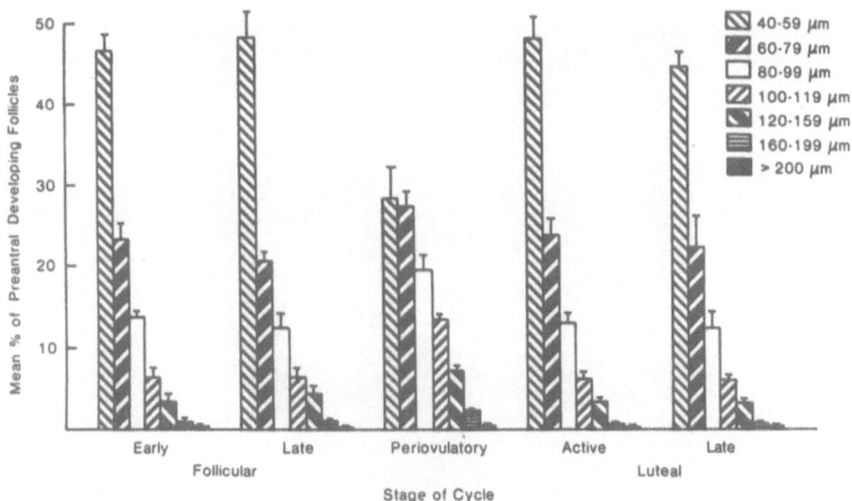

Fig. 8. Status of developing preantral follicles throughout the cycle in the rhesus monkey. The mean percentage of developing follicles in various size categories is depicted at different stages of the cycle. There was a significant increase (P<0.05) in follicles·100-200 μm in diameter during the periovulatory period. (Reprinted with permission of Alan R. Liss, Inc.)

ovarian vein blood draining the ovary with the dominant follicle (3). At the same time, there is an increase in the percentage of atretic medium-size follicles (7). At this stage, elevated exogenous levels of gonadotropins fail to stimulate more follicles (13), suggesting that the dominant follicle has an inhibitory effect on the other follicles. This is supported by additional evidence that estradiol has gonadotropin-suppressing activity (15) which normally interferes with folliculogenesis following selection of the dominant follicle.

At ovulation in the macaque ovary, the remaining developing follicles are 1.0 mm in diameter, and there is an abundance of interstitial gland tissue (Fig. 11) that is derived from the theca interna of late atretic follicles (8). If these cells are capable of hormone synthesis, they may be responsible for the secretion of androstenedione and estrogen as has been shown in less degenerate follicles in the human (16).

During the luteal phase, antral nonatretic follicles can attain diameters up to 1 mm but no mitosis is observed (8). The inhibition is attributed to the presence of progesterone (10), a speculation that is further supported by data showing that follicle growth is resumed earliest in areas most distant from the corpus luteum (17).

Atresia

The majority of developing follicles degenerate: only about 200 ovulate during reproductive life in macaques and about 400 in the human. Although the atretic process is characterized morphologically by cell death, it should be remembered that the theca interna of some atretic follicles may become involved in folliculogenesis. In these atretic follicles, the theca interna hypertrophies and forms interstitial gland tissue (8,2). This tissue is abundant during ovulation in macaque ovaries (2), in late pregnancy in the human (18) and in some new-world monkeys (Fig. 5) and may have secretory activity (2).

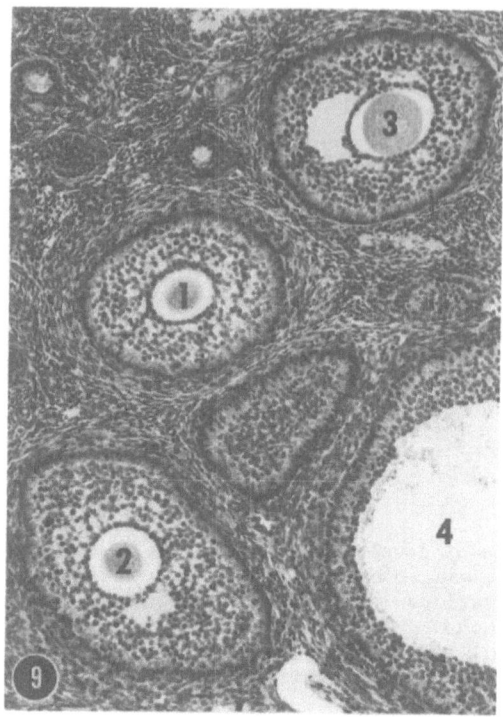

Fig. 9. A portion of the inner cortex of an
ovary from a rhesus monkey depicting three
stages of antral follicle development. The
preantral follicle (1) shows a separation
between adjacent granulosa cells. As
follicular fluid increases (2), small antra
form until there is a distinct antrum (3),
which then enlarges (4). 124x. (Reprinted
with permission of Alan R. Liss, Inc.)

To recognize atresia, certain morphological criteria have been
established, even though it is likely that the initial cellular stages of
degeneration have already occurred at the molecular level. For preantral
follicles, the best indicator is degenerative changes in the oocyte, since
the granulosa cells appear normal (19-21,6). In the rhesus monkey,
preantral follicle atresia is minimal (6). In antral follicles, the best
evidence for regression is the presence of pyknotic nuclei in granulosa
cells lining the lumen (Fig. 10, 12). Such a nuclear change has been
utilized to identify cellular degeneration in other tissues (22).
However, it has been shown that larger developing follicles can have a
small percentage of granulosa cells with pyknotic nuclei in both the human
(23) and monkey (24). With advancing regression, the number of degen-
erating granulosa cells increases (Fig. 12). The basement (glassy)
membrane thickens as the follicle collapses. Finally, the glassy membrane
is the only visual remnant of atretic follicles (Fig. 12).

Morphological signs of regression can occur in developing follicles
as a result of chemical and mechanical trauma and during the later stages
of the maturation process. Therefore, investigators should be aware of
these conditions so proper evaluation of the tissue can be made. Poor
tissue preparation techniques can lead to a breakdown of the oocyte in
smaller follicles (2), so the follicles appear atretic. In addition,

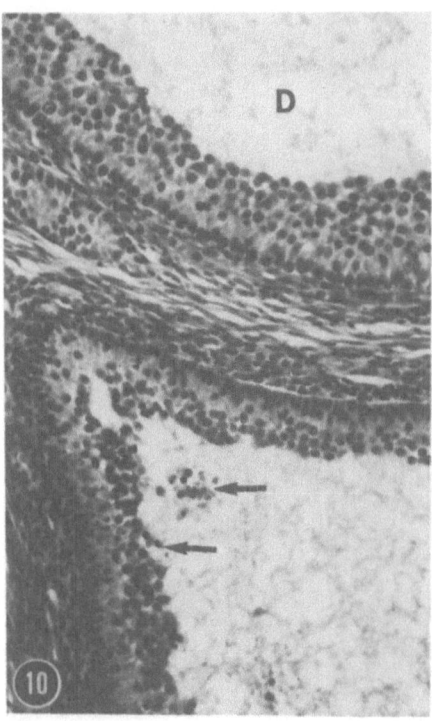

Fig. 10. A portion of two antral follicles with a distinct theca interna,
from a rhesus monkey ovary at day 8 of
the menstrual cycle. The dominant follicle (D) has been selected, and the
competing follicles have become atretic.
Numerous granulosa cells with pyknotic
nuclei (arrows) are located along the
luminal border.   225x

granulosa cells in antral follicles that have been crushed can show signs
of regression. Such granulosa cells have pyknotic nuclei, and the cells
are located along the basement membrane (Fig. 13, 14) of the follicle.
This is in contrast to normal regression, in which granulosa cells with
pyknotic nuclei first appear along the luminal border (Fig. 12). Following mechanical trauma, cells can lose their normal appearance in
minutes (25) and, therefore, the result can be seen in the tissue sections. Incorrect classification can also occur in the later stages of
follicle maturation. In these follicles, more than one area should be
evaluated because granulosa cells with pyknotic nuclei can be unequally
distributed (24). Depending on where the section is made, no cells with
pyknotic nuclei or numerous cells with pyknotic nuclei might be present.

In macaque ovaries, early atresia is most prevalent in medium-sized
(0.5-1.0 mm) antral follicles (Fig. 11, 22, 28). Similarly, atretic
follicles are most common in an equivalent size range in the human (26).
After selection of the dominant follicle in the monkey, the percentage of
medium-sized follicles increases (7), which suggests that the competing
follicles can no longer survive in the new microenvironment where the
dominant follicle has taken control.

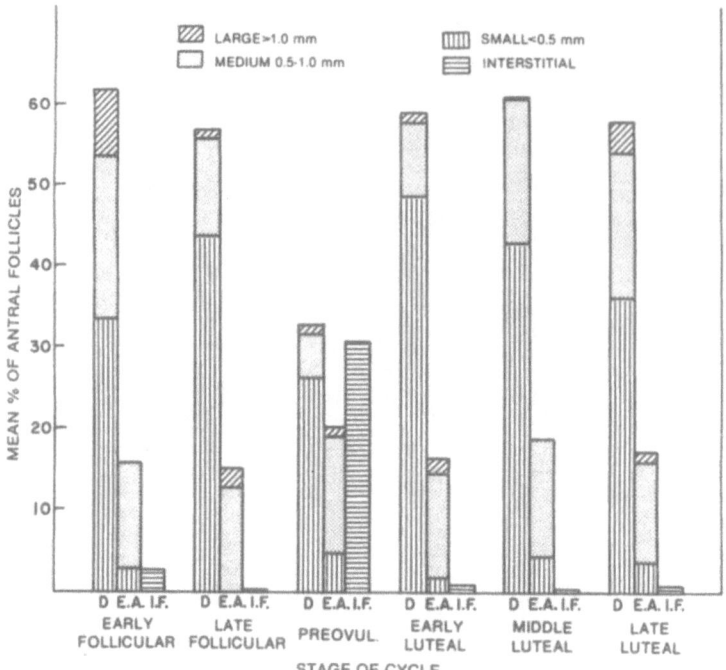

Fig. 11. Status of antral follicles throughout the menstrual cycle in the rhesus monkey. Mean percentages of developing (D), early atretic (E.A.) and late atretic follicles with interstitial gland tissue (I.F.) in various size categories are related to stage in cycle. Modified from (8).

Luteinization

As the wall of the ruptured dominant follicle becomes luteinized, progesterone is introduced into the intraovarian environment. In monkeys and the human, the single corpus luteum is composed of a minimum of two secretory cell types (27,8) and the structure secretes both progesterone and estrogen. During the period of corpus luteum activity, follicular development is arrested with follicles being maintained in the medium-size range in monkeys (8) and human (28). This effect has been attributed directly to progesterone (9) or indirectly to the suppression of gonadotropins (29).

In addition to the typical corpus luteum, two other types of corpora lutea, aberrant and accessory, may be present in ovaries. In some rhesus monkeys, normal regression of the corpus luteum does not always occur (Fig. 1, 2). These structures are retained and are referred to as aberrant corpora lutea (30). Up to five can reside in one ovary (8). They should not be confused with the corpus luteum of the last cycle. Similarly, accessory corpora lutea may appear. These are luteinized follicles that did not ovulate and can be of any size. They can also occur as the result of hyperstimulation during ovulation induction (Fig. 26).

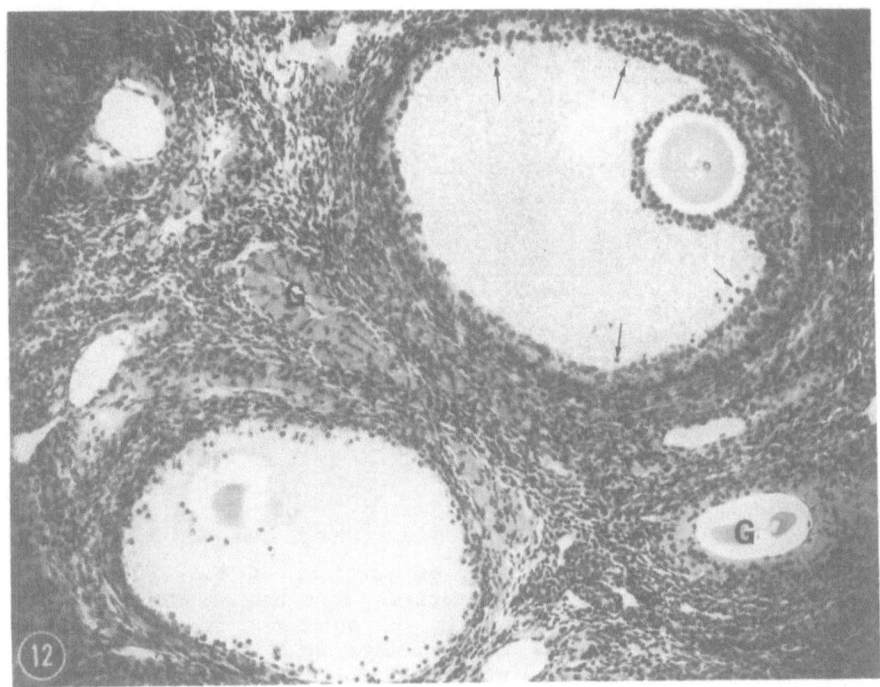

Fig. 12. Portion of a rhesus monkey ovary showing two atretic antral follicles. The largest follicle is in early atresia, as only a few granulosa cells with pyknotic nuclei (arrows) are present along the luminal border. In the other follicle, all granulosa cells have degenerated. Remnants of late atretic follicles are represented by the presence of the glassy membrane (G). 128x. (Reprinted with permission of Alan R. Liss, Inc.)

HORMONAL STIMULATION AND FOLLICLE MATURATION AND ATRESIA

It is known that FSH stimulates the growth of antral follicles in the primate, but the question arises as to what hormones/factors stimulate preantral follicles. In primates, it is also known that preantral and early antral follicle development occurs prior to the induction of normal cyclic behavior (31), an indication that follicle stimulation is not directly related to hypothalamic-pituitary function (32). However, the ovaries of juvenile monkeys are responsive to exogenous FSH (33). In addition, at this age, the neuroendocrine unit is refractory to the administration of estrogen (34,35), which has a possible augmentative effect with FSH. In rodents, estrogens stimulate preantral follicle development (36). These observations on the role of the ovarian-hypothalamic-pituitary interactions in juvenile monkeys led to their use as a model for determining the effects of estrogen, estrogen priming and FSH on follicle maturation and atresia.

Effects of Estrogen

To determine the effects of estrogen on follicle development in a primate, juvenile (12-22 months of age) cynomolgus monkeys (~1.5 kg) were given 30 mg of diethylstilbestrol (DES) in sesame oil for 14 days (Fig. 15). Blood was removed on alternate days, and perineal skin was evaluated as an index of estrogen level. Uterine size was measured before and at

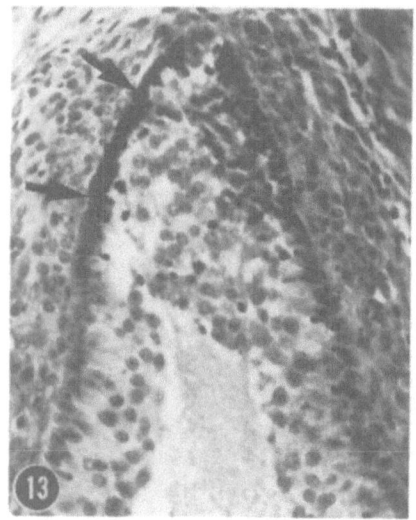
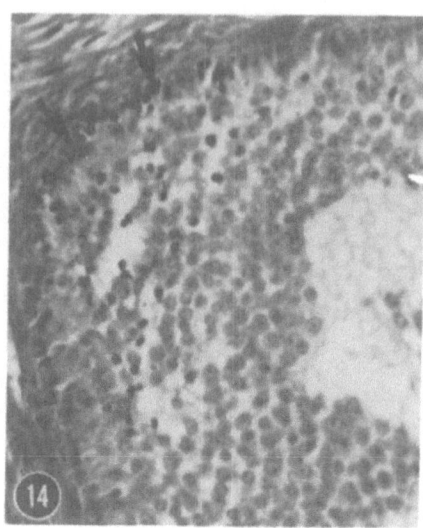

Figures 13 and 14. Sections of portions of two developing follicles from rhesus monkey ovaries. Each has granulosa cells with pyknotic nuclei located in the outermost granulosa cell layer (arrows). Contrast this process, which is likely due to tissue trauma, with normal atresia (Fig. 12). 335x

the end of the treatment period. The left ovary was removed prior to treatment and used as a control since follicle status (number and type) is basically the same in both ovaries (8,6) (Table 1). The right ovary was removed after 14 days of DES treatment. Both ovaries were prepared for light microscopic evaluation. The ovaries were serially sectioned, and the antral follicles on every tenth section were classified and measured. All preantral follicles with more than two layers of granulosa cells and a nucleus present in the oocyte on that section were measured on every fifth section. To determine the percentage of area occupied by preantral follicles, three sections taken at equal distances throughout the ovary were used. All measurements and sorting were obtained with the Bioquant Image Analysis System.

Results indicated that the doses of DES administered caused edema and redness in the perineal region. The width of the uterus increased from 0.5 to 1.5 mm following DES exposure. The results for preantral follicles showed slight variations after treatment, but no significant differences were seen (Fig. 16). The mean percentage of developing follicles de-

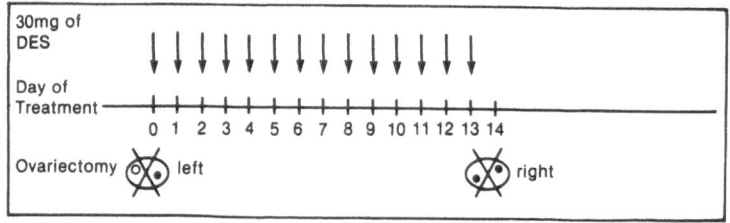

Fig. 15. Schema for the sequence of administration of diethylstilbestrol (DES) in juvenile cynomolgus monkeys and times of ovariectomies.

Table 1. Status following DES treatment.

Monkey Number	Number of Primordial Follicles		Number of Preantral Follicles		Percent of Preantral Follicles *	
	Left	Right	Left	Right	Left	Right
442D	227,370	200,480	100	61	0.04	0.03
MK3	389,527	443,315	370	233	0.09	0.05
MK4	58,530	59,972	831	822	1.42	1.37
				$\bar{x}$	0.51±0.5	0.48±0.4

*percent of area occupied by preantral follicles

creased as size increased in all categories, starting with the 80 μm size group. The reason the percentage is lower for size groups <80 μm is because follicles with less than two layers of granulosa cells were not included in this study. The percentage of area occupied by preantral follicles after treatment also did not vary (Table 1).

Examination of the status of developing antral follicles (Fig. 17) shows a slight decrease in the number of developing follicles following treatment, but it was not significant. Even less variation was seen in early atretic follicles. These data suggest that DES at the doses administered did not have a significant effect on stimulating development of preantral and antral follicles.

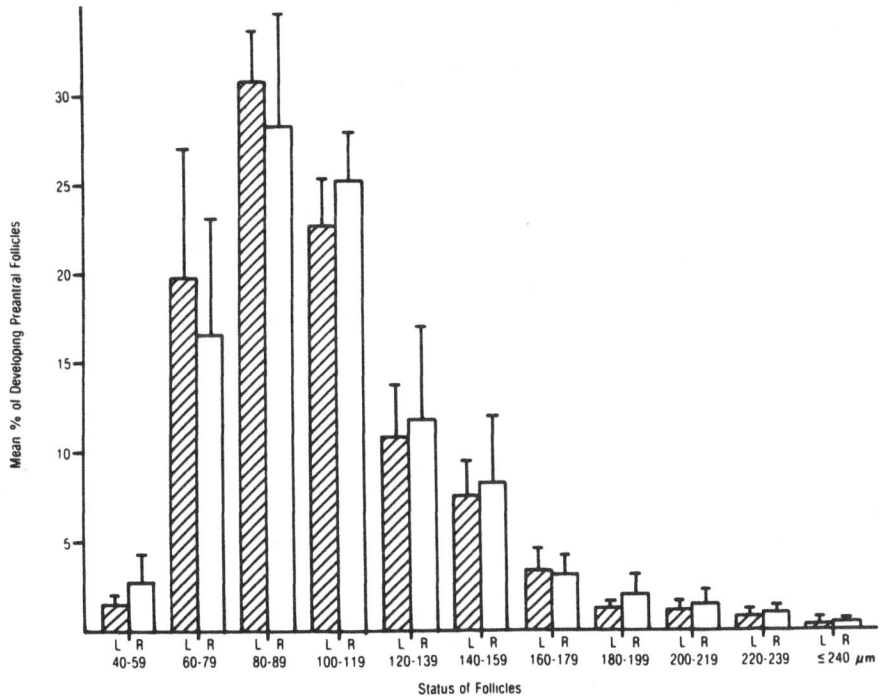

Fig. 16. Status of developing preantral follicles following DES treatment in juvenile cynomolgus monkeys. Mean percentage of follicles before treatment in left (L) ovary is compared with that after treatment in the right (R) ovary in various size categories. No significant changes were detected.

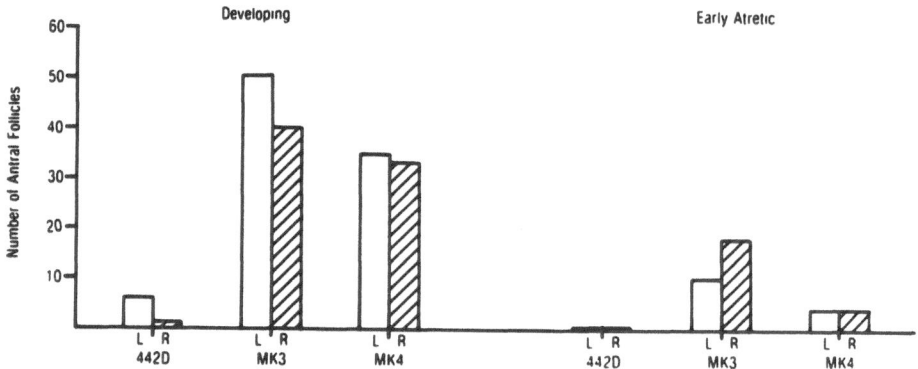

Fig. 17. The number of developing and early atretic antral follicles in the left (L) ovary before and in the right (R) ovary after DES treatment in 3 monkeys (442D, MK3, MK4).

Effect of Estrogen and FSH Treatment

The interest in understanding the possible augmentative effect of estradiol on FSH-induced follicular maturation was stimulated by the observations (37) that DES administered to acutely hypophysectomized rats resulted in increased ovarian response to FSH.

To determine the effect of estrogen priming on follicle maturation, 8 juvenile cynomolgus monkeys were assigned to one (N=4) of two groups: those receiving vehicle-filled capsules and FSH injections or those receiving estradiol-filled capsules and FSH injections (Fig. 18). Blood was removed on alternate days throughout the study and later assayed for estradiol, progesterone and FSH. Silastic capsules (2.5 cm) containing estradiol or vehicle were inserted sc intrascapularly on day 1 (Fig. 18). One capsule was added each day for 4 days (days 1-4) as a means of elevating intraovarian estradiol levels. The capsules were removed on day 6. On day 4, each monkey began receiving daily injections (25 IU) of FSH (Metrodin®, Serono Laboratories). The left ovary was removed 4 days after the beginning of FSH treatment in the first cycle and acted as a control.

On the day following the last FSH injection and if estradiol levels were elevated, 1000 IU of hCG was administered to induce ovulation. The resulting luteal phase lasted 12+2 days. On the day of menses, the capsules were reinserted and FSH given in the same time sequence as previously described for the first treatment cycle. The right ovary was removed after the fourth FSH injection in the second treatment cycle. Both ovaries were prepared for light microscopic examination. The ovaries were serially sectioned, and all antral follicles were classified and measured on every tenth section. Preantral follicles with more than two layers of granulosa cells and with a visible oocyte nucleus on that section were measured on every fifth section. All measurements were made using the Bioquant Image Analysis System.

The hormone assays revealed that exogenous estradiol levels in peripheral blood attained 1300 pg/ml or more, and endogenous levels reached 900 pg/ml (Fig. 19 and 20). Progesterone levels were also elevated due to the hyperstimulation of the ovary, resulting in the presence of numerous corpora lutea (Fig. 24).

14

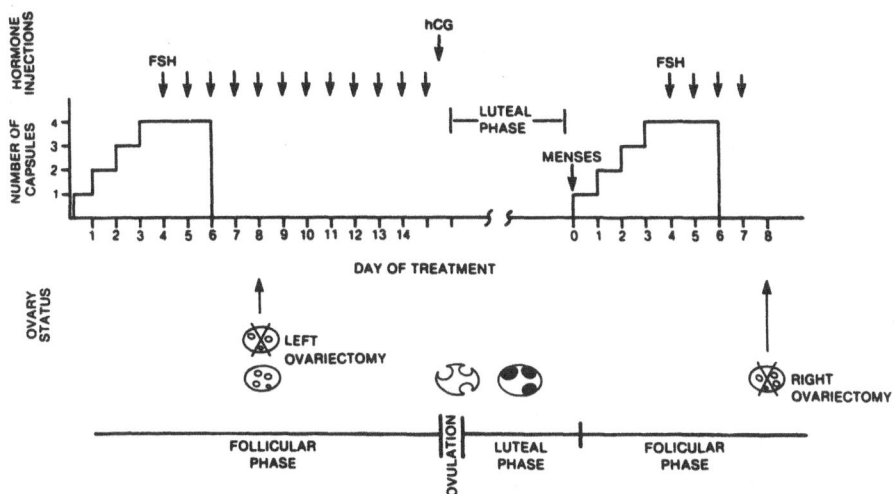

Fig. 18. Protocol for estradiol and FSH treatment. Schema showing administration of hormones, status of ovary and time of ovariectomy for juvenile cynomolgus monkeys. One group of 4 monkeys received capsules that contained only vehicle, and the second group of 4 monkeys received capsules with estradiol. The left ovary was used as a control and removed on day 8 of the first treatment cycle. The right ovary passed one cycle and was removed on day 8 of the second treatment cycle.

When examining the status of antral follicles in groups that received vehicle-filled capsules and FSH, a significant decrease (P<0.05) in the mean percentage of developing follicles occurred after one cycle of treatment (Fig. 21). It is most pronounced in the follicles >1 mm in diameter (Fig. 27). With the loss of developing follicles that occurs in the second cycle (Fig. 23, 24), there was a significant increase (P<0.01) in the mean percentage of early atretic follicles (Fig. 21). The majority of early atretic follicles were in the medium-size category (Fig. 22), which is consistent with what was previously observed in other studies (8,7).

Data obtained after estradiol and FSH treatment revealed similar trends. There was a significant decrease (P<0.05) in the mean percentage of developing antral follicles in the second cycle (Fig. 25) which was also seen in each monkey and was evident in follicles 1 mm in diameter (P<0.05) (Fig. 27). This was accompanied by a significant increase (P<0.05) in the mean percentage of early atretic follicles (Fig. 25) of which the majority were medium sized (Fig. 26). In contrast, when evaluating the mean percentage of developing preantral follicles (Fig. 28), only slight variations were seen after treatment. A significant increase was present in the 80-99 μm category, while the majority of other categories showed decreases.

When comparing the 2 groups, those that received vehicle-containing capsules and FSH versus estradiol and FSH, there is a significantly less (P<0.05) mean percentage of developing follicles >1 mm in diameter (Fig. 27) in the estradiol-primed monkeys. This is in contrast to the overall developing and early atretic groups, which have similar mean percentages in the right and left ovaries (Fig. 21, 25).

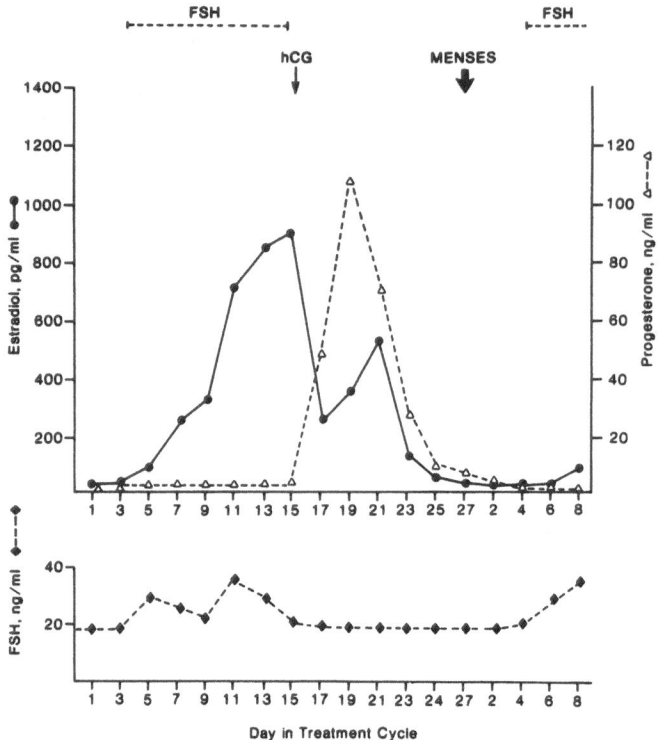

Fig. 19. Exogenous and endogenous hormone levels during the treatment period for monkeys receiving FSH and capsules containing either vehicle.

SUMMARY

These data show that supraphysiological levels of estradiol, either exogenously administered or endogenously induced, cause a decrease in the mean percentage of developing antral follicles, which was accompanied by an increase in early atretic follicles. In addition, there was a decrease in the mean percentage of developing follicles <1 mm in diameter, and this becomes more dramatic when comparing the estradiol-primed with the FSH-only group. There was also an overall lower mean percentage of these follicles in the estrogen-primed group, suggesting that an estrogenic effect was already occurring in the first treatment cycle. In contrast, no differences were seen in preantral follicle activity following elevated peripheral estradiol levels.

These data support earlier work on the atretogenic effect of supraphysiological amounts of exogenous estrogen on preovulatory follicles in the adult rhesus monkey (38). More recently, it was shown that atresia is generally an all or none phenomenon (39). The question remains as to whether this regression is a direct effect on the follicle or is mediated through the hypothalamic-pituitary axis. However, in the present studies, the neuroendocrine unit in juvenile primates is incapable of supporting sufficient estrogen production (32). Therefore, the atresia observed is more likely due to effects of elevated estrogen levels within an ovary achieved through exogenous administration or FSH-induced endogenous secretion of estradiol. Alternatively, the action of exogenous FSH, while promoting the maturation of a few follicles during ovulation induction, ultimately results in failure to stimulate more follicles in the second treatment cycle. This suggests that the recruitment pool of available follicles may be depleted when compared to the first treatment cycle.

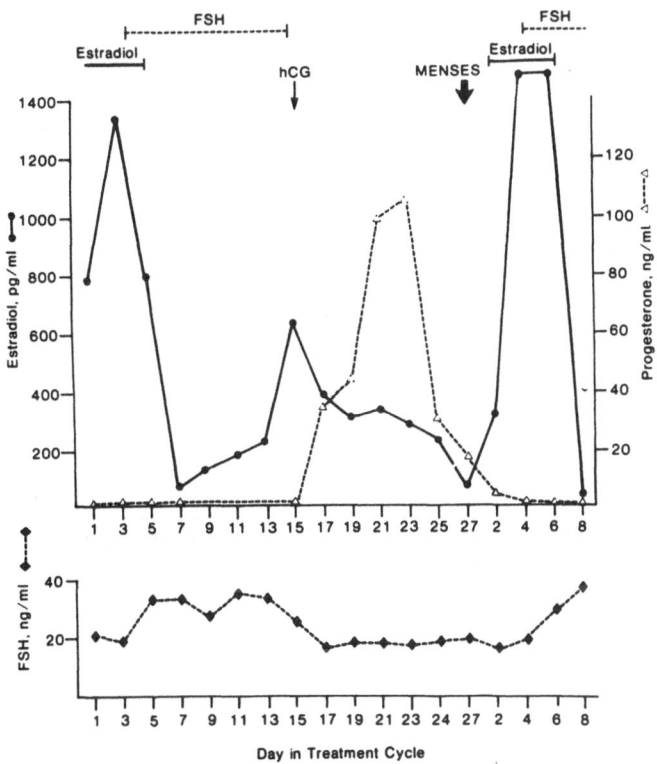

Fig. 20. Exogenous and endogenous hormone levels during the treatment period for monkeys receiving FSH and capsules containing estradiol.

The lack of stimulation of preantral follicle growth by estrogen could be explained simply by its inability to promote follicular development. However, another aspect must be considered and that is whether sufficient intraovarian amounts of estrogen reached the primordial and early preantral follicles. It is possible that the high peripheral exogenous levels did not achieve sufficient elevation within the ovarian compartments to induce development. This could be attributed to rate of blood flow or lack of sufficient vasculature in the ovarian cortex where these follicles are located. Therefore, before totally eliminating estrogen as an augmentative hormone, studies must be done to correlate the morphology of the circulatory system in the primate ovary with blood flow and to demonstrate estrogen access to the ovarian stroma.

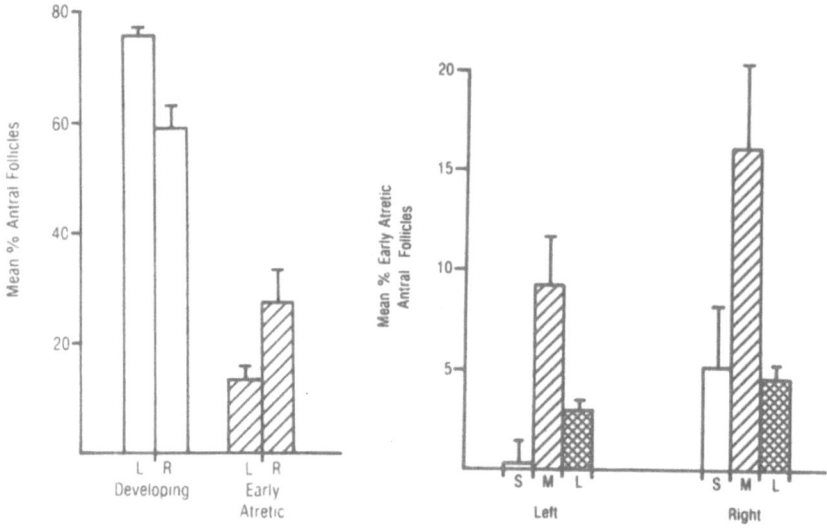

Figures 21 and 22. Fig. 21 (left). Relationship of the mean percentage of developing and early atretic follicles in the left (L) ovary on day 8 of the first treatment cycle and in the right (R) ovary on day 8 of the second cycle. Each monkey received capsules containing vehicle and FSH injections.

Fig. 22 (right). FSH treatment. Relationship between the mean percentage of small (S) (<0.5 mm), medium (M) (0.5-1.0 mm) and large (L) (>1 mm) early atretic follicles from the left ovary on day 8 of the first treatment cycle and from the right ovary on day 8 of the second cycle.

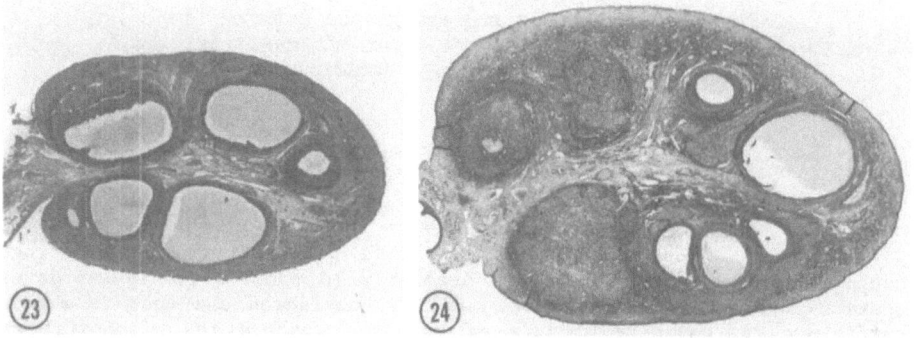

Figures 23 and 24. Sections from a pair of ovaries from a juvenile cynomolgus monkey (B52A). Each ovary has a distinct cortex, and all antral follicles are projecting into the medulla. The left ovary (Fig. 23), removed on day 8 of the first cycle, has 4 follicles >1 mm in diameter. The right ovary (Fig. 24), removed on day 8 of the second treatment cycle, has fewer developing follicles >1 mm than the left ovary but has numerous corpora lutea (CL). 10x

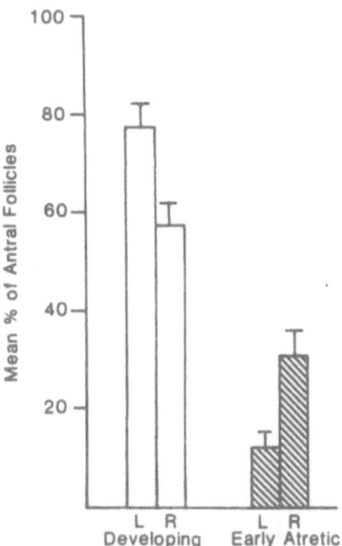

Fig. 25. Relationship of the mean percentage of developing and early atretic follicles in the left (L) ovary on day 8 of the first treatment cycle and in the right (R) ovary on day 8 of the second cycle. Each monkey received estradiol-containing capsules and FSH.

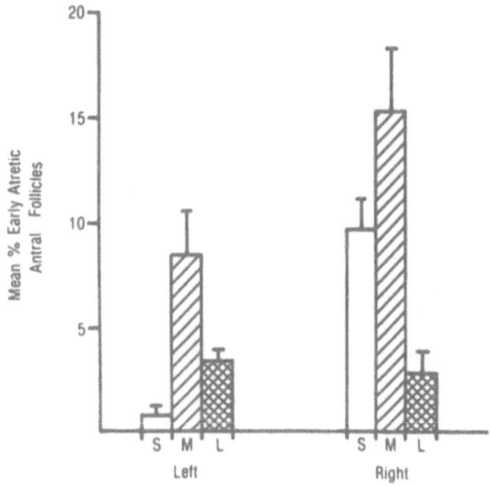

Fig. 26. Estradiol and FSH treatment. Relationship between the mean percentage of small (S) (<0.05), medium (M) (0.5-1 mm) and large (L) (>1.0 mm) early atretic follicles from the left ovary on day 8 of the first treatment cycle and from the right (R) ovary on day 8 of the second cycle.

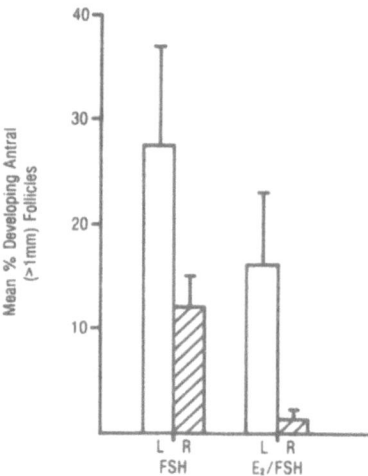

Fig. 27. Relationship between the mean
percentage of developing antral follicles >1
mm in diameter in the FSH treatment group
and the estradiol (E₂) and FSH group. There
is a significant decrease (P<0.05) in mean
percentage of follicles when comparing the
left (L) ovary from the first treatment
cycle to the right (R) ovary of the second
cycle in both groups.

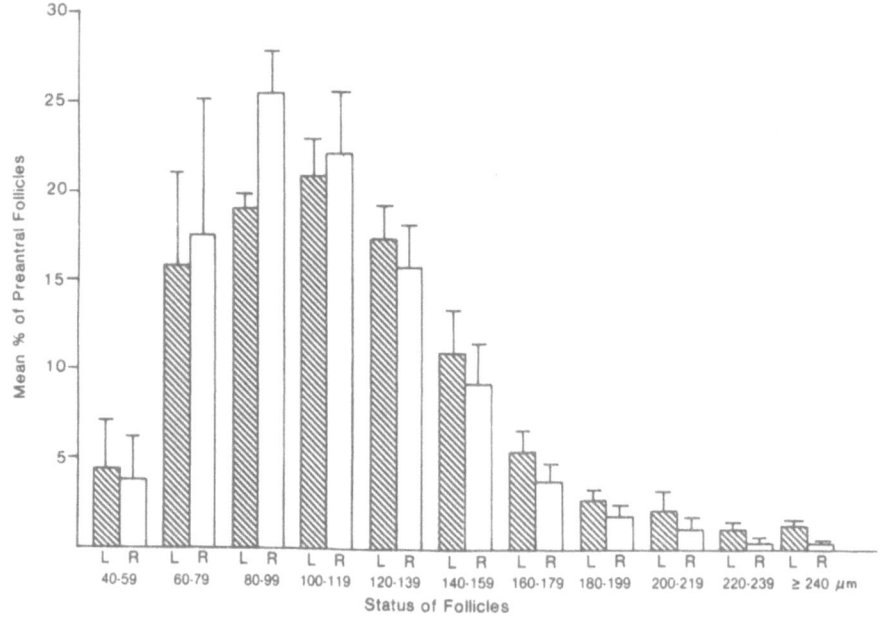

Fig. 28. Status of developing preantral follicles following
estradiol and FSH treatment in juvenile cynomolgus monkeys.
Mean percentage of follicles before treatment in left (L) ovary
is compared with that after treatment in the right (R) ovary for
various size categories.

ACKNOWLEDGMENTS

Recent experimental data incorporated were obtained in studies supported in part by NIH Grant R01-HD-15180 and performed in collaboration with Dr. Gary Hodgen and Dr. Douglas Danforth at the Jones Institute for Reproductive Medicine at Eastern Virginia Medical School, Norfolk. The author is grateful to Shirley Wicklander and Lynn Sharpe for their technical assistance and to Marian Thor and Linda Baldwin for manuscript preparation.

REFERENCES

1. Knobil E. The neuroendocrine control of the menstrual cycle. Recent Prog Horm Res 1980; 36:53–88.
2. Koering MJ. Ovarian architecture during follicle maturation. In: Dukelow WR, Erwin J, eds. Comparative primate biology. New York: Alan R. Liss, Inc., 1986:215–62.
3. Goodman AL, Hodgen GD. The ovarian triad of the primate ovarian cycle. Recent Prog Horm Res 1983; 39:1.
4. Block E. Quantitative morphological investigations of the follicular system in women. Variations in the different phases of the sexual cycle. Acta Endocrinol (Copenh) 1951b; 8:33–54.
5. Green SH, Zuckerman S. Further observations on oocyte numbers in mature rhesus monkeys (Macaca mulatta). J Endocrinol 1954; 10:284–90.
6. Koering MJ. Preantral follicle development during the menstrual cycle in the Macaca mulatta ovary. Am J Anat 1983; 166:429–43.
7. Koering MJ, Baehler EA, Goodman AL, Hodgen GD. Developing morphological asymmetry of ovarian follicular maturation in monkeys. Biol Reprod 1982; 27:989–98.
8. Koering MJ. Cyclic changes in ovarian morphology during the menstrual cycle in Macaca mulatta. Am J Anat 1969; 126:73–101.
9. diZerega GS, Hodgen GD. Cessation of folliculogenesis during the primate luteal phase. J Clin Endocrinol Metab 1980; 158–60.
10. Zeleznik AJ, Resko JA. Progesterone does not inhibit gonadotropin-induced follicular maturation in the female rhesus monkey (Macaca mulatta). Endocrinology 1980; 106:1820–6.
11. diZerega GS, Nixon WE, Hodgen GD. Intercycle serum follicle-stimulating hormone elevations: significance in recruitment and selection of the dominant follicle and assessment of corpus luteum normalcy. J Clin Endocrinol Metab 1980; 50:1046–8.
12. Nass TE, Dierschke DJ, Clark JE, Wolf RD. The role of FSH and the corpus luteum in folliculogenesis and ovulation in rhesus monkeys. In: Schwartz NB, Hunzicker-Dunn M, eds. Dynamics of ovarian function. New York: Raven, 1980; 135–40.
13. diZerega GS, Hodgen GD. The primate ovarian cycle: suppression of human menopausal gonadotropin-induced follicular growth in the presence of the dominant follicle. J Clin Endocrinol Metab 1980; 50:819–25.
14. Stouffer RL, Hodgen GD. Induction of luteal phase defects in rhesus monkeys by follicular fluid administration at the onset of the menstrual cycle. J Clin Endocrinol Metab 1980; 51:669–71.
15. Zeleznik AJ, Hutchison JS, Schuler HM. Interference with the gonadotropin-suppressing actions of estradiol in macaques overrides the selection of a single preovulatory follicle. Endocrinology 1985; 117:991–9.
16. Brailly S, Gougeon A, Milgrom E, Bomsel-Helmreich O, Papiernik E. Importance of changes in the transformation of progestin into androgen during preovulatory development and atresia of human follicles. In: Rolland R, van Hall EV, Hillier SG, McNatty KP,

Schoemaker J, eds. Follicular maturation and ovulation. Amsterdam: Excerpta Medica, 1982:180-7.

17. diZerega GS, Hodgen GD. The interovarian progesterone gradient: a spatial and temporal regulator of folliculogenesis in the primate ovarian cycle. J Clin Endocrinol Metab 1982; 54:495-9.

18. Mossman HW, Koering MJ, Ferry D. Cyclic changes of interstitial gland tissue of the human ovary. Am J Anat 1964; 115:235-56.

19. Vermande-Van Eck GJ. Neo-ovogenesis in the adult monkey. Anat Rec 1956; 125:207-24.

20. Byskov AG. Atresia. In: Midgley AR, Sadler WA, eds. Ovarian follicular development and function. New York: Raven, 1979; 41-57.

21. Gougeon A. Cinetique de la croissance et de l'involution des follicules ovariens pendant le cycle menstruel chez la femme. These de doctorat d'etat es sciences naturelles, University of Paris, 1981.

22. Leuchtenberger C. A cytochemical study of pycnotic nuclear degeneration. Chromosoma 1950; 3:449-73.

23. Brailly S, Gougeon A, Milgrom E, Bomsel-Helmreich O, Papiernik E. Androgens and progestins in the human ovarian follicle: differences in the evolution of preovulatory, healthy nonovulatory, atretic follicles. J Clin Endocrinol Metab 1981; 53:128-34.

24. Koering MJ, Goodman AL, Williams RF, Hodgen GD. Granulosa cell pyknosis in the dominant follicle of monkeys. Fertil Steril 1982; 37:837-44.

25. Searle J, Kerr JFR, Bishop CJ. Necrosis and apoptosis: distinct modes of cell death with fundamentally different significance. Pathol Annu 1982; 17:229-59.

26. Chikazawa K, Araki S, Tamada T. Morphological and endocrinological studies on follicular development during the human menstrual cycle. J Clin Endocrinol Metab 1986; 62:305-13.

27. Corner GW, Hartman CG, Bartelmez GW. Development, organization and breakdown of the corpus luteum in the rhesus monkey. Contr Embry Carneg Inst 1945; 31:117-46.

28. Block E. Quantitative morphological investigations of the follicular system in women. Variations at different ages. Acta Anat (Basel) 1952; 14:108-23.

29. Baird DT, Backstrom T, McNeilly AS, Smith SK, Wathen CG. Effect of enucleation of the corpus luteum at different stages of the luteal phase of the human menstrual cycle on subsequent follicular development. J Reprod Fertil 1984; 70:615-24.

30. Corner GW, Bartelmez GW, Hartman CG. On normal and aberrant corpora lutea of the rhesus monkey. Am J Anat 1936; 59:433-57.

31. van Wagenen G, Simpson ME. Postnatal development of the ovary in Homo sapiens and Macaca mulatta. New Haven: Yale University Press, 1973.

32. Wildt L, Marshall G, Knobil E. Experimental induction of puberty in the infantile female rhesus monkey. Science 1980; 207:1373-5.

33. Kenigsberg D, Littman BA, Williams RF, Hodgen GD. Medical hypophysectomy: II. Variability of ovarian response to gonadotropin therapy. Fertil Steril 1984; 42:116-26.

34. Dierschke DJ, Karsch FJ, Weick RF, Weiss G, Hotchkiss J, Knobil E. Hypothalamic-pituitary regulation of puberty: feedback control of gonadotropin secretion in the rhesus monkey. In: Grumbach MM, Grave GD, Mayer FE, eds. Control of the onset of puberty. New York: Wiley, 1974; 104-14.

35. Williams RF, Turner CK, Hodgen GD. The late pubertal cascade in perimenarchial monkeys: onset of asymmetrical ovarian estradiol secretion and bioassayable luteinizing hormone release. J Clin Endocrinol Metab 1982; 55:660-5.

36. Pencharz RI. Effect of estrogens and androgens alone and in combination with chorionic gonadotropin on the ovary of the hypophysectomized rat. Science 1940; 91:554-5.

37. Goldenberg RL, Vaitukaitis JL, Ross GT. Estrogen and follicle stimulating hormone interactions on follicle growth in rats. Endocrinology 1972; 90:1492-8.
38. Clark JR, Dierschke DJ, Wolf RC. Hormonal regulation of ovarian folliculogenesis in rhesus monkeys: III. Atresia of the preovulatory follicle induced by exogenous steroids and subsequent follicular development. Biol Reprod 1981; 25:332-41.
39. Dierschke DJ, Hutz RJ, Wolf RC. Induced follicular atresia in rhesus monkeys: strength-duration relationships of the estrogen stimulus. Endocrinology 1985; 117:1397-403.

REGULATION OF FOLLICLE DEVELOPMENT BY GONADOTROPINS AND GROWTH FACTORS

David W. Schomberg, Ph.D.

Professor, Departments of Obstetrics and Gynecology
and Physiology
Duke University Medical Center
Durham, NC 27710

INTRODUCTION

The hypothesis that growth factors interact with reproductive hormones to modulate cellular function is attractive because it extends our
concepts of reproductive endocrinology to the level of cell-cell regulation. In the most general sense, one could propose three working hypotheses by which growth factors and reproductive hormones could interact to
modulate reproductive function: (1) reproductive hormones might modulate
the production of and/or cellular responsiveness to growth factors; (2)
growth factors might modulate the production of and/or cellular responsiveness to reproductive hormones; and, (3) target cells for certain
growth factors or reproductive hormones may respond directly only to their
specific regulators, but interact with each other via gap-junction-
mediated second messenger systems.

Testing of the above hypotheses is particularly appropriate and
challenging in the case of the ovarian follicle, since during its maturation, simultaneous regulation of both growth and differentiative processes
occurs in a properly balanced developmental context. In this chapter,
results from our laboratory as well as those of others, will be reviewed
which support the concept of growth factor-gonadotropin interaction in
ovarian function. Since this area is truly in its infancy, several of
these observations hold exciting promise for future avenues of research.

PROPERTIES OF SELECTED GROWTH FACTORS AND FOLLICULAR CELLS
WHICH DETERMINE SUITABLE EFFECTOR-TARGET CELL COMBINATIONS

In the past few years, literally dozens of putative growth factors
have been isolated from as many different tissues or fluids. A consensus
is growing, however, that many of these factors will prove to be identical
in amino acid sequence to several of the growth factors already identified. Thus, most of the putative factors excluding angiogenesis factors
and those regulating the immune system can likely be categorized into
approximately five major groups with identical or near-identical homology
to the following: (1) Insulin-Like Growth Factors (IGFs), (2) Fibroblast
Growth Factors (FGFs), (3) Epidermal Growth Factor (EGF), (4) Transforming

Growth Factors (TGFs), and (5) Platelet-Derived Growth Factor (PDGF). Factors from all of these classes have already been studied in combination with isolated follicular cells or intact follicle preparations in vitro and to a very limited extent in some in vivo models.

Growth Factor Responsiveness

Even though members of all the growth factor "families" mentioned above have been studied with respect to regulation of growth and/or differentiation of various follicular cell types, bona fide ovarian cellular receptors have not yet been demonstrated for all of the factors for which a biological response has been demonstrated experimentally. Somatomedin-C (SmC) or IGF-1 receptors have been demonstrated in rat and porcine granulosa cell preparations (1-3). Likewise, EGF receptors have been demonstrated on cells of the same two species as well as on bovine cells (4-6). Some regulation of these receptor populations has been reported, but much more needs to be done to establish the extent to which the receptors for either of these factors is regulated by the classical reproductive hormones. An examination of the only two reports available thus far with respect to the in vitro effect of FSH upon EGF receptor binding by rat and porcine granulosa cells (marked increase vs. slight decrease, respectively; 7,8) points to a need to understand these phenomena in a developmental context.

The effects of FGF and TGF-β upon cultured granulosa cells have been well documented (9-13), but the binding characteristics of their putative receptors have not yet been published because of scarcity of pure labeled ligands. An investigation of the receptor population(s) for TGF-β might prove quite interesting given several recent discoveries regarding its action, e.g., (1) its structural homology with inhibin (14), (2) its physiological similarity to activin and FSH Releasing Protein (FRP) in enhancing FSH production by cultured pituitary cells (15,16), (3) its ability to facilitate FSH-dependent steroidogenesis and LH receptor induction in rat granulosa cells (11-13,17); and, (4) its ability to enhance ^{3}H-thymidine incorporation into porcine granulosa cells when combined with EGF and IGF-1 (18). Thus, with respect to granulosa cells, this compound has potential mitotic activity different from that reported for other epithelial cells, and it potentiates different responses depending upon the state of cell maturation and/or the presence of other effectors in the environment. It is difficult to explain how the same compound could exert such different functional responses. Some possibilities have been reviewed (19). In rat liver and mink lung epithelial cells, up to 3 TGF-β binding proteins have been identified which meet the criterion of receptor binding on the basis of affinity (20). The form which is "coupled" to the mitogenic response has not been identified unequivocally. The possibility that different receptor forms might be functionally coupled to different cellular responses is an attractive idea for future research. Granulosa cells, which mature from a relatively undifferentiated, mitotically active state to a very highly differentiated, non-mitotic form may constitute a unique model system for investigation of this issue.

Among the various growth factor-gonadotropin-follicular cell interrelationships, the role of PDGF is the most problematical. We initially reported that PDGF potentiated FSH-mediated LH receptor induction in the rat granulosa cell model and postulated that PDGF may contribute somehow to the terminal differentiation of granulosa cells into luteal cells at the corpus hemorrhagicum stage following follicle rupture (10). The experimental observations were confirmed by Knecht and Catt (21). We subsequently noted that different and successively more highly purified PDGF preparations diverged widely with respect to mitogenic activity and differentiating activity (22), leading to the hypothesis that the component of PDGF preparations responsible for potentiating LH receptor induction may not be PDGF itself. Further work in our laboratory shows that the active material from human platelet preparations purified through ion-exchange, hydrophobic interaction, and molecular sieving (Bio-Gel P-60) procedures essentially according to Heldin et al. (23) is not, in fact, PDGF (unpublished observations). The active moiety from P-60 fractions does not migrate at Mr 30–32,000 on SDS polyacrylamide gel electrophoresis but instead migrates at Mr 25,000. Thus, it is reasonable to conclude that the effects upon rat granulosa cells previously ascribed to PDGF (10,21), are due to other components of the platelet preparation, a prime candidate being TGF-β. Efforts are currently underway in our laboratory to establish definitely whether this growth factor is, in fact, the active component.

The above findings still leave open the question of the role of pure PDGF. Studies in progress in our laboratory by Dr. I-C. Kim indicate that fractions from the "PDGF only" region of Bio-Gel P-60 eluates which were very potent in stimulating ^{3}H-thymidine incorporation in BALB/c-3T3 fibroblasts did not potentiate FSH-dependent LH receptor induction in rat granulosa cell cultures. The results shown in Figure 1 indicate that very high doses of this PDGF preparation did not contain sufficient amounts of contaminating activity to potentiate induction; impure preparations of 0.3–120 U/ml PDGF have been previously shown to potentiate induction (22).

Before concluding that PDGF has no role in granulosa or luteal cell physiology, studies should be performed with the pure compound at different stages of cell development, particularly at the corpus hemorrhagicum stage where platelet products come into direct contact with the cells. Human granulosa cells from in vitro fertilization (IVF) protocols should be uniquely appropriate for these studies. From a theoretical point of view, Westermark et al. have argued that granulosa cells are an epithelial cell type based on classical morphology, and thus should not contain PDGF receptors (24). However, granulosa cells are, in fact, an interesting "hybrid" cell type based upon cytoskeletal immunocytochemical staining for intermediate filaments and cytokeratins. Based upon these studies, Czernobilsky et al. (25) have shown that human granulosa cells possess both specific cytokeratins, characteristic of epithelial cells, and vimentin, characteristic of mesenchymal cells; porcine and rat granulosa cells contain significant amounts of vimentin. Therefore, granulosa cells can be considered as a cell type which theoretically could contain PDGF receptors, the expression and/or function of which may be developmentally dependent.

As indicated previously, human granulosa cells from IVF procedures constitute a useful model system for certain experimental objectives. Utilizing culture techniques, a good deal of information has been obtained with respect to production of and responsiveness to reproductive hormones. Estrogen and progesterone secretion, at least under basal conditions, has been characterized in short (hours), moderate (up to 6 days) and long-term (up to 12 days) culture (26–28). Responsiveness to FSH and hCG has been documented (27); binding studies have demonstrated bona fide high-affinity hCG receptor sites (29). Steroid production and microfilament and/or microtubule changes can also be elicited by agents which enhance intracellular cAMP levels (30). A striking feature of steroidogenesis is the sustained, high-level production of estrogen by these cells in the absence of exogenous gonadotropin. Estrogen production from androstenedione is maintained at the same level from 3 to at least 12 days of culture. This level of synthetic capability is not diminished by the systematic withholding of androgen substrate for up to 9 days of culture; progesterone production is likewise maintained at a very high level for the same period (28). Cell viability, attachment, and steroid production are not maintained, however, when the cells are cultured under serum-free conditions in a medium containing low-density lipoprotein (unpublished observations). Other non-gonadotropic serum constituents, therefore, must play a significant role in maintaining normal cellular function. As in the case of the nonprimate cell models, growth factors can be considered as one class of effectors which could facilitate normal function.

Using Scatchard analysis (31), high-affinity, low-capacity binding sites for IGF-1 can be demonstrated on IVF derived cells (unpublished observations), suggesting that cellular responsiveness could be demonstrated under the appropriate conditions. Perhaps because of the high rate and level of steroid production demonstrated above, we have been unable to demonstrate potentiation of basal or hCG-stimulated progesterone secretion by IGF-1 under serum step-down conditions from days 3-6 of culture (Fig. 2). Using serum-free conditions, Garzo and Dorrington (32) demonstrated that insulin augmented FSH-stimulated aromatase activity by granulosa cells from normally developing follicles 0.4-1.5 cm in diameter. In addition to the issue of prior hormonal stimulation, issues such as growth factor content of serum, serum binding proteins, duration of culture, and selection of the proper response parameter may be important considerations in assessing the influence of growth factors upon granulosa/luteal cell responsiveness in vitro.

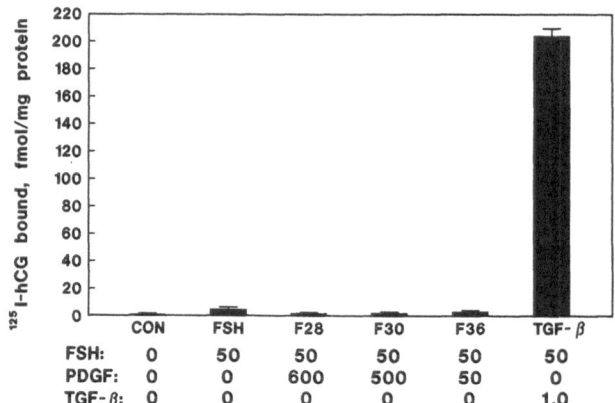

Fig. 1. Comparison of very highly purified PDGF and TGF-β upon FSH-mediated LH receptor induction in rat granulosa cell cultures. These experiments were carried out according to previously published procedures wherein the test substances were added to insulin-containing nutrient medium from days 3-6 of culture; the cultures were established in 3% serum (22). The dose of hFSH (LER 1577; 50 ng/ml) was selected to give a marginal inductive effect. TGF-β (1 ng/ml) markedly stimulated the response. TGF-β alone does not stimulate induction in this system (data not shown). PDGF prepared free of TGF-β by electrophoretic analysis using silver staining did not potentiate induction at levels of 50-600 units/ml. The "F" numbers refer to fraction numbers of a Bio-Gel P-60 column purification. PDGF activity (units/ml) was determined by ^{3}H-thymidine incorporation into Balb/C-3T3 cells.

Growth Factor Production

The production of immunoreactive IGF-1 by the rat ovary in response to growth hormone and by cultured porcine granulosa cells in response to FSH and estradiol has been demonstrated (33,34). In the latter study, Hsu and Hammond (34) also demonstrated that FSH and estradiol increase the production of an IGF-1 binding protein.

No information is available as to whether reproductive hormones modulate EGF production in the ovary. This is not an issue that can be easily resolved because of the facts that: (1) antisera have not been generated to EGF from species other than the human and the mouse, and (2) even with appropriate antibodies for radioimmunoassay (RIA) or immunoprecipitation, the presence of EGF binding proteins may complicate the results, as has been a problem for quantitation of IGF-1. Prepro EGF mRNA has been detected in mouse ovarian tissue (35).

Using anti-porcine TGF-β in RIA and immunoprecipitation procedures, and soft-agar bioassay, Skinner et al. have recently identified TGF-β in conditioned medium of bovine and rat thecal cultures; granulosa cell conditioned medium contained smaller amounts of activity (36). This is an exciting observation, because coupled with the previously demonstrated effects of TGF-β upon granulosa cell steroidogenesis and LH receptor induction, it establishes a paracrine or autocrine role for TGF-β in the ovarian follicle. Since TGF-β shares significant sequence homology with inhibin, activin, FRP, and Mullerian Inhibiting Substance (MIS), all of which are found in the follicle, it heightens the need to study the regulation of this gene family in order to understand more thoroughly the cellular mechanisms underlying follicle development, selection, and atresia.

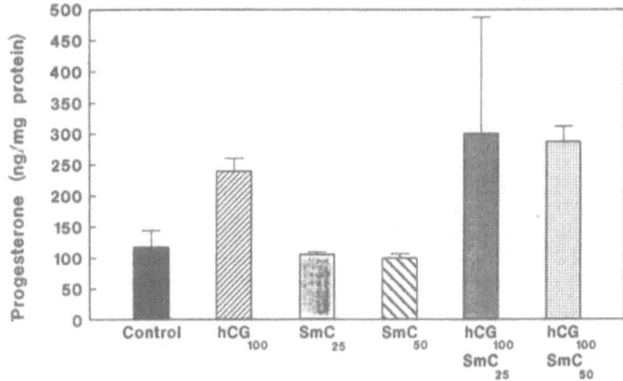

Fig. 2. Lack of effect of SmC upon basal or hCG-stimulated (100 ng/ml) progesterone production by human granulosa/luteal cells obtained during IVF protocols. Cells were cultured in 10% serum with or without SmC (25 ng/ml) for 3 days. The presence of SmC during this preincubation had no effect upon progesterone production (data not shown). Serum-free medium (Ham's F12:DMEM, 1:1) containing 10 µg/ml human low-density lipoprotein or medium containing hCG and/or SmC (25 or 50 ng/ml) as indicated was added at day 3 and cultures were maintained for an additional 3 days. Bars and associated lines represent the mean and associated standard deviation of 3 cultures. These results are representative of 3 experiments with cells from 3 different patients.

FGF has been shown to modulate granulosa cell growth, steroidogenesis and LH receptor induction similarly to EGF (10,37). Because of its angiogenic properties, it is also likely to play a role in neovascularization of the corpus luteum. Corpus luteum-derived capillary endothelial cells respond to acidic and basic FGF similarly to those derived from large vessels (38). Corpus luteum tissue has been demonstrated to be a rich source of angiogenesis factors (39). Angiogenic activity has also been associated with the follicle and with the nonluteal ovary (40). Conditioned medium from rat granulosa cell cultures contains activities which are mitogenic to endothelial cells (41). Follicular fluid from patients undergoing IVF contains an enriched amount of angiogenic material, but this activity has not been demonstrated to be acidic or basic FGF (42). These results constitute indirect evidence supporting the concept that granulosa and luteal cells produce angiogenic factors and that the level of production is modulated by reproductive hormones. With specific reference to the FGFs, however, the biochemical evidence is that they are not cell secretory products since the bFGF gene sequence does not provide for a signal peptide or internal hydrophobic domain designating secretion (43). Rather, the concept is emerging that cellular FGFs are not secreted but are released secondary to injury and then act in an autocrine fashion to facilitate angiogenesis. Thus, even though the hypothesis that granulosa or luteal cells produce FGFs in a hormonally regulated fashion is most attractive, it must await more direct testing by immunocytochemical techniques and/or other approaches which demonstrate unequivocally that these cells contain FGFs.

CONCLUSION

Taken collectively, the experiments reviewed in the previous sections demonstrate unequivocally that growth factors are able to modulate the production of reproductive hormones as well as the differentiated functions of reproductive hormone target cells. Much more work is needed, however, to establish that growth factors are produced by the steroidogenic cells of the ovary, and, if so, whether production is constitutive or is variably regulated.

The issue of paracrine regulation between putative growth factor producing and growth factor responsive cellular subpopulations has not been examined as yet and to some extent must await refinements in techniques of cell isolation, receptor distribution, and cellular sites of synthesis. These issues can, however, be examined more rapidly from a compartmental standpoint, e.g., theca, granulosa, cumulus interactions.

Lastly, the most difficult issues of all will be to address the physiological significance of the experimental results obtained utilizing model systems in vitro, and to evaluate the conclusions of such studies by appropriately designed studies in vivo. With respect to EGF, some studies in vivo have confirmed (44,45) while others have contradicted (46) the results of studies in vitro. In this context, I am reminded of the phrase used some 20 years ago by Dr. Kenneth Ryan, one of the contributors to this symposium, "in vivo veritas" (47).

ACKNOWLEDGMENTS

Supported in part by Grants HD 11827 and HD 21261 from the NICHD, NIH. I wish to acknowledge Dr. L. E. Reichert, Jr., for the gift of highly purified human FSH (LER 1577), Drs. Richard Assoian and M. Sporn for providing pure human Transforming Growth Factor-β, and The Center for Population Research of NICH, NIH for providing hCG 11B01. I also want to acknowledge the invaluable technical expertise of Ms. Sharon Townsend and the expert secretarial assistance of Ms. Lynn Honeycutt.

REFERENCES

1. Adashi EY, Resnick CE, D'Ercole AJ, Svoboda ME, Van Wyk JJ. Insulin-like growth factors as intraovarian regulators of granulosa cell growth and function. Endocr Rev 1985; 6:400.

2. Adashi EY, Resnick CE, Svoboda ME, Van Wyk JJ. Follicle-stimulating hormone enhances Somatomedin C binding to cultured rat granulosa cells. J Biol Chem 1986; 261:3923.

3. Veldhuis JD, Furlanetto RW, Juchter D, Garmey J, Veldhuis P. Trophic actions of human Somatomedin C/Insulin-like Growth Factor I on ovarian cells: in vitro studies with swine granulosa cells. Endocrinology 1985; 116:1235.

4. Jones PBC, Welsh TH Jr, Hsueh AJW. Regulation of ovarian progestin production by epidermal growth factor in cultured rat granulosa cells. J Biol Chem 1982; 257:11268.

5. Buck PA, Schomberg DW. ^{125}I-iodo-epidermal growth factor binding and mitotic responsiveness of porcine granulosa cells is modulated by differentiation and FSH. Endocrinology (in press).

6. Vlodavsky I, Brown KD, Gospodarowicz D. A comparison of the binding of epidermal growth factor to cultured granulosa and luteal cells. J Biol Chem 1978; 253:3744.

7. Feng P, Knecht M, Catt KJ. Hormonal control of epidermal growth factor receptors by gonadotropins during granulosa cell differentiation. Endocrinology 1987; 120:1121.

8. Buck PA. Modulation of cultured porcine granulosa cell responsiveness to Follicle-Stimulating Hormone and Epidermal Growth Factor [Ph.D. Thesis]. Duke University, 1986.

9. Gospodarowicz D, Ill CR, Birdwell CR. Effects of fibroblast and epidermal growth factors on ovarian cell proliferation in vitro. I. Characterization of the response of granulosa cells to FGF and EGF. Endocrinology 1977; 100:1108.

10. Mondschein JS, Schomberg DW. Growth factors modulate gonadotropin receptor induction in granulosa cell cultures. Science 1981; 211:1179.

11. Dodson WC, Schomberg DW. The effect of Transforming Growth Factor-β on follicle-stimulating hormone-induced differentiation of cultured rat granulosa cells. Endocrinology 1987; 120:512.

12. Feng P, Catt KJ, Knecht M. Transforming Growth Factor β regulates the inhibitory actions of epidermal growth factor during granulosa cell differentiation. J Biol Chem 1986; 261:14167.

13. Knecht M, Feng P, Catt K. Bifunctional role of Transforming Growth Factor-β during granulosa cell development. Endocrinology 1987; 120:1243.

14. Mason AJ, Hayflick JS, Ling N, et al. Complementary DNA sequences of ovarian follicular fluid inhibin show precursor structure and homology with transforming growth factor-β. Nature 1985; 318:659.

15. Ling N, Ying S-Y, Ueno N, et al. Pituitary FSH is released by a heterodimer of the β-subunits from the two forms of inhibin. Nature 1986; 321:779.

16. Vale W, Rivier J, Vaughn J, et al. Purification and characterization of an FSH releasing protein from porcine ovarian follicular fluid. Nature 1986; 321:776.

17. Adashi EY, Resnick CE. Antagonistic interactions of transforming growth factors in the regulation of granulosa cell differentiation. Endocrinology 1986; 119:1879.

18. May JV, Schomberg DW. Synergistic action of EGF, TGF-β, and Sm-C on initiation of DNA synthesis in porcine granulosa cells maintained in

serum-free medium [Abstract]. Program of the 69th annual meeting of the Endocrine Society, 1987.

19. Sporn MB, Roberts AB, Wakefield LM, Assoian RK. Transforming growth factor-β: biological function and chemical structure. Science 1986; 233:532.

20. Cheifetz S, Weatherbee JA, Tsang M L-S, et al. The transforming growth factor-β system, a complex pattern of cross-reactive ligands and receptors. Cell 1987; 48:409.

21. Knecht M, Catt KJ. Modulation of cAMP-mediated differentiation in ovarian granulosa cells by epidermal growth factor and platelet-derived growth factor. J Biol Chem 1983; 258:2789.

22. Mondschein JS, Schomberg DW. Effects of partially and more highly purified platelet-derived growth factor preparations on luteinizing hormone receptor induction in granulosa cell cultures. Biol Reprod 1984; 30:603.

23. Heldin C-H, Westermark B, Wasteson A. Platelet-derived growth factor: purification and partial characterization. Proc Natl Acad Sci USA 1979; 76:3722.

24. Westermark B, Heldin C-H, Ek B, et al. Biochemistry and biology of platelet-derived growth factor. In: Guroff G, ed. Growth and maturation factors; vol 1. New York: John Wiley & Sons, 1983:73.

25. Czernobilsky B, Moll R, Levy R, Franke WW. Co-expression of cytokeratin and vimentin filaments in mesothelial, granulosa and rete ovarii cells of the human ovary. Eur J Cell Biol 1985; 37:175.

26. Hillier SG, Wickings EJ, Afnan M, Margara RA, Winston RML. Oocyte developmental potential and granulosa cell steroidogenesis in the human ovulatory follicle. In: Toft DO, Ryan RJ, eds. Proceedings of the fifth ovarian workshop. Champaign: Ovarian Workshops, 1985:255.

27. Wickings EJ, Hillier SG, Reichert LE Jr. Gonadotropic control of human granulosa-lutein cell function in vitro. In: Toft DO, Ryan RJ, eds. Proceedings of the fifth ovarian workshop. Champaign: Ovarian Workshops, 1985:375.

28. Bernhisel MA, Holman JF, Haney AF, Schomberg DW. Estrogen and progesterone production by granulosa cell monolayers derived from in vitro fertilization procedures: lack of evidence for modulation by androgen. J Clin Endocrinol Metab 1987; 64:1251-6.

29. Schomberg DW, Haney AF, Holman JF. Differential expression of hCG receptor binding patterns in granulosa cell (GC) monolayers following in vitro fertilization (IVF) protocols: clomiphene/human menopausal gonadotropic (C/HMG) vs. HMG only [Abstract]. Society for Gynecologic Investigation, 1984:91.

30. Soto EA, Kliman HJ, Strauss JF III, Paavola LG. Gonadotropins and cyclic adenosine 3'5'-monophosphate (cAMP) alter the morphology of cultured human granulosa cells. Biol Reprod 1986; 34:559.

31. Scatchard G. The attraction of proteins for small molecules and ions. Ann NY Acad Sci 1949; 51:660.

32. Garzo VG, Dorrington JH. Aromatase activity in human granulosa cells during follicular development and the modulation by follicle-stimulating hormone and insulin. Am J Obstet Gynecol 1984; 148:657.

33. Ja X-C, Kalmijn J, Hsueh AJW. Growth hormone enhances follicle-stimulating hormone-induced differentiation of cultured rat granulosa cells. Endocrinology 1986; 118:1401.

34. Hsu CJ, Hammond JM. Gonadotropins and estradiol stimulate immunoreactive insulin-like growth factor-I production by porcine granulosa cells in vitro. Endocrinology 1987; 120:198.

35. Rall LB, Scott J, Bell GI. Mouse preproepidermal growth factor synthesis by the kidney and other tissues. Nature 1985; 313:228.

36. Skinner MK, Keski-Oja J, Osteen KG, Moses HL. Ovarian theca cells produce transforming growth factor-β which can regulate granulosa cell growth. Endocrinology 1987; 121:786-92.

37. Gospodarowicz D, Bialecki H. Fibroblast and epidermal growth factors are mitogenic for cultured granulosa cells of rodent, porcine, and human origin. Endocrinology 1979; 104:757.

38. Gospodarowicz D, Massoglia S, Cheng J, Fujii DK. Effect of fibroblast growth factor and lipoproteins on the proliferation of endothelial cells derived from bovine adrenal cortex, brain cortex, and corpus luteum capillaries. J Cell Physiol 1986; 127:121.

39. Gospodarowicz D. The control of proliferation of ovarian cells by the epidermal and fibroblast growth factors. In: Spilman CH, Wilks JW, eds. Novel aspects of reproductive physiology. New York: SP Medical and Scientific Books, 1978:107.

40. Makris A, Ryan KJ, Yasumizu T, Hill CL, Zetter BR. The nonluteal porcine ovary as a source of angiogenic activity. Endocrinology 1984; 115:1672.

41. Koos RD. Stimulation of endothelial cell proliferation by rat granulosa cell-conditioned medium. Endocrinology 1986; 119:481.

42. Frederick JL, Shimanuki T, DiZerega GS. Initiation of angiogenesis by human follicular fluid. Science 1984; 224:389.

43. Abraham JA, Mergia A, Whang JL, et al. Nucleotide sequence of a bovine clone encoding the angiogenic protein, basic fibroblast growth factor. Science 1986; 233:545.

44. Gospodarowicz D, Mescher AL, Birdwell CR. Control of cellular proliferation by the fibroblast and epidermal growth factors. In: Third decennial review conference: cell, tissue, and organ culture. National Cancer Institute monograph 48. Bethesda: USPHS, NIH, 1978:109.

45. Shaw G, Jorgenson GI, Tweendale R, Tennison M, Waters MJ. Effect of epidermal growth factor on reproductive function of ewes. J Endocrinol 1985; 107:429.

46. Lintern-Moore S, Moore GPM, Panaretto BA, Robertson D. Follicular development in the neonatal mouse ovary: effect of epidermal growth factor. Acta Endocrinol (Copenh) 1981; 96:123.

47. Short RV. Ovarian steroid synthesis and secretion in vivo. Recent Prog Horm Res 1964; 20:303.

RECENT ADVANCES IN INHIBIN RESEARCH

Thomas A. Bicsak and Aaron J. W. Hsueh

Department of Reproductive Medicine, M-025
University of California, San Diego
La Jolla, California 92093

INTRODUCTION

The first evidence for the presence of a gonadal hormone which regulates pituitary cell function arose from the pioneering work of Mottram and Cramer (1). In their study, irradiation of adult rats' testes resulted in the hypertrophy of their pituitary cells, similar to that observed in castrated animals. These animals had normal Leydig cells, but their germinal epithelium had been destroyed. It was, therefore, suggested that an unknown testicular factor(s) derived from a non-Leydig cell component is necessary for normal pituitary cell function. Shortly thereafter, McCullagh (2) reported that administration of a water-soluble extract of bovine testes to such irradiated animals was able to prevent the formation of the so-called "castration cells" in the anterior pituitary. McCullagh chose "inhibin" as the name for this putative hormone, in order to differentiate it from the lipid-soluble steroid hormone called androitin, better known to us today as testosterone.

It was not until the mid 1970s, with the advent of radioimmunoassays (RIA) for the gonadotropins, that this testicular inhibin was shown to possess follicle stimulating hormone (FSH)-suppressing activity (3,4). Subsequent to these reports, follicular fluid was also shown to contain inhibin activity capable of suppressing FSH production in vivo (5,6). Experiments by Lee et al. (7) showed that gonadotropins increase ovarian inhibin bioactivity in the ovarian vein, while Uilenbroek et al. (8) demonstrated that ovaries transplanted into castrated rats of either sex caused a decrease in their serum FSH levels. By using a pituitary cell bioassay to measure inhibin bioactivity in conditioned media of gonadal cells, the source of inhibin was localized to the testis Sertoli cells (9) and ovarian granulosa cells (10). All of these experiments pointed toward a similar mechanism of FSH regulation in males and females.

Detailed studies of inhibin structure and function have been hampered by the difficulties encountered in its purification and assay (11). The present review summarizes recent advances in the purification and characterization of ovarian inhibin. We also summarize work done in our laboratory concerning the hormonal regulation of inhibin in both ovarian granulosa and testicular Sertoli cells.

35

PURIFICATION AND CHARACTERIZATION OF INHIBIN

Major breakthroughs in the study of inhibin came with the application of reversed-phase high performance liquid chromatography (RP-HPLC; 12) and fast protein liquid chromatography (FPLC; 13) techniques to the fractionation of follicular fluid. The hydrophobic nature of inhibin has necessitated the use of relatively harsh conditions during purification. Robertson et al. (14) used a combination of gel filtration chromatography under denaturing conditions and RP-HPLC to purify inhibin from bovine follicular fluid. The final product, purified 3,300-fold with respect to the starting material, had a molecular weight of 56,000 and was composed of two dissimilar subunits bound to each other by cysteine disulfide bonds. The smaller beta subunit had a molecular weight of 14,000, while the larger alpha subunit had a molecular weight of 44,000. Several other groups subsequently reported the purification of inhibin from both bovine (15,16) and porcine (17-20) follicular fluid using similar methods. Ling et al. (19) isolated two forms of inhibin which they called A and B. The two forms differed only in the sequence of the beta chains but not the alpha chains. Therefore, the beta chains are designated beta-A and beta-B. While these studies also suggested that inhibin is a disulfide-linked dimer, the molecular weight of the alpha subunit was apparently 18-20,000, resulting in a dimer molecular weight of approximately 32,000. Regardless of molecular weight, the purified inhibin preparations all had an EC_{50} of approximately 10 pM in the in vitro pituitary cell bioassay.

Later studies by Miyamoto et al. (21) used monoclonal antibodies raised against purified inhibin subunits to demonstrate that follicular fluid does contain, in addition to the 32,000 and 56,000 mol wt inhibins, larger forms of biologically-active inhibin. McLachlan et al. (22) subsequently showed that a protease present in serum but not in follicular fluid is capable of converting the 56,000 mol wt bovine follicular fluid inhibin into the 32,000 mol wt form, suggesting that the inhibin is synthesized as a precursor molecule. Data from our laboratory (23) suggest that rat granulosa cells in culture produce both high (48,000) and low (30,000) molecular weight forms of inhibin in response to FSH, but that only the 30,000 form is biologically active (24). All of these results helped to explain the previous confusion regarding the "true" molecular weight of inhibin (11).

CLONING AND SEQUENCE OF INHIBIN SUBUNITS

Conclusive evidence that both inhibin subunits are synthesized as high molecular weight precursors became available with the cloning of porcine (25,26), human (26-28) and bovine (29) inhibins. The beta subunit cDNA coded for a protein of 47,000 mol wt, while the alpha subunit cDNA contained an open reading frame which could code for a 39,000 mol wt protein (25). Potential proteolytic processing sites were identified in several parts of the precursor sequence, suggesting that differential processing may give rise to the multiple molecular weight forms of the protein. Also identified were several potential N-glycosylation sites. The cDNA sequence analyses by Mason et al. (25) confirmed an earlier observation (19) which suggested that there are two forms of the 32,000 mol wt inhibin, referred to as A and B. Indeed, while there is only one gene coding for the inhibin alpha subunit, there are two coding for the beta, corresponding to the two forms observed in follicular fluid. A summary of inhibin secondary structure, as deduced from both protein and cDNA sequences, is presented in Figure 1.

A surprising finding from the cloning studies is the sequence homology observed between the beta subunit of inhibin and two other protein

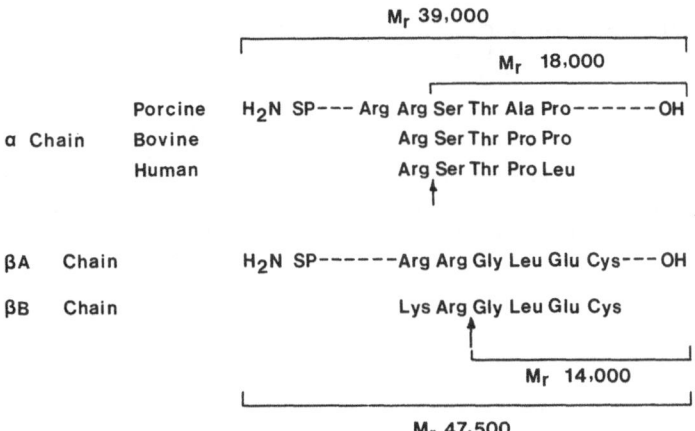

Fig. 1. Schematic representation of inhibin subunit structure. The data presented are derived from references 14-18, 24-28. SP, signal peptide; arrow, probable site of proteolytic processing to form 18,000 mol wt (Mr) α-chain and 14,000 mol wt (Mr) β-chain(s).

hormones, transforming growth factor-beta (25) and Mullerian inhibiting substance (MIS; 27). Also unique is the extreme conservation of the inhibin beta subunit. The beta-A subunits for human, porcine, and bovine inhibins are identical, and there is only one amino acid difference in the beta-B subunits when comparing human and porcine sequences. The cross-species homology between alpha subunits (85%) is lower, but still striking.

HORMONAL REGULATION OF INHIBIN PRODUCTION

Ovarian Studies

Most studies of inhibin have relied upon the use of a pituitary cell bioassay. In this assay, samples containing putative inhibin are incubated in monolayer cultures of dispersed anterior pituitary cells. Specific decreases in basal FSH release, as measured by FSH RIA, are considered to be due to the presence of inhibin. Therefore, although there have been recent improvements in the in vitro pituitary cell bioassay for inhibin (30), investigations of the hormonal regulation of inhibin production could not effectively be pursued without an RIA because exogenously added hormones (e.g., FSH itself) might affect FSH measurement. Also, an improved inhibin bioassay using ovine pituitary cells may still be interfered with by estrogens in the tested sample (31) because these steroids also suppress FSH release.

Our laboratory (24) has used an RIA based on an antibody raised against a synthetic peptide which mimics the 26 amino acids at the N-terminal of the porcine inhibin alpha subunit. This antibody, prepared by immunizing rabbits with the peptide coupled to human alpha-globulin (18), was shown to be specific for inhibin, with no cross-reactivity against related proteins such as TGF-β. Examination of serum-free cultures of granulosa cells obtained from hypophysectomized, estrogen-treated immature rats (32) demonstrated that FSH increases inhibin production by these cells in a dose-dependent fashion (Fig. 2). This effect could be reproduced with the adenyl cyclase activator forskolin or with dibutyryl cAMP, consistent with FSH acting through a cAMP-mediated pathway. The role of cAMP as the second messenger in the stimulation of inhibin production was further substantiated by the observation that a phosphodiesterase inhibitor (MIX) augmented the action of FSH (Fig. 2). Conditioned media from forskolin-treated cells were fractionated by FPLC and were shown to contain bioactive and immunoreactive inhibin with a molecular weight of 32,000, similar to the molecular weights reported for purified inhibin. Also of interest was the observation that both estradiol and Δ^4-androstenedione were capable of enhancing the FSH-stimulated inhibin production, while having no effect on basal inhibin levels. This latter finding suggested that the granulosa cells can exert an autocrine effect on inhibin production via estrogens.

Other experiments using granulosa cells which were treated with FSH for 2 days to induce luteinizing hormone (LH) receptors showed that these "granulosa-luteal" cells respond to either LH or human chorionic gonadotropin (hCG) with increased inhibin production (Fig. 3). In contrast, inhibin synthesis by these cells was not affected by prolactin, even though there are receptors for prolactin on the cell surface.

Since several growth factors and regulatory peptides have been shown to influence granulosa cell function (32), their role in inhibin regulation was also investigated. We found that gonadotropin-releasing hormone (GnRH) and epidermal growth factor (EGF) both inhibited FSH-stimulated

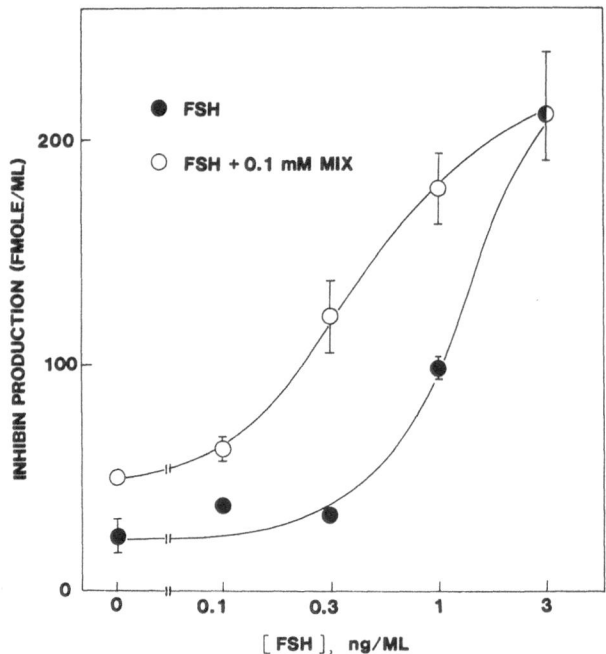

Fig. 2. Dose-dependent stimulation of granulosa cell inhibin by FSH. Rat granulosa cells were treated for 2 days with increasing concentrations of FSH, both with and without the phosphodiesterase inhibitor, MIX. Inhibin production was measured by RIA. Reprinted with permission from Bicsak et al., Endocrinology 1986; 119:2711.

production of inhibin, while fibroblast growth factor had no effect. Insulin and insulin like growth factor-I (IGF-I) both stimulated inhibin production, with insulin only showing an effect in the presence of FSH. Interestingly, a subsequent investigation by another laboratory (33) has revealed a similar stimulation of granulosa cell inhibin bioactivity by IGF-I, both in the presence and absence of FSH. Finally, vasoactive intestinal peptide (VIP) showed a low level of stimulation. An overview of granulosa cell inhibin regulation is presented in Figure 4. Because the hormones which have action at the granulosa cell level act through diverse pathways, including protein kinase A (FSH, LH, VIP), protein kinase C (GnRH), and tyrosine kinase (EGF, IGF-I), it is possible that the granulosa cell will provide a good model system for studies of inhibin gene regulation.

We have also shown that injections of FSH into hypophysectomized, estrogen-treated rats doubles the circulating levels of inhibin (24). These studies, together with data showing that injection of inhibin antibodies into cycling female rats causes an increase in circulating FSH levels (34) and data correlating age-related increases in inhibin with concomitant decrease of FSH (35), validate the existence of a feedback loop between ovarian inhibin and pituitary FSH.

Using an RIA based on an antibody directed against bovine follicular fluid inhibin (22), it was shown that plasma inhibin levels were elevated in patients treated with FSH to hyperstimulate their ovaries (36).

Mason et al. (25) measured the amounts of inhibin subunit mRNA from porcine ovary and found that the alpha subunit mRNA is 10 times more abundant than the beta-A and twentyfold higher than the beta-B. It was shown subsequently that porcine inhibin alpha mRNA levels could be

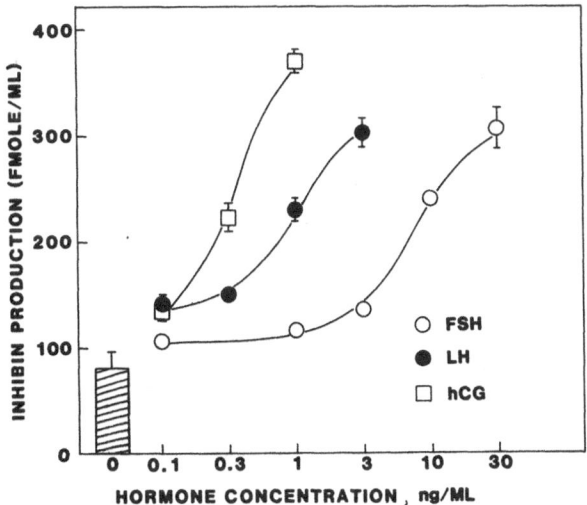

Fig. 3. Stimulation of inhibin production in FSH-primed granulosa cells by FSH, LH, and hCG. Rat granulosa cells were cultured for 2 days in the presence of FSH, followed by increasing doses of FSH, LH, or hCG. Inhibin production was measured by RIA. Reprinted with permission from Bicsak et al., Endocrinology 1986; 119:2711.

increased fivefold by treating the animals with pregnant mare's serum
gonadotropin (PMSG) prior to mRNA extraction (26).   Davis et al. (37)
employed a cDNA probe specific for the inhibin alpha subunit (29) in order
to demonstrate that inhibin mRNA levels in the ovaries of immature female
rats were increased by treatment with PMSG, suggesting that FSH or LH can
act at the ovarian level to increase inhibin production.   They also found
that rat uterus and placenta did not contain inhibin mRNA, while human
placenta did (38).   This unusual finding pointed out that while inhibin
structure is very highly conserved across species boundaries, differences
in its regulation may exist, especially in nongonadal tissues.

Testicular Studies

Most recent research has focused on purification of inhibin from
follicular fluid, largely because the concentration of inhibin in follicular fluid is high when compared with rete testis fluid.   Less attention
has been paid to testicular inhibin, even though the hormone was first
detected in the male.   It was reported several years ago that a 31 amino
acid peptide purified from seminal plasma had inhibin activity (39), but
more recent attempts to reproduce these studies have been less than
successful (40).

We have recently used the same inhibin RIA which was employed to
study granulosa cell inhibin to investigate the production of this hormone
by Sertoli cells (41).   We employed serum-free cultures of immature rat
Sertoli cells and found that FSH elicited a dose-dependent stimulation of
inhibin production, while hCG and prolactin were ineffective, even at high
concentrations (Fig. 5).   Inclusion of a phosphodiesterase inhibitor
enhanced the FSH-stimulated inhibin production, consistent with a cAMP-
mediated pathway for FSH action.   The fact that forskolin, cholera toxin,
and dibutyryl cAMP could all increase inhibin biosynthesis by Sertoli
cells confirmed cAMP as the second messenger for FSH-stimulated inhibin
production.   Unlike the case of the granulosa cells, inhibin production by
Sertoli cells was not enhanced by the addition of androgens or estradiol.
This is consistent with the recent data of Au et al. (42) which showed
that during postnatal development of the male rat, increased inhibin

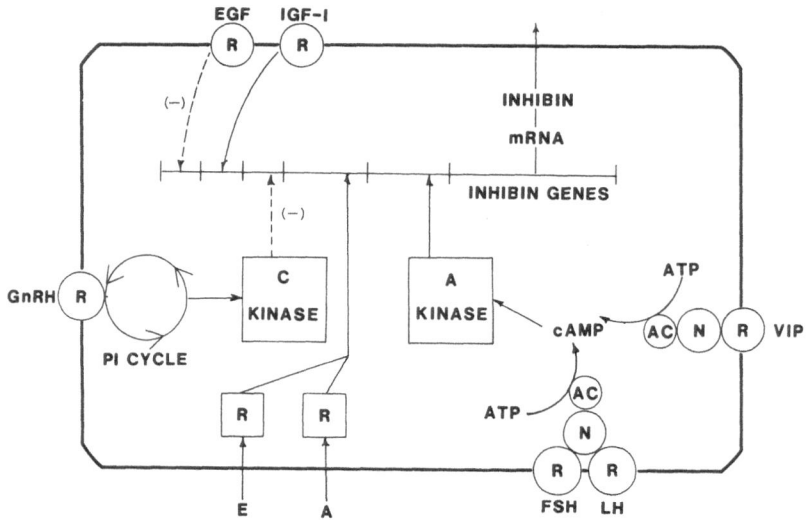

Fig. 4. Summary of the hormonal regulation of
granulosa cell inhibin biosynthesis.

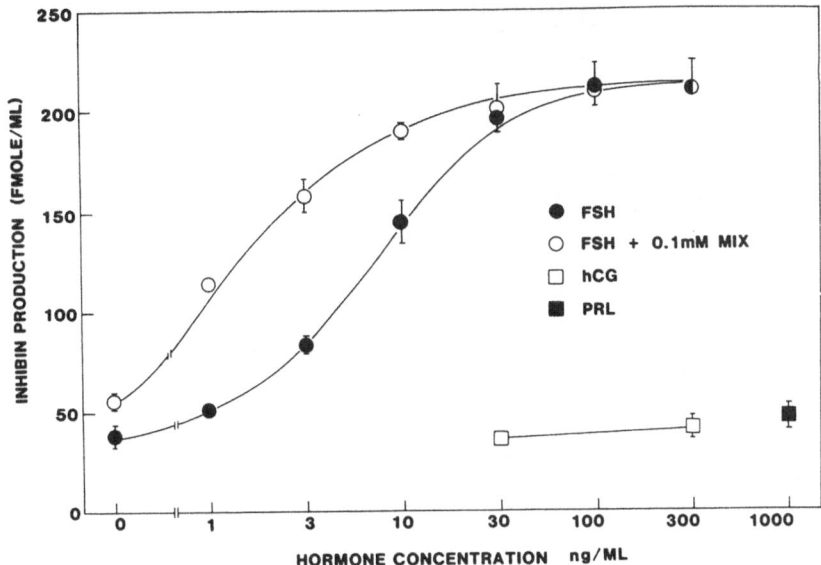

Fig. 5. Stimulation of Sertoli cell inhibin production by FSH.
Rat Sertoli cells were cultured with increasing doses of FSH,
both with and without the phosphodiesterase inhibitor MIX.
Cells were also treated with high doses of hCG or prolactin
(PRL). Inhibin production was measured by RIA. Reprinted with
permission from Bicsak et al., Mol Cell Endocrinol 1987; 49:211.

production is correlated with increased FSH levels, but not with increased
testosterone. Therefore, pituitary FSH stimulates Sertoli cell inhibin,
which in turn blocks FSH release. Thus, as in the female, FSH and inhibin
constitute a closed-loop feedback system along the pituitary-gonadal axis
(Fig. 6).

In the Sertoli cell study, we also fractionated conditioned media
from forskolin-treated cells on an FPLC gel filtration column and measured
inhibin by both RIA and pituitary cell bioassay. One peak of immunoreactive inhibin was detected, coincident with a peak of bioactivity eluting
with a molecular weight of 32,000. It is likely, therefore, that the
granulosa cell and Sertoli cell inhibins are similar proteins under
similar regulation. A recent study (43) demonstrated that Sertoli cells
from cynomolgus monkeys produce bioactive inhibin of molecular weight
40,000, suggesting that testicular inhibins from different species are
also quite similar. However, further characterization awaits the
availability of a purified testicular inhibin.

INHIBIN-RELATED PROTEINS

During the course of purifying follicular fluid inhibin, Rivier et
al. (18) noted the presence of an FSH-releasing factor with physical
properties similar to inhibin itself. This factor was subsequently
purified and shown to be either a homodimer of the inhibin beta-A subunit
(FSH-releasing protein [FRP]; 44) or a heterodimer of the inhibin beta-A
and beta-B subunits ("Activin;" 45). Because the beta-A homodimer and the
beta-A heterodimer possess similar biological activity, these hormones
were named "homoactivin-A" and "heteroactivin," respectively (46). A
homodimer of beta-B subunits with similar function may exist but has not

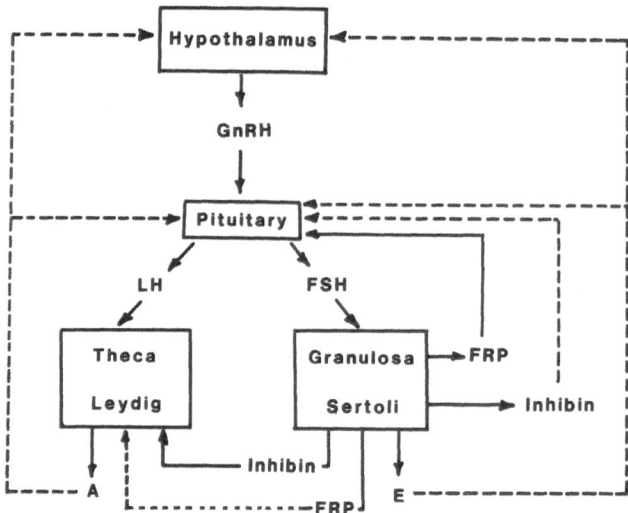

Fig. 6. Closed-loop feedback along the hypothal-
amus-pituitary-gonadal axis. In response to GnRH,
FSH from the pituitary stimulates granulosa
(female) and Sertoli (male) cells to produce both
estrogen (E) and inhibin. Estrogen acts at both
the pituitary and hypothalamic levels to suppress
FSH release, while inhibin acts only at the
pituitary to inhibit FSH, but not LH release.
FRP, possibly gonadal in origin, acts at the
pituitary to stimulate FSH, but not LH, secretion.
Within the gonad, inhibin and FRP have opposite
effects on theca (female) and Leydig (male) cell
androgen (A) production. While inhibin augments
LH-stimulated androgen production, FRP is inhibitory in this respect.

yet been discovered. The factors which influence beta-beta dimer formation versus alpha-beta dimerization at the ovarian level remain to be
elucidated. A summary of the different possible combinations of inhibin
subunits is presented in Table 1.

The high degree of structural homology among the members of the
inhibin gene family suggested that there may also be a functional similarity between inhibin, FRP, TGF-β, and MIS. It has been shown, for example,
that TGF-β is capable of stimulating FSH release by cultured pituitary
cells (47), much as FRP does. It has also been observed that inhibin
exerts an autocrine effect by inhibiting granulosa cell aromatase activity
(48) while TGF-β is stimulatory in the same respect (48,49). In contrast,
Maraud et al. (50) have shown that inhibin does not possess MIS activity
in a chick embryo system, and this suggests that there are limits to the
degree of functional overlap between these hormones.

PARACRINE EFFECTS OF INHIBIN AND FRP

Current studies by our laboratory have investigated the possible
roles of inhibin and FRP in gonadal function (51). It was found that
purified preparations of inhibin augment the LH-stimulated androgen
production by rat testicular Leydig and ovarian theca cells maintained in

Table 1. Subunit combination and
nomenclature of inhibin and
inhibin-related proteins.

Inhibin	α–βA
	α–βB
FRP	βA–βA
Homoactivin A	βA–βA
Homoactivin B	βB–βB
Heteroactivin	βA–βB

vitro under serum-free conditions. In contrast, when these cells were cultured in the presence of LH and FRP, androgen production was inhibited. Neither inhibin nor FRP had any effect in the absence of LH. However, FRP was capable of reversing the stimulatory effect of inhibin, and both proteins exhibited an EC_{50} of approximately 50 pM, suggesting that their action was mediated through a common receptor.

It is conceivable that inhibin from the Sertoli or granulosa cells acts to increase secretion of androgens, which can in turn function at the hypothalamic and pituitary levels to decrease production of GnRH and LH, respectively. FRP, if produced by the granulosa or Sertoli cells, may have the opposite effect. Therefore, the in vivo effects of inhibin and FRP may not be restricted to the pituitary. The concerted action of both inhibin and FRP could thus modulate androgen production directly and LH secretion indirectly. These postulated actions of inhibin and FRP are summarized in Figure 6.

A recent investigation has described a protein factor of molecular weight greater than 10,000 which is produced by rat Sertoli cells in response to FSH, and which can stimulate Leydig cell androgen production in vitro (52). Given that Sertoli cells produce inhibin in response to FSH, and since we have shown that inhibin does augment LH-stimulated androgen production by Leydig cells, it is possible that the unknown Sertoli cell factor which was under study is inhibin. This, however, remains to be shown conclusively.

CONCLUSIONS AND FUTURE DIRECTIONS

The result of recent inhibin research is an improved understanding of the regulation of gonadal function. The elusive inhibin has finally been purified and shown not only to exert an effect on the anterior pituitary, but to also act at the granulosa cell level to lower estrogen production. A whole gene family of inhibin-like proteins has been uncovered, with the most surprising finding of all being that of the FRP. Whether or not such variable subunit combinations (in this case, inhibin $\alpha\beta$ versus FRP $\beta\beta$) alter the function of other hetero-dimeric hormones is unknown. The recent finding that an erythroid differentiation factor purified from a human leukemia cell line is identical to FRP (53) suggests that the beta subunit of inhibin plays an important role apart from its more obvious function at the pituitary level.

With the availability of an inhibin RIA, it has become possible to study the hormonal regulation of inhibin by both the ovary and testis.

The long-suspected role of FSH in modulating inhibin has been conclusively demonstrated in both sexes and, in the female at least, several novel regulators of inhibin production have been identified. We have also shown that both inhibin and FRP exert paracrine effects on ovarian theca and testicular Leydig cells within the gonads.

While a recent immunohistochemical study has shown that inhibin is present in ovarian granulosa cells and in seminiferous tubules (54), more detailed immunocytochemical studies of inhibin, especially during postnatal development and in nongonadal tissues, are warranted. Also of interest will be studies of how and when the high molecular weight precursors of inhibin are processed to the smaller species. On the more clinical side, further exploration of the value of inhibin and inhibin-like peptides as contraceptives or in the treatment of various gonadal dysfunctions is certainly of importance. Such studies should serve to increase our understanding of gonadal function even further.

ACKNOWLEDGMENTS

This work was supported by NIH Program Project Grant HD-13527. TAB is the recipient of NIH Postdoctoral Fellowship HD-06939.

REFERENCES

1. Mottram JC, Cramer W. On the general effects of exposure to radium on metabolism and tumour growth in the rat and the special effects on testis and pituitary. Q J Exp Physiol 1923; 13:209-29.
2. McCullagh DR. Dual endocrine control of the testes. Science 1932; 76:19-20.
3. Franchimont P, Chari S, Hagelstein MT, Duraiswami S. Existence of a follicle-stimulating hormone inhibiting factor "inhibin" in bull seminal plasma. Nature 1975; 257:402-4.
4. Baker HWG, Bremner WJ, Burger HG, et al. Testicular control of follicle-stimulating hormone secretion. Recent Prog Horm Res 1976; 32:429-76.
5. deJong FH, Sharpe RM. Evidence of inhibin-like activity in bovine follicular fluid. Nature 1976; 263:71-2.
6. Schwartz NB, Channing CP. Evidence for ovarian "inhibin": suppression of the secondary rise in serum follicle stimulating hormone levels in proestrous rats by injection of porcine follicular fluid. Proc Natl Acad Sci USA 1977; 74:5721-4.
7. Lee VWK, McMaster J, Quigg H, Findlay J, Leversha L. Ovarian and peripheral blood inhibin concentrations increase with gonadotropin treatment in immature rats. Endocrinology 1981; 108:2403-5.
8. Uilenbroek JTJ, Tiller R, deJong FH, Vels F. Specific suppression of follicle-stimulating hormone secretion in gonadectomized male and female rats with intrasplenic ovarian transplants. J Endocrinol 1978; 78:399-406.
9. Steinberger A, Steinberger C. Secretion of an FSH-inhibiting factor by cultured Sertoli cells. Endocrinology 1976; 99:918-21.
10. Erickson GF, Hsueh AJW. Secretion of "inhibin" by rat granulosa cell in vitro. Endocrinology 1978; 103:1960-3.
11. deJong FH, Robertson DM. Inhibin: 1985 update on action and purification. Mol Cell Endocrinol 1985; 42:95-103.
12. Dobos M, Burger HG, Hearn MTW, Morgan FJ. Isolation of inhibin from bovine follicular fluid using reversed phase liquid chromatography. Mol Cell Endocrinol 1983; 31:187-98.
13. van Dijk S, deJong FH, van der Molen HJ. Use of fast protein liquid chromatography in the purification of inhibin from bovine follicular

fluid. Biochem Biophys Res Commun 1984; 125:307-14.

14. Robertson DM, Foulds LM, Leversha L, et al. Isolation of inhibin from bovine follicular fluid. Biochem Biophys Res Commun 1985; 126:220-6.

15. Fukuda M, Miyamoto K, Hasegawa Y, et al. Isolation of bovine follicular fluid inhibin of about 32 kDa. Mol Cell Endocrinol 1986; 44:55-60.

16. Robertson DM, de Vos FL, Foulds LM, et al. Isolation of a 31 kD form of inhibin from bovine follicular fluid. Mol Cell Endocrinol 1986; 44:271-7.

17. Miyamoto K, Hasegawa Y, Fukuda M, et al. Isolation of porcine follicular fluid inhibin of 32K daltons. Biochem Biophys Res Commun 1985; 129:396-403.

18. Rivier J, Spiess J, McClintock R, Vaughan J, Vale W. Purification and partial characterization of inhibin from porcine follicular fluid. Biochem Biophys Res Commun 1985; 133:120-7.

19. Ling N, Ying S-Y, Ueno N, Esch F, Denoroy L, Guillemin R. Isolation and partial characterization of a Mr 32,000 protein with inhibin activity from porcine follicular fluid. Proc Natl Acad Sci USA 1985; 82:7217-21.

20. Gordon WL, Liu W-K, Ward DN. Inhibin fractionation: a comparison of human and porcine follicular fluid, with particular reference to protease activation. Biol Reprod 1986; 35:209-18.

21. Miyamoto K, Hasegawa Y, Fukuda M, Igarashi M. Demonstration of high molecular weight forms of inhibin in bovine follicular fluid (bFF) by using monoclonal antibodies to bFF 32K inhibin. Biochem Biophys Res Commun 1986; 136:1103-9.

22. McLachlan RI, Robertson DM, Burger HG, de Kretser DM. The radioimmunoassay of bovine and human follicular fluid and serum inhibin. Mol Cell Endocrinol 1986; 46:175-85.

23. Bicsak TA. Biosynthetic labelling and immunoprecipitation of inhibin in cultured rat granulosa cells [Abstract]. The 69th Annual Meeting of the Endocrine Society, Indianapolis, IN, 1987.

24. Bicsak TA, Tucker EM, Cappel S, et al. Hormonal regulation of granulosa cell inhibin biosynthesis. Endocrinology 1986; 119:2711-9.

25. Mason AJ, Hayflick JS, Ling N, et al. Complementary DNA sequences of ovarian follicular fluid inhibin show precursor structure and homology with transforming growth factor-beta. Nature 1985; 318:659-63.

26. Mayo KE, Cerelli GM, Spiess J, et al. Inhibin A-subunit cDNAs from porcine ovary and human placenta. Proc Natl Acad Sci USA 1986; 83:5849-53.

27. Mason AJ, Niall HD, Seeburg PH. Structure of two human ovarian inhibins. Biochem Biophys Res Commun 1986; 135:957-64.

28. Stewart AG, Milborrow HM, Ring JM, Crowther CE, Forage RG. Human inhibin genes—genomic characterization and sequencing. FEBS Lett 1986; 206:329-34.

29. Forage RG, Ring JW, Brown RW, et al. Cloning and sequence analysis of cDNA species coding for the two subunits of inhibin from bovine follicular fluid. Proc Natl Acad Sci USA 1986; 83:3091-5.

30. Robertson DM, Giacometti MS, de Kretser DM. The effects of inhibin purified from bovine follicular fluid in several in vitro pituitary cell culture systems. Mol Cell Endocrinol 1986; 46:29-36.

31. Tsonis CG, McNeilly AS, Baird DT. Measurement of exogenous and endogenous inhibin in sheep serum using a new and extremely sensitive bioassay for inhibin based on inhibition of ovine pituitary FSH secretion in vitro. J Endocrinol 1986; 110:341-52.

32. Hsueh AJW, Adashi EY, Jones PBC, Welsh TH Jr. Hormonal regulation of the differentiation of cultured ovarian granulosa cells. Endocr Rev 1984; 5:76-127.

33. Zhiwen Z, Carson RS, Herington AC, Lee VWK, Burger HG. Follicle-stimulating hormone and somatomedin-C stimulate inhibin production by

rat granulosa cells in vitro. Endocrinology 1987; 120:1633-8.

34. Rivier C, Rivier J, Vale W. Inhibin-mediated feedback control of follicle-stimulating hormone secretion in the female rat. Science 1986; 234:205-8.

35. Rivier C, Vale W. Inhibin: measurement and role in the immature female rat. Endocrinology 1987; 120:1688-90.

36. McLachlan RI, Robertson DM, Healy DL, de Kretser DM, Burger HG. Plasma inhibin levels during gonadotropin-induced ovarian hyperstimulation for IVF: a new index of follicular function? Lancet 1986; 1:1233-4.

37. Davis SR, Dench F, Nikoaidis I, et al. Inhibin A-subunit gene expression in the ovaries of immature female rats is stimulated by pregnant mare serum gonadotropin. Biochem Biophys Res Commun 1986; 138:1191-5.

38. McLachlan RI, Healy DL, Robertson DM, Burger HG, de Kretser DM. The human placenta: a novel source of inhibin. Biochem Biophys Res Commun 1986; 140:485-90.

39. Ramasharma K, Sairam MR, Seidah MG, et al. Isolation, structure, and synthesis of a human seminal plasma peptide with inhibin-like activity. Science 1984; 223:1199-202.

40. Liu L, Booth J, Merriam GR, et al. Evidence that synthetic 31-amino acid inhibin-like peptide lacks inhibin activity. Endocr Res 1985; 11:191-7.

41. Bicsak TA, Vale W, Vaughan J, Tucker EM, Cappel S, Hsueh AJW. Hormonal regulation of inhibin production by cultured Sertoli cells. Mol Cell Endocrinol 1987; 49:211-7.

42. Au CL, Robertson DM, de Kretser DM. Measurement of inhibin and an index of inhibin production by rat testes during postnatal development. Biol Reprod 1986; 35:37-43.

43. Noguchi K, Keeping HS, Winters SJ, Saito H, Oshima H, Troen P. Identification of inhibin secreted by cynomolgus monkey Sertoli cell cultures. J Clin Endocrinol Metab 1987; 64:783-8.

44. Vale W, Rivier J, Vaughan J, et al. Purification and characterization of an FSH releasing protein from porcine ovarian follicular fluid. Nature 1986; 321:776-9.

45. Ling N, Ying S-Y, Ueno N, et al. Pituitary FSH is released by a heterodimer of the beta-subunits from the two forms of inhibin. Nature 1986; 321:779-82.

46. Ling N, Ying S-Y, Ueno N, et al. A homodimer of the beta-subunits of inhibin A stimulates the secretion of pituitary follicle stimulating hormone. Biochem Biophys Res Commun 1986; 138:1129-37.

47. Ying S-Y, Becker A, Baird A, et al. Type beta transforming growth factor (TGF-β) is a potent stimulator of the basal secretion of follicle-stimulating hormone (FSH) in a pituitary monolayer system. Biochem Biophys Res Commun 1986; 135:950-6.

48. Ying S-Y, Becker A, Ling N, Ueno N, Guillemin R. Inhibin and beta type transforming growth factor (TGF-β) have opposite modulating effects on the follicle stimulating hormone (FSH)-induced aromatase activity of cultured rat granulosa cells. Biochem Biophys Res Commun 1986; 136:969-75.

49. Adashi EY, Resnick CE. Antagonistic interactions of transforming growth factors in the regulation of granulosa cell differentiation. Endocrinology 1986; 119:1879-81.

50. Maraud R, Vergnaud O, Franchimont P. Absence of anti-Mullerian activity of inhibin in the chick embryo. Horm Res 1987; 25:56-9.

51. Hsueh AJW, Dahl KD, Vaughan J, et al. Hetero- and homo-dimers of inhibin subunits have different paracrine actions in the modulation of LH stimulated androgen biosynthesis. Proc Natl Acad Sci USA 1987 (in press).

52. Verhoeven G, Cailleau J. A factor in spent media from Sertoli cell-enriched cultures that stimulates steroidogenesis in Leydig

cells. Mol Cell Endocrinol 1985; 40:57-68.

53. Eto Y, Tsuji T, Takezawa M, Takano S, Yokogawa Y, Shibai H. Purification and characterization of erythroid differentiation factor (EDF) isolated from human leukemia cell line THP-1. Biochem Biophys Res Commun 1987; 142:1095-103.

54. Cuevas P, Ying S-Y, Ling N, Ueno N, Esch F, Guillemin R. Immunohistochemical detection of inhibin in the gonad. Biochem Biophys Res Commun 1987; 142:23-30.

FOLLICLE REGULATORY PROTEIN: AN INTRAOVARIAN REGULATOR

OF FOLLICULAR RESPONSE TO GONADOTROPIN STIMULATION

Gregor Westhof, Katsuhiko Fujimori, Sharon A. Tonetta, Karin
Westhof, James Ireland, Jeffrey Fay, and Gere S. diZerega

Livingston Reproductive Biology Laboratory, University of
Southern California School of Medicine, Los Angeles,
California 90033; Department of Animal Science, Michigan
State University, East Lansing, Michigan 48823; Department
of Obstetrics and Gynecology, University of Colorado Health
Sciences Center, Denver, Colorado 80262

INTRODUCTION

Follicular fluids from various species contain inhibitor(s) of
aromatase activity. Fractions of bovine follicular fluid inhibited the
induction of aromatase activity in granulosa cells in proportion to their
concentration in the culture medium (1). Furthermore, equine follicular
fluid was shown to inhibit porcine granulosal production of estradiol and
progesterone (2,3), and steroid-free, bovine follicular fluid inhibited
FSH-induced secretion of estrogen by ovine granulosa cells collected from
follicles more than 3 mm in diameter (4). Guthrie found that charcoal-
extracted, porcine follicular fluid blocked the recruitment of medium-
sized follicles into preovulatory development after the administration of
exogenous FSH (5). When administered to intact ewes, ovine follicular
fluid, with or without the addition of pregnant mare serum (PMS), reduced
the number of follicles more than 4 mm in diameter as well as the relative
proportion of follicles less than 2 mm (6). These studies in vivo were
extended by observations in vitro that treatment with ovine follicular
fluid inhibited aromatase activity as well as mitotic activity in granulosa cells. It was suggested that ovine follicular cells produce an
endogenous inhibitor of granulosal aromatase which they secrete into the
follicular fluid. Fractions of human follicular fluid which bound to dye
Matrix gel Orange A inhibited human menopausal gonadotropin (hMG)-
stimulated secretion of estradiol by rats in vivo as well as production of
estrogen by porcine granulosa cells in vitro (7). Saito and Hiroi (8)
treated PMS-stimulated mice with human follicular fluid recovered from
women who were undergoing in vitro fertilization-embryo transfer therapy
(IVF-ET). Human follicular fluid inhibited the PMS-induced increase in
mouse ovarian weight and the number of ova shed in a dose-dependent
manner. Mice treated with human follicular fluid from mature follicles
had a greater inhibition in ovarian weight and a decrease in the number of
ovulations per cycle compared to mice treated with human follicular fluid
from immature follicles. Thus, a growing body of data derived from
experiments on a variety of species and from different laboratories
supports the theory that follicular fluid contains a direct inhibitor of
aromatase activity. Follicular fluid also contains factors which stim-

ulate aromatase activity, e.g., insulin-like growth factors (IGF, 9), transforming growth factor β (TGFβ, 10) and other factor(s) which have yet to be defined (11, Numazaki, Chari, diZerega, unpublished observation). However, the findings in various species that steroid-free follicular fluid inhibits estrogen production or estrogen-dependent biological functions suggest that aromatase inhibitor(s) may possess sufficient potency to overcome the stimulatory effects of other factors in vivo.

FOLLICLE REGULATORY PROTEIN

Using inhibition of aromatase activity in granulosa cells as the reference bioassay, we identified a protein, referred to as follicle regulatory protein (FRP), which was subsequently purified to homogeneity from human (Chari, unpublished data) and porcine (11,12) follicular fluid. These follicular proteins have similar molecular weights (15,000) and isoelectric points (pH 4.5). When FRP was tested in vitro for inhibin activity (Channing, Wehrenberg and Campeau, personal communications) or injected into male rats (13), no reduction in levels of FSH was detected. In addition, FRP demonstrates biochemical and biological properties different from those of growth factors which are known to influence ovarian steroidogenesis, e.g., IGFI, IGFII, EGF, TGFα and TGFβ.

Steroidogenesis in Granulosa Cells

FRP inhibits aromatase activity in porcine granulosa cells from medium- and small-sized follicles. However, FRP does not appear to have an effect on the secretion of estrogen by cells from large follicles (14). Inhibition of FSH-inducible aromatase activity by FRP occurred in granulosa cells from small- and medium-sized, but not large, porcine follicles. Increases in intrafollicular levels of androgens enhance the sensitivity of FSH-responsive steroidogenic enzymes to FRP in granulosa cells. Testosterone appears to sensitize granulosa cells to FRP-related alterations in the secretion of progesterone. Although atretic follicles contain higher ratios of androgen to estrogen than nonatretic follicles (15-17), the cause and effect relationship between androgens and atresia is unclear. Intrafollicular androgens may enhance the sensitivity of follicles to FRP, causing a reduction in the extent of FSH-mediated events which leads to irreversible atresia. Indeed, FRP itself may account, at least in part, for the persistently low levels of estrogens in atretic follicles. Conversely, these findings suggest that, once the follicle begins to grow, its ability to aromatize its own androgens reduces the sensitivity of the growing follicle to FRP and, thus, reduces the likelihood of it becoming atretic.

FRP induces a biphasic effect on the secretion of progesterone by granulosa cells from sows (18) and rats (19). At low doses, FRP stimulates the secretion of progesterone while, at higher doses, it is inhibitory. When FRP is added to hMG-treated human and porcine granulosa cells, there is a dose-dependent decrease in the concentrations of progesterone in culture media and cytosol as well as microsomal 3β-hydroxysteroid dehydrogenase activity (20,21). FRP-enriched fractions of follicular fluid stimulate basal levels of progesterone secretion by porcine granulosa cells from small- and medium-sized follicles, but not by granulosa cells from large follicles. The biphasic pattern of the effect of FRP on 3β-hydroxysteroid dehydrogenase activity (3β-HSD) may have several potential explanations. The increase in secretion of progesterone by granulosa cells treated with higher doses of FRP may result from an inhibition of the 17-hydroxylase/17-20 desmolase enzymes, which may provide an increase in the levels of substrate, rather than an actual increase in 3β-HSD activity per se. It is unlikely that the effects of

FRP on granulosal secretion of progesterone are due to toxicity of FRP, since FSH in high concentration is able to overcome the FRP-induced inhibition of progesterone secretion (19). As estrogen and androgen inhibit 3β-HSD activity in granulosa cells, the apparent biphasic effects of FRP on the secretion of progesterone by granulosa cells may be indirectly mediated by alterations in aromatase activity (22,24). It is unlikely that the action of FRP on the secretion of progesterone simply reflects a local reduction in the production of estradiol, since Veldhuis and co-workers (25) found that estradiol itself blocks the synthesis of progesterone by human granulosa cells. Aromatizable androgens inhibit FSH-stimulated synthesis of progesterone in porcine granulosa cells at a step distal to the formation of cAMP (24). Furthermore, aromatizable androgens markedly increase the accumulation of pregnenolone in FSH-treated cultures. Since FRP is an effective inhibitor of aromatase activity, the possibility remains that the buildup of endogenous intracellular androgen, caused by the FRP-mediated inhibition of aromatase activity, may alter 3β-HSD activity.

These studies on the interactions of FRP with rat and swine granulosa cells offer possible explanations for findings in the human ovary. Previously, we described a negative correlation between the concentration of progesterone in follicular fluid and FRP activity (26,27). This agrees with the findings that FRP inhibits the synthesis of progesterone in vitro, irrespective of the concentration of FSH in rat granulosa cells in culture (19). Although FRP inhibited the production of estradiol by isolated granulosa cells, we found a positive correlation between the activity of FRP and the concentrations of estradiol in follicular fluid from human follicles. This suggests that the amount of FRP secreted by a growing follicle is directly related to the number of intact granulosa cells in that particular follicle. Human follicles with the highest concentration of estradiol in their follicular fluid also contain the highest concentrations of FSH (15,28). High levels of FSH can overcome the inhibitory effect of FRP on estrogen production in the rat (19). Therefore, the positive correlation between estrogen levels and FRP activity in the human follicle may reflect the ability of a locally high concentration of FSH to block the potentially inhibitory effect of FRP. Since withdrawal of stimulation by estrogen induces follicular atresia (29), FRP may induce atresia by blocking FSH-induced aromatase activity. The dominant follicle would be protected from the deleterious effect of FRP by the locally high levels of FSH and estrogen.

The effects of FRP on steroidogenesis in granulosa cells are reversible unless aromatase activity is inhibited by more than 85-90%. If inhibition by FRP exceeded 85-90%, full aromatase activity did not return after the removal of FRP (19). This may explain another feature of the preovulatory follicle, namely, that if the dominant ovarian structure (follicle or corpus luteum) is destroyed, no other follicle (30,31) can soon take its place (32-37). Thus, FRP may irreversibly suppress the ability of nonovulatory follicles to produce estrogen.

A preparation of follicular fluid with enriched concentrations of FRP (50 to 200 μg/ml) inhibited aromatase activity in porcine granulosa cells, while stimulating 3β-HSD activity (18). When the concentration of crude FRP was increased to 500 μg/ml, both aromatase and 3β-HSD activities were inhibited. Importantly, increasing doses of FSH selectively reversed the inhibition of 3β-HSD, but not of aromatase activity. When granulosa cells were exposed to FSH in the relative absence of FRP, they produced more estradiol and less progesterone. However, when granulosa cells were exposed to FSH in the presence of FRP, they produced more progesterone and less estradiol. These observations suggest that FRP alters the dose-response relationship between FSH and the activities of 3β-HSD and aromatase in granulosa cells. Thus, FRP may play a role in modulating the relative levels of progesterone and estrogen secreted by granulosa cells in response to stimulation by FSH. These results demonstrate that the effects of FRP on ovarian steroidogenesis are complex and depend on: (1) the concentration of gonadotropins; (2) the concentration of FRP; and, (3) the availability of substrate.

Thecal Steroidogenesis

From studies utilizing individual rat follicles (38) and human ovarian homogenates (39), it appears that thecal 17α-hydroxylase/C17, 20-lyase is active in small antral follicles and maximal in preovulatory follicles. Therefore, it appears that this enzyme activity increases as the follicle obtains more substrate for estrogen production. In addition, thecal cells from large- and medium-sized porcine follicles (40,41) have an active aromatase system sufficient to contribute significant amounts of estrogen to the peripheral circulation. Estrogen and progesterone administered to porcine thecal cells in vitro inhibit thecal aromatase and 3β-HSD activities (40,42). Granulosal FRP has little effect on aromatase activity in thecal cells from medium-sized follicles, but enhances the hCG-induced decrease in aromatase activity. In contrast, in large follicles, FRP inhibited thecal aromatase activity and prevented the hCG-induced increase in aromatase activity. This effect of FRP on thecal cells is also dependent upon the extent of follicular maturation.

FRP alone had little effect on 3β-HSD activity, but inhibited hCG-stimulated 3β-HSD activity at 72 h in thecal cells from medium-sized follicles. In theca from large follicles, FRP inhibited the hCG-induced increase in 3β-HSD activity while having little effect by itself. Thus, FRP appears to inhibit gonadotropin-stimulated enzyme activity in thecal cells. Theca cells from large follicles concomitantly treated with hCG do respond to FRP, in contrast to FSH-treated granulosa cells from large follicles. Thus, granulosa cells in large follicles can fully express their estrogen and progestin synthesis, despite the presence of FRP, whereas thecal synthesis of progestin and estrogen in large follicles could be suppressed by FRP. In large preovulatory follicles, FRP may thus facilitate the separation of the steroidogenic functions of theca and granulosa cells (43,44).

Secretion of FRP

FRP is secreted by granulosa cells, from small- and medium-sized porcine follicles, but not by thecal cells, as determined by both biological (27) and immunological assays. Enlargement of the porcine follicle to preovulatory size (8-10 mm in diameter) leads to a marked reduction in the secretion of FRP. FRP activity was determined in bovine follicular fluid from heifers 3-72 h after prostaglandin $F_{2\alpha}$ administration. As found in other species, there was a positive correlation between estradiol levels in follicular fluid and follicular diameter. Additionally, there was a positive correlation between FRP activity in follicular fluid and increasing follicular diameter. However, there was no correlation between FRP activity or levels of steroid and gonadotropin in follicular fluid from either ovulatory or nonovulatory follicles. Whether these results are due to low levels of FRP in bovine follicular fluid or the lack of the porcine antibody to recognize bovine FRP remains to be determined. In contrast to the cow, follicles from horses had FRP activity measurable by both bioassay and immunoassay. Levels of FRP in follicular fluid from follicles destined to ovulate were highest in the medium-size range and demonstrated a decreasing trend when the ovulatory follicle increased in size (Fig. 1, lower panel). Medium-sized, nonovulatory follicles had similar FRP levels in follicular fluid as ovulatory follicles of the same

size range. However, smaller, nonovulatory follicles contained low levels
of FRP (Fig. 1, upper panel). Taken together with the findings in porcine
preovulatory follicles, these data obtained from the horse support the
assumption that the secretion of FRP by granulosa cells in large (presumably preovulatory) follicles is decreased when compared with medium-sized
ones. Provided that nonovulatory follicles become smaller in size with
the progress of atresia (45,46), the decreasing trend in FRP levels in
those follicles seems to reflect the decreasing number of intact granulosa
cells which is a hallmark of ongoing atresia.

Levels of FRP in human urine rise, beginning in the midfollicular
phase and reach their zenith by the midluteal phase (Fig. 2). Immunohistochemical evaluation of porcine ovaries in the follicular phase demonstrated binding of antibodies by FRP to granulosa cells and no staining
of theca cells in medium- and small-sized follicles. Staining was
restricted to the perifollicular components outside of the basal lamina in
large-viable and in atretic follicles. In porcine ovaries obtained during
the luteal phase, staining was restricted to the large cells of the corpus
luteum. Large luteal cells are thought to be successors of the granulosa
cells from the preceding preovulatory follicle. During luteolysis,
however, no or very little immunostaining of FRP was found in luteal
cells. Thus, the majority of FRP is derived from the active corpus luteum
during the luteal phase. Several possibilities exist which could explain
the accumulation of FRP during the late follicular phase: FRP could be
derived from: (1) the granulosa cells of small antral follicles which may
represent a relatively large population during this time, together secreting a relatively large quantity of FRP. After ovulation, this population
of small viable follicles is markedly reduced, perhaps due, in part, to
the increasing amount of FRP secreted by the corpus luteum. (2) The
possibility exists that theca cells which showed an intense immunostaining
in preovulatory follicles do secrete FRP in vivo but not in vitro. A

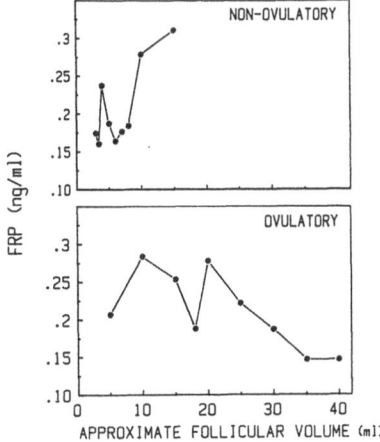

Fig. 1. Equine FRP levels. Immunoreactive
levels of follicle regulatory protein (FRP)
in follicular fluid obtained from mares.
Determination of ovulatory vs. nonovulatory
status of the aspirated follicle was made on
the basis of follicular fluid steroid
levels. (Fay and Douglas, Biol Reprod 1983;
28:110a.) An ELISA assay with a monoclonal
antibody prepared against porcine FRP was
used to quantitate the FRP levels.

direct release of FRP from theca cells into the blood stream could account
for low levels of FRP in follicular fluid. (3) FRP secreted by granulosa
cells from large follicles could immediately leave the follicle and
therefore accumulate in the intracellular space between theca cells before
entering the blood stream. (4) FRP could be secreted by atretic follicles
during the late follicular phase, since atretic follicles also demonstrated an intense staining of their theca cells. Overall, the highest
levels of FRP were found during the luteal phase, a time when most ter-
tiary follicles are atretic (30,47). The decrease of FRP levels in late
luteal phase reaching a nadir in the early follicular phase coincides with
the critical period of recruitment of the dominant follicle(s) (48). The
small number of healthy follicles available for recruitment during the
rise in serum levels of FSH in the late luteal to early follicular phase
may be determined by the number of follicles which survive the early to
midluteal phase. McNatty reported a marked increase in FSH-responsive
aromatase activity in granulosa cells aspirated from human follicles
collected during the mid to late luteal phase (49). Thus, FRP produced
during the periovulatory interval and the subsequent luteal phase may play
a role in the reduction of the size of the potential follicular population
to that number which is consistent with the ovulatory quota.

Recruitment and selection of the preovulatory follicle may occur as a
result of an FRP-mediated reduction in the number of healthy follicles

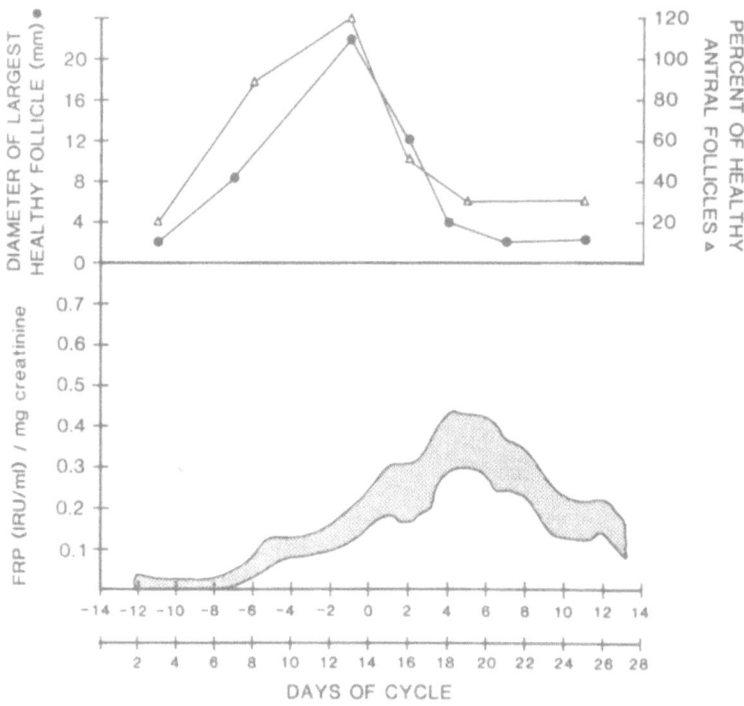

Fig. 2. Top panel: Diameter of largest healthy
follicle and percent of healthy antral follicles
determined from human ovaries collected throughout the
normal menstrual cycle. Bottom panel: Urinary levels
of follicle regulatory protein (expressed in IRU:
immunoreactive units) determined by the ELISA assay in
daily collections throughout the cycle from normally
menstruating women. Shaded area represents 2 standard
errors of the mean.

during the luteal phase, followed by an FSH-mediated stimulation of the remaining viable follicle(s) in the subsequent intercycle interval. Within the follicle, FRP may mediate a dose-response set-point for FSH, which increasing exposure of the follicle to FSH can override, to allow the recruitment of ovulatory follicles. When intrafollicular levels of FRP are low, multiple follicles are recruited. However, when intrafollicular levels of FRP are high, ovarian dysfunction (i.e., anovulation) may ensue. High levels of intrafollicular FSH can reduce the action of FRP in granulosa cells which may, in turn, allow for enhanced granulosal aromatization and the production of estrogen. If FSH is unable to overcome the intrafollicular effects of FRP, the follicle becomes atretic. Thus, FRP may be an active promoter of atresia within the ovary.

Inappropriate exposure to FRP may limit the ability of follicles to respond to FSH, resulting in suppressed follicular maturation and reduced production of estradiol. A group of anovulatory patients was recently found to have elevated serum concentration of FRP when compared with levels in normally cycling women in the follicular phase of the cycle (50). A differential ovarian response to clomiphene citrate therapy by anovulatory patients with elevated serum levels of FRP was observed on days 22-23 of the menstrual cycle (Fig. 3). There appeared to be abnormalities of follicular recruitment during the intercycle interval, as demonstrated by reduced levels of estradiol in serum and concomitant elevations in serum levels of FRP 3-5 days after the onset of the last menstrual period. From these limited data, it is tempting to speculate that anovulation in these patients may be the result of an overproduction of FRP and the subsequent reduction in follicular responsiveness to stimulation by gonadotropin. That additional exposure to gonadotropin was not successful in overcoming this putative, FRP-induced block in follicular maturation is suggested by the elevated levels of FRP in other anovulatory patients, 22-23 days after the onset of the last menstrual period, even after receipt of clomiphene citrate therapy on days 3-7 of the cycle. A separate group of anovulatory patients was identified by relatively low concentrations of estradiol in serum and low levels of FRP determined on days 3-5 of the cycle (50). Follicles in these patients who did respond to clomiphene citrate therapy by increasing their peripheral serum levels of estradiol and presumably ovulated—as evidenced by elevated levels of progesterone in serum on days 22-23—did not have elevated FRP values during these intervals as shown in Figure 3. Thus, follicular dysfunction expressed clinically as anovulatory cycles may result from abnormalities in ovarian protein as well as steroid hormone secretion.

PERSPECTIVE

The studies described here indicate that FRP alters 3β-HSD and aromatase activities in porcine, human, and rat granulosa cells. FRP also inhibits the induction by FSH of granulosal receptors for LH (51) and adenylate cyclase activity (52), as well as hCG-responsive steroidogenesis in thecal cells. The inhibitory effects of FRP on granulosal aromatase activity depend upon the response of the cell to FSH: large amounts of FSH can partially overcome the inhibition by FRP while relatively small amounts of FSH sensitize the granulosal aromatase system to FRP. Although androgens potentiate FSH-mediated granulosal functions, they also sensitize the steroidogenic enzymes in granulosa cells to inhibition by FRP. The demonstration that FRP acts primarily on granulosa cells of less mature, antral follicles to inhibit aromatase activity supports the hypothesis that FRP may facilitate the selection of follicles and suggests a role for FRP in atresia. In response to increased exposure to FSH, the preovulatory follicle may decrease its own sensitivity to FRP, in contrast

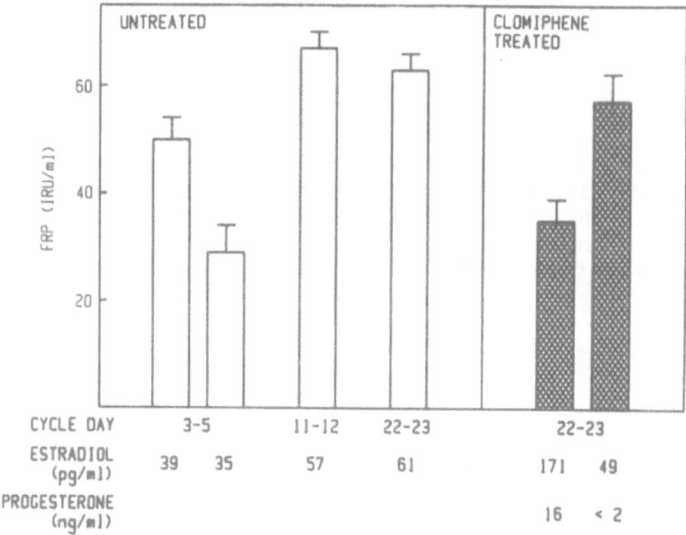

Fig. 3. Serum levels of follicle regulatory protein (FRP) determined by an ELISA from anovulatory patients untreated or treated with clomiphene citrate on menstrual cycle days 5-9 (data are expressed as means ± SEM; IRU, immunoreactive unit, from reference 50).

to events in other follicles, thereby potentiating an advantage in the selection process which is expressed, in part, as enhanced synthesis of estrogen. Other follicles would rapidly undergo atresia as a result of the FRP-mediated reduction in FSH-responsiveness. Most of the effects of FRP on granulosal activities reflect an interplay between the systemic endocrine and local paracrine systems. That FRP functions, at least in part, by modulating the follicular response to FSH is consistent with the hypothesis that paracrine effectors are the principal mediators of folliculogenesis in the presence of gonadotropins (26,33,53,54).

Many investigators have hypothesized that a timely induction or activation of the granulosal aromatase system and the concomitant changes in the profiles of the sex steroids in follicular cells are major determinants of the dominant follicle during its selection, early in the ovarian cycle (55-61). Adashi and Hsueh (62) suggested that intrafollicular estrogen can enhance the actions of FSH through stimulation of aromatase activity. Once a chosen follicle is producing a significant amount of estrogen, it then would have the capacity to produce more estrogen than neighboring follicles and the selection of the dominant follicle would be assured. In contrast, follicles destined to undergo atresia may not be able to produce enough estrogen to counteract the adverse effects of deprivation of FSH. Moor (63), Carson (64) and Tsonis et al. (65) concluded that reduced aromatase activity in atretic follicles is due to a loss of existing aromatase activity rather than a failure to acquire this activity initially, and that a decrease in aromatase activity is an early event in the atretic degeneration of antral follicles. It is the lack of granulosal aromatase and not androgen substrate per se which limits the production of estrogen in atretic follicles. Thus, atresia appears to be, at least in part, an active event, mediated by the intraovarian suppression of FSH-responsive aromatase activity.

ACKNOWLEDGMENT

This research was supported, in part, by a grant from the National Institute for Child Health and Human Development, number R01-18602.

REFERENCES

1. Hillier SG, Van Hall EV, Van Den Boogaard AJM, et al. Activation and modulation of the granulosa cell aromatase system: experimental studies with rat and human ovaries. In: McNatty KP, Schoemaker J, eds. Follicular maturation and ovulation. Amsterdam: Excerpta Medica, 1982:51-70.

2. Channing CP, Anderson LD, Hoover DJ, et al. Comparison of follicular maturation. Recent Prog Horm Res 1987; 38:331-404.

3. Tonetta SA, DeVinna RS, Fay J, et al. Comparison of follicular regulatory protein activity in porcine, equine and bovine follicular fluid [Abstract]. Ovarian Workshop, Ithaca, New York, 1986.

4. McNatty KP, Gibb M, Bodson C, et al. Preovulatory follicular development in sheep treated with PMSG and/or prostaglandin. J Reprod Fertil 1982; 65:111-23.

5. Guthrie HD, Bold DJ, Kiracafe GH, et al. Effects of charcoal-extracted porcine follicular fluid and porcine FSH on recruitment of medium follicles on gilts. Biol Reprod 1986; 34:71a.

6. Cahill LP, Driancourt MA, Chamley WA, et al. Role of intrafollicular regulators and FSH in growth and development of large antral follicles in sheep. J Reprod Fertil 1985; 75:1-9.

7. Chari S, Daume E, Sturm G, et al. Regulators of steroid secretion and inhibin activity in human ovarian follicular fluid. Mol Cell Endocrinol 1985; 41:137-45.

8. Saito H, Hiroi M. Correlation between the follicular gonadotropin inhibitor and the maturity of the ovum-corona-cumulus complex. Fertil Steril 1986; 46:66-72.

9. Adashi EY, Resnick CE, D'Ercole AJ, et al. Insulin-like growth factors as intraovarian regulators of granulosa cell growth and function. Endocr Rev 1985; 6:400-20.

10. Adashi EY, Resnick CE. Antagonistic interactions of transforming growth factors in the regulation of granulosa cell differentiation. Endocrinology 1986; 119:1879-81.

11. Holmberg EA, Campeau JD, Ono T, et al. Comparison of isoelectric focusing in sephadex vs immobiline flat beds for the preparative purification of follicular fluid. Prep Biochem 1986; 16:275-95.

12. Ono T, Campeau JD, Holmberg EA, et al. Biochemical and physiological characterization of follicle regulatory protein: a paracrine regulator of folliculogenesis. Am J Obstet Gynecol 1986; 154:709-16.

13. Isutsumi I, Fujimori K, Ono T, et al. Inhibition of spermatogenesis in the rat with follicle regulatory protein. Biol Reprod 1987; 36:451-61.

14. Kling OR, Roche PC, Campeau JD, et al. Identification of protein(s) in porcine follicular fluid which suppress follicular response to gonadotropins. Biol Reprod 1984; 30:564-72.

15. McNatty KP, Hunter WM, McNeilly AS, et al. Changes in the concentration of pituitary and steroid hormones in the follicular fluid of human Graafian follicles throughout the menstrual cycle. J Endocrinol 1975; 64:555-71.

16. McNatty KP, Makris A, DeGrazie C, et al. The production of progesterone, androgens and estrogens by granulosa cells, thecal tissue and stromal tissue from human ovaries in vitro. J Clin Endocrinol Metab 1979; 49:851-60.

17. McNatty KP, Moore, Smith D, et al. The microenvironment of the human follicle: interrelationships among the steroid levels in antral

fluid, the population of granulosa cells and the status of the oocyte in vivo and in vitro. J Clin Endocrinol Metab 1984; 49:851-60.

18. Battin DA, diZerega GS. Effect of follicular fluid protein(s) on gonadotropin modulated secretion of progesterone in porcine granulosa cells. Am J Obstet Gynecol 1985; 60:1116-9.

19. Schreiber JR, diZerega GS. Porcine follicular fluid protein(s) inhibit rat ovary granulosa cell steroidogenesis. Am J Obstet Gynecol 1986; 155:1281-8.

20. Battin DA, diZerega GS. Effect of hMG and follicle regulatory protein on 3β-ol-dehydrogenase activity in human granulosa cells. J Clin Endocrinol Metab 1985; 153:432-8.

21. Chicz R, Campeau JD, diZerega GS. Follicular regulatory protein noncompetively inhibits microsomal aromatase activity. In: Ryan RJ, Toaf D, eds. Proceedings of the 5th Ovarian Workshop, 1985:351-6.

22. Leung PCK, Armstrong DT. Interactions of steroids and gonadotropins in the control of steroidogenesis in the ovarian follicle. Annu Rev Physiol 1980; 42:71-95.

23. Leung PCK, Goff AK, Armstrong DT. Stimulatory effect of androgen administration in vivo on ovarian responsiveness to gonadotropins. Endocrinology 1979; 1204:1119-23.

24. Lischinsky A, Armstrong DT. Granulosa cell stimulation of thecal androgen synthesis. Can J Pharmacol 1983; 61:472-7.

25. Veldhuis JD, Klase PA, Sandow BA, et al. Progesterone secretion by highly differentiated human granulosa cells isolated from preovulatory Graafian follicles induced by exogenous gonadotropins and human chorionic gonadotropin. J Clin Endocrinol Metab 1983; 57:87-93.

26. diZerega GS, Campeau JD, Ujita EL, et al. Possible role for a follicular fluid protein in the intraovarian regulation of folliculo- genesis. Sem Reprod Endocrinol 1983; 11:309-22.

27. diZerega GS, Marrs RP, Campeau JD, et al. Human granulosa cell secretion of protein(s) which suppress follicular response to gonad- otropins. J Clin Endocrinol Metab 1983; 56:147-55.

28. McNatty KP, Baird DT. Relationship between follicle-stimulating hormone, androstenedione and oestradiol in human follicular fluid. J Endocrinol 1981; 76:527-31.

29. diZerega GS, Turner CK, Stouffer RL, et al. Suppression of FSH dependent folliculogenesis during the primate ovarian cycle. J Clin Endocrinol Metab 1981; 52:451-6.

30. Chikazawa K, Araki S, Tamada I. Morphological and endocrinological studies on follicular development during the human menstrual cycle. J Clin Endocrinol Metab 1986; 62:305-13.

31. Gougeon A. Dynamics of follicular growth in the human: a model from preliminary results. Human Reprod 1986; 1:81-7.

32. Baird DT, Backstrom T, McNeilly AS, et al. Effect of enucleation of the corpus luteum at different stages of the luteal phase of the human menstrual cycle on subsequent follicular development. J Reprod Fertil 1984; 70:615-24.

33. diZerega GS, Hodgen GD. Initiation of asymmetrical ovarian estradiol secretion in the primate ovarian cycle after lutectomy. Endocrinol- ogy 1981; 108:1233-6.

34. diZerega GS, Ross GT. Regulation of follicle growth. In: Taymor MC, Nelson J, eds. Progress in gynecology, vol 7. New York: Grune and Stratton, 1983:21-42.

35. Goodman AL, Hodgen GD. Systemic versus intraovarian progesterone replacement after luteectomy in rhesus monkeys: differential pat- terns of gonadotropins and follicle growth. J Clin Endocrinol Metab 1977; 45:837-43.

36. Goodman AL, Nixon WE, Johnson DL, et al. Regulation of folliculo- genesis in the rhesus monkey: selection of the dominant follicle. Endocrinology 1977; 100:155-63.

37. Nilsson L, Wikland M, Hamberger L. Recruitment of an ovulatory follicle in the human following follicle-ectomy and luteectomy. Fertil Steril 1984; 37:30-4.
38. Bogavich K, Richards JS. Androgen biosynthesis in developing ovarian follicles: evidence that luteinizing hormone regulates thecal 17α-hydroxylase and C17,20-lyase activities. Endocrinology 1982; 111:1201-8.
39. Sano Y, Suzuki K, Arai K, et al. Changes in enzyme activities on human ovaries during the menstrual cycle. J Clin Endocrinol Metab 1981; 52:994-8.
40. Tonetta SA, DeVinna RS, diZerega GS. Modulation of porcine thecal cell aromatase activity by human chorionic gonadotropin, progesterone, estradiol-17β and dihydrotestosterone. Biol Reprod 1986; 35:785-91.
41. Tsang BK, Ainsworth L, Downey BR, et al. Differential production of steroids by dispersed granulosa and theca interna cells from developing preovulatory follicles of pigs. J Reprod Fertil 1985; 74:459-71.
42. Tonetta SA, DeVinna RS, diZerega GS. Thecal cell 3β-hydroxysteroid dehydrogenase activity: modulation by hCG, progesterone, estradiol, and DHT. J Steroid Biochem (in press).
43. Liu Y-X, Hsueh AJ. Synergism between granulosa and theca-interstitial cells in estrogen biosynthesis by gonadotropin-treated rat ovaries: studies on the two-cell, two-gonadotropin hypothesis using steroid antisera. Biol Reprod 1986; 35:27-36.
44. Fortune JE. Bovine theca and granulosa cells interact to promote androgen production. Biol Reprod 1986; 35:292-9.
45. Choudary J, Gier H, Marion G. Cyclic changes in bovine vesicular follicles. J Anim Sci 1968; 27:468-71.
46. Driancourt MA, Fry RC, Clark IJ, Cahill LP. Follicular growth and regression during the 8 days after hypophysectomy in sheep. J Reprod Fertil 1987; 79:635-41.
47. McNatty KP. Ovarian follicular development from the onset of luteal regression in humans and sheep. In: Rolland R, VanHall EV, Hillier SG, McNatty KP, Schoemaker J, eds. Follicular maturation and ovulation. Proceedings of the IVth Reinier De Graff Symposium. Amsterdam: Elsiever, 1982:1-18.
48. Hodgen GD. The dominant ovarian follicle. Fertil Steril 1982; 38:281-300.
49. McNatty KP, Hillier SG, van den Boogaard AMJ, et al. Follicular development during the luteal phase of the human menstrual cycle. J Clin Endocrinol Metab 1983; 56:1022-31.
50. Lew NW, Katt EL, Rogers KE, et al. Alteration of follicle regulatory protein levels in human reproductive disorders and anovulation. Obstet Gynecol 1987; 70:157-62.
51. Montz FJ, Ujita EL, Campeau JD, et al. Inhibition of luteinizing hormone/human chorionic gonadotropin binding to porcine granulosa cells by a follicular fluid protein. Am J Obstet Gynecol 1984; 148:436-41.
52. Ujita EL, Campeau JD, diZerega GS. Inhibition of porcine granulosa cell adenylate cyclase activity by an ovarian protein. Exp Clin Endocrinol 1987 (in press).
53. diZerega GS, Hodgen GD. The primate ovarian cycle. Suppression of human menopausal gonadotropin-induced follicular growth in the presence of the dominant follicle. J Clin Endocrinol Metab 1980; 50:819-25.
54. Lindner HR, Amsterdam A, Salomon Y, et al. Intraovarian factors in ovulation: determinants of follicular response to gonadotropins. J Reprod Fertil 1977; 51:215-35.
55. Baird DT. Factors regulating the growth of the preovulatory follicle in the sheep and human. J Reprod Fertil 1983; 69:343-53.

56. Erickson GF, Hsueh AJW. Stimulation of aromatase activity by follicle stimulating hormone in rat granulosa cells in vivo and in vitro. Endocrinology 1978; 102:1275-82.

57. Goodman AL, Hodgen GD. The ovarian triad. Recent Prog Horm Res 1983; 39:1-73.

58. Goodman AL, Hodgen GD. Between-ovary interaction in the regulation of follicle growth, corpus luteum function and gonadotropin secretion in the primate ovarian cycle II. Effects of luteectomy and hemiovariectomy during the luteal phase in cynomolgus monkeys. Endocrinology 1979; 104:1310-8.

59. Hillier SG. Sex steroid metabolism and follicular development in the ovary. Oxf Rev Reprod Biol 1985; 7:168-222.

60. Hsueh AJW, Adashi EY, Jones PBC, et al. Hormonal regulation of the differentiation of cultured ovarian granulosa cells. Endocr Rev 1984; 5:76-127.

61. Veldhuis JD, Klase PA, Strauss JF, et al. The role of estradiol as a biological amplifier of the actions of follicle-stimulating hormone: in vitro studies in swine granulosa cells. Endocrinology 1982; 111:144-51.

62. Adashi EY, Hsueh ASW. Estrogens augment the stimulation of ovarian aromatase activity by follicle-stimulating hormone in cultured rat granulosa cells. J Biol Chem 1982; 257:6077-83.

63. Moor RM, Hay MF, Dott HM, et al. Macroscopic identification and steroidogenic function of atretic follicles in sheep. J Endocrinol 1978; 77:306.

64. Carson RS, Findlay JK, Clarke IJ, et al. Estradiol, testosterone and androstenedione in ovine follicular fluid during growth and atresia of ovarian follicles. Biol Reprod 1981; 24:105-12.

65. Tsonis CG, Carson RG, Findlay JK. Relationships between aromatase activity, follicular fluid oestradiol-17β and testosterone concentrations, and diameter and atresia of individual ovine follicles. J Reprod Fertil 1984; 72:153-63.

66. diZerega GS, Tonetta SA, Westhof G. Role of follicle regulatory protein in follicle selection. In: Hazeltine F, First N, eds. Molecular control of meiosis. New York: Alan Liss Publications, 1987 (in press).

GRANULOSA CELL DIFFERENTIATION IN PRIMATE OVARIES: THE

MARMOSET MONKEY (Callithrix jacchus) AS A LABORATORY MODEL

Stephen G. Hillier, Christopher R. Harlow[1], Helen J. Shaw[2],
E. Jean Wickings, Alan F. Dixson[3], and J. Keith Hodges[2]

Department of Obstetrics and Gynecology, and [3]MRC Unit of
Reproductive Biology, University of Edinburgh Center for
Reproductive Biology, Edinburgh EH3 9EW, Scotland;
[1]Institute of Obstetrics and Gynecology, Royal Postgraduate
Medical School, Hammersmith Hospital, DuCane Road, London
W12 OHS; [2]MRC/AFRC Comparative Physiology Research Group,
Institute of Zoology, Zoological Society of London,
Regent's Park, London NW1 4RY

SUMMARY

The ovarian cycle of the common marmoset (Callithrix jacchus) is
intermediate with those of laboratory rats and human beings. There are
also qualitative and quantitative similarities between preovulatory
granulosa cell function in marmosets and women. Cyclic and acyclic
(reproductively suppressed) marmoset ovaries are packed with multiple
immature follicles, and these contain granulosa cells which respond
biochemically and morphologically to human FSH in vitro. Hormone-
dependent differentiation can, therefore, be studied systematically using
primary cell cultures, the strategy which has contributed so much to
current concepts of nonprimate folliculogenesis. Our experience establishes the marmoset monkey as a valid laboratory model for studies. of
cellular aspects of folliculogenesis in primates.

INTRODUCTION

Most information on cellular aspects of folliculogenesis in mammals
has come from work with nonprimates, mainly the laboratory rat (see
references 1-5 for major reviews of the literature). The data which have
been obtained support the following precepts:

(1) Follicle-stimulating hormone (FSH) stimulates growth and differentiation of granulosa cells in immature ovarian follicles.

(2) FSH-stimulated granulosa cells undertake altered patterns of
protein synthesis and phosphorylation leading to the development of
steroidogenic enzymes, including aromatase, and LH receptors which are
functionally coupled to steroidogenesis.

(3) Luteinizing hormone (LH) stimulates androgen biosynthesis in
theca/interstitial cells, and androgen amplifies FSH action on immature

granulosa cells; intrafollicular regulators (steroids and peptides) modify granulosa cell responsiveness throughout preovulatory follicular development.

(4) In the preovulatory follicle, granulosa cell endocrine function (estradiol biosynthesis) becomes directly responsive to LH and dependence on FSH declines; after ovulation, granulosa-lutein cell endocrine function (progesterone biosynthesis) remains dependent on LH and independent of FSH.

Since rats are polyovular with short ovarian cycles, there are difficulties in extrapolating these findings to man or other primate species which have much longer ovarian cycles and lower ovulation rates. To obtain new insights on primate folliculogenesis, a laboratory primate is needed which is as open to experimentation as rodents, and that provides access to follicular tissues for systematic experimental studies in vitro. To this end, we have begun to examine cellular aspects of folliculogenesis in a laboratory monkey, the common marmoset (Callithrix jacchus). This highly fecund primate species thrives in captivity and has relevance to human beings and existing nonhuman primate models in terms of its ovarian cycle and its basic reproductive physiology (6). Moreover, marmoset monkeys can be maintained in sufficient numbers to allow systematic study of granulosa cell function at progressive stages of preovulatory follicular development. This article summarizes basic aspects of folliculogenesis in marmoset ovaries and describes the results of initial studies on the control of marmoset granulosa cell function in vitro.

THE MARMOSET OVARIAN CYCLE

Relevant details of the reproduction, growth and development of marmoset monkeys in captivity are outlined in Table 1. The ovarian cycle lasts about 28 days and there are usually two or three ovulations. Cyclic changes in ovarian steroid levels in plasma and urine, and the mid-cycle LH surge are well documented (7-9). The preovulatory or follicular phase (defined as that period of the cycle during which peripheral plasma progesterone levels remain below 10 ng/ml) is characterized by increasing levels of estradiol in both peripheral and utero-ovarian vein blood and lasts approximately 8 or 9 days (8,9). The luteal phase (progesterone between 10 and 150 ng/ml) lasts for approximately 19 days (8,9). Since the follicular phase is relatively short, it has been suggested that preovulatory follicular growth might be initiated during the previous luteal phase (9). However, this is uncertain because no published information exists on FSH levels in the marmoset.

The luteal phase comprises roughly two-thirds of the marmoset ovarian cycle; therefore, it is relatively easy to obtain luteal-phase ovaries. To obtain accurately staged follicular-phase tissue, precise control over the onset of preovulatory follicular development is required. This can be achieved by a single injection of synthetic prostaglandin-F2α given during the preceding luteal phase (10). The prostaglandin causes luteolysis which initiates a new wave of preovulatory follicular development, culminating in ovulation approximately 11 days later. Ovaries removed at progressive periods after prostaglandin-induced luteal regression are ideal for systematic studies of granulosa cell function in relation to preovulatory follicular development (11).

When marmoset monkeys are caged together as families or peer groups, usually only one behaviorally-dominant adult female has regular ovarian cycles and breeds (6,12). Behaviorally-subordinate adult females in the

Table 1. The common marmoset monkey in captivity.*

Social Groups	Adult pair + 1-4 offspring
Ovarian cycle:	28 days
Follicular phase	9 days
Luteal phase	19 days
Weight at:	
Birth	25-35 g
Social/sexual maturity	400-600 g
Age at:	
Weaning	40-80 days
Puberty	8 months
Maturity	18-24 months
Longevity:	10-16 years

*Based on reference 6.

group remain acyclic in her presence. The ovaries in reproductively suppressed animals contain multiple immature follicles which yield granulosa cells ideal for in vitro studies on the control of hormone-dependent differentiation (13).

FOLLICLE-SIZE DISTRIBUTION IN MARMOSET OVARIES

Typically, there are up to 100 antral follicles ≥0.5 mm in diameter present in a pair of cyclic marmoset ovaries (13). The size distribution of follicles dissected from marmoset ovaries during the mid-follicular (7 days postprostaglandin-induced luteolysis) and luteal phases of the cycle is illustrated in Figure 1. "Small" follicles (0.5-1.0 mm in diameter) constitute approximately 90% of the total population of antral follicles. Of these follicles, 70-80% appear to be nonatretic based on macroscopic appearance and microscopic assessment of membrana granulosa integrity. However, medium-sized follicles (1.0-1.9 mm in diameter) are relatively rare and form <10% of all follicles ≥0.5 mm in diameter. This implies that only a limited number of "small" follicles ever grow beyond about 1.0 mm in diameter to begin preovulatory stages of development (11). Two or three "large" follicles ≥2.0 mm in diameter are usually present in mid-follicular phase ovaries. These are the preovulatory follicles which normally grow to a maximum diameter of about 4.0 mm before ovulating. After ovulation, there are no large follicles other than the postovulatory follicles or corpora lutea (Fig. 1). The proportion of small follicles present in luteal phase follicles remains high at approximately 90%; medium-sized follicles continue to be rare.

AROMATASE ACTIVITY AND GRANULOSA CELL NUMBER IN MARMOSET FOLLICLES

Increases in granulosa cell aromatase activity accompany preovulatory follicular growth and development; measurement in vitro of aromatase activity provides an index of granulosa cell maturity (14). Granulosa cell number and aromatase activity as functions of preovulatory follicular development in marmoset ovaries are shown in Figure 2. Consistent with observations in other species, including rat and man (5), large preovulatory follicles contain many more granulosa cells with higher levels of aromatase than smaller nonovulatory follicles (4,12). The aromatase activity of marmoset preovulatory granulosa cells is quantitatively similar to the level measured in human preovulatory granulosa

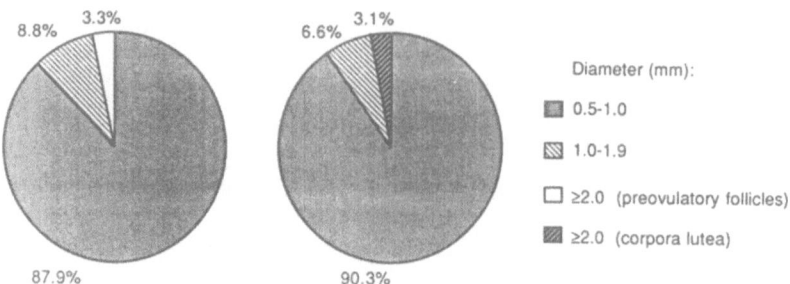

Fig. 1. Follicle-size distribution in cyclic marmoset
ovaries. Follicular phase: data from 429 follicles
dissected from the ovaries of 6 cyclic marmosets 7 days
after prostaglandin-induced luteolysis (redrawn from reference 11). Luteal phase: data from 791 follicles
dissected from the ovaries of 10 animals at various stages
of the luteal phase.

cells under similar assay conditions (11,13,14). When differences in mean
granulosa cell number are taken into account, the total follicular aromatase capacity (i.e., estrogenic potential) of large preovulatory follicles is approximately 2,000 times higher than that of nonovulatory
follicles. The human preovulatory follicle has similar characteristics,
further highlighting qualitative and quantitative similarities which exist
between preovulatory granulosa cell function in marmoset monkeys and human
beings.

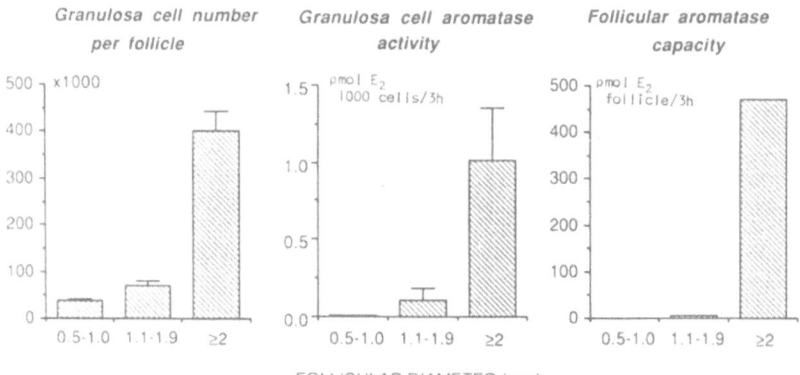

Fig. 2. Granulosa cell number per follicle (left panel),
granulosa cell aromatase activity (center panel) and follicular aromatase capacity (right panel) in relation to follicular diameter in cyclic marmoset ovaries. The data are mean
± SE from observations on ovaries removed from 5 animals 7
days after prostaglandin-induced luteolysis. Granulosa cell
isolation and measurement of extant aromatase activity was
carried out as described previously (13). "Follicular
aromatase capacity" is the product of mean granulosa cell
aromatase activity and mean granulosa cell number from
observations on all of the follicles in each follicle-size
category. (Redrawn from reference 11.)

MARMOSET GRANULOSA CELL CULTURES

The "small" antral follicles in cyclic marmoset ovaries are functionally immature and contain FSH-responsive granulosa cells with a low level of extant steroidogenic capacity (11). These follicles are easy to dissect from the ovary and provide tissue which can be used for studies on the initiation and control of preovulatory granulosa cell development in vitro. Marmoset granulosa cells at all stages of preovulatory development adapt well to primary culture and show functional and morphological responses to human FSH (Fig. 3). The choice of culture medium influences FSH-stimulated steroidogenesis (progesterone production) as shown in Figure 4. Relatively high basal levels of steroidogenesis are expressed in medium 199 containing 5% calf serum but serum suppresses responsiveness to FSH, similar to its effect on cultured rat granulosa cells (3,16). Serum-free McCoy's modified 5a medium, popular for culturing rat granulosa cells (3,16), allows greater responsiveness to FSH but with low maximal levels of steroid production. By deleting serum from medium 199 and using serum-precoated culture dishes (17), both responsiveness to FSH and overall rates of steroid production are satisfactory. We, therefore, use these conditions routinely.

Development-Dependent Changes in FSH Responsiveness

Granulosa cell responsiveness to FSH (cyclic AMP production, steroid biosynthesis, etc.) increases during preovulatory follicular development in rat ovaries (1-5). This change is induced by FSH itself and is subject to modulation by locally produced factors such as sex steroids and peptides (1-5,18). Work with cultures of marmoset granulosa cells confirms that equivalent development-related changes occur in primates (11,13). Figure 5 shows the dose-related effects of a human pituitary FSH preparation on aromatase activity and progesterone production in granulosa cell cultures from small (0.5-1.0 mm diameter) and large (>2 mm diameter) follicles present in marmoset ovaries at mid-follicular phase. Granulosa cells from immature follicles are highly responsive to the gonadotropin, giving rise to FSH-stimulated maxima more than 30 times greater than control values within 2 days of culture. Granulosa cells from large follicles have higher basal levels of steroidogenesis, commensurate with their more advanced state of preovulatory development. They are also far more sensitive to FSH as shown by ED_{50} values of <1 ng/ml compared with approximately 10 ng/ml for the less mature granulosa cells. The finding that primate granulosa cells become increasingly sensitive to FSH during preovulatory development in vivo is in accord with the experimental evidence from work with macaques, showing that the growing preovulatory follicle has a progressively diminished requirement for FSH stimulation during the late follicular phase (19). This may be one of the mechanisms whereby the human preovulatory follicle once selected is capable of continued growth and estrogen secretion, despite the reduction in circulating FSH levels which occurs during the late follicular phase. Further work with marmoset granulosa cell cultures should help elucidate the cellular mechanisms which underlie the preovulatory increase in granulosa cell sensitivity to FSH in primates.

Development-Dependent Changes in LH Responsiveness

Preovulatory biochemical changes in granulosa cells include the expression of a membrane-associated LH receptor system which is functionally coupled to steroid hormone biosynthesis (1-5,16). Granulosa cells in preovulatory follicles thereby become directly responsive to LH in anticipation of the ovulation-inducing LH surge. This means that aromatization (hence, estradiol biosynthesis) and progesterone biosynthesis both fall under direct LH control.

Evidence that marmoset granulosa cells acquire direct responsiveness to LH during advanced preovulatory follicular development is shown in Figure 6. Only granulosa cells from preovulatory follicles undertake LH-responsive progesterone biosynthesis and have an LH-responsive aromatase system. Granulosa cells from immature follicles in follicular- and luteal-phase ovaries show responsiveness to FSH but not LH in vitro. These data agree with autoradiographic evidence from rhesus monkey ovaries

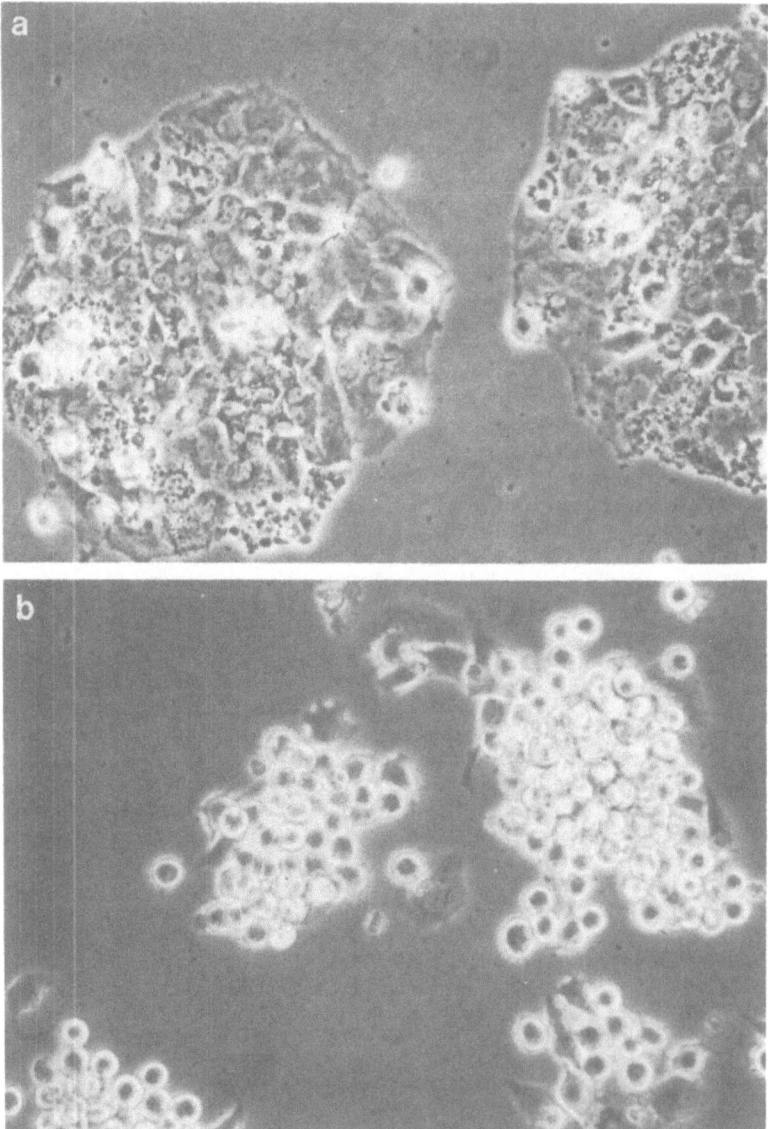

Fig. 3. Marmoset granulosa cells after culture for 48 h in serum-free medium 199 using serum-precoated culture dishes (17): (a) control; (b) in the presence of human FSH (LER 8/116, 30 ng/ml). The cells were harvested from a 4-mm diameter preovulatory follicle. Note the rounded, refractile appearance of cells cultured in the presence of FSH. (Light micrographs [x200].)

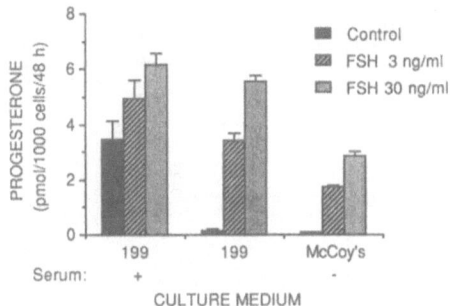

Fig. 4. Basal and FSH-stimulated progesterone production by marmoset granulosa
cells: variation with culture conditions.
The culture media were McCoy's (5a modified
without serum) or medium 199 with (+) or
without (-) 5% donor calf serum (Gibco).
The culture wells used to culture granulosa
cells in serum-free medium 199 were pre-
coated (overnight incubation at 37°C) with
serum and then washed with Dulbecco's
phosphate-buffered saline before use (17).
Granulosa cells were pooled from 33 0.5-1.0
mm diameter follicles obtained from a single
marmoset ovary at an indeterminate stage of
the ovarian cycle. Replicate cultures (1.4
x 10^4 cells/0.5 ml medium) were incubated
for 48 h at 37°C in a humidified tissue
culture incubator gassed with 5% CO_2 in air.
The FSH was hFSH LER 8/116 at 3 ng/ml and 30
ng/ml as indicated. Progesterone accumulation was measured in culture medium by
radioimmunoassay. Data are mean ± SE from
incubations in quadruplicate. (Unpublished
results.)

that granulosa cells in immature follicles do not possess specific binding
sites for human chorionic gonadotropin (hCG), whereas preovulatory
granulosa cells show high levels of specific hCG binding (20), similar to
the situation in nonprimates (1-5,16).

FSH Induction of LH/hCG Responsiveness

The induction of the LH/hCG receptor system is known to be under
direct FSH control in nonprimate granulosa cells (1-5). Our work with the
marmoset monkey has provided experimental evidence that FSH induces LH/hCG
responsiveness in primate granulosa cells as well. As shown in Figure 7,
cells isolated from immature (0.5-1.0 mm diameter) follicles in mid-follicular phase ovaries show minimal steroidogenic responsiveness to hCG
after culture for 2 days in the absence of FSH. However, after culture
for 2 days in the presence of FSH (30 ng/ml), they express hCG-responsive
aromatase activity. This implies that FSH acts directly to induce LH/hCG
receptors on primate granulosa cells, similar to its well-documented
action on nonprimate cells (16,21). Direct measurement of LH/hCG receptors on marmoset granulosa cells is required to verify this.

67

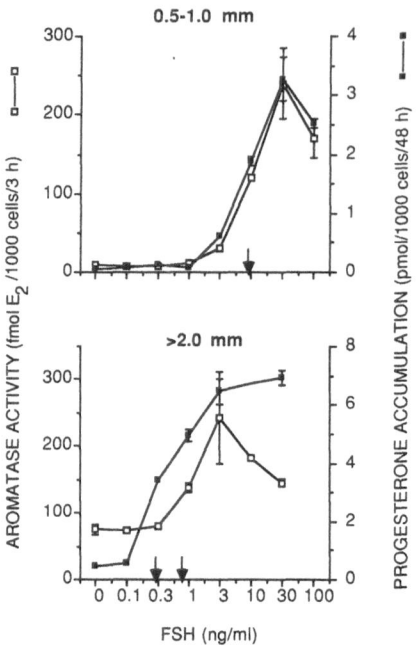

Fig. 5. Dose-related effects of FSH on progesterone accumulation and aromatase activity in marmoset granulosa cell cultures. The granulosa cells were obtained from "small" (0.5-1.0 mm diameter, upper panel) and "large" (>2.0 mm diameter, lower panel) follicles 7 days after prostaglandin-induced luteolysis. The FSH was human FSH LER 8/116. Progesterone accumulation was measured in culture medium collected at 48 h. Aromatase activity was measured at 48 h by determining estradiol production (radioimmunoassay) during a further 3-h (37°C) incubation of washed cell monolayers in the presence of 1.0 μM testosterone as an exogenous aromatase substrate (13). Data are mean ± SE from incubations in quadruplicate (progesterone) or triplicate (aromatase). Arrows on the abscissa indicate approximate ED_{50} values. (Redrawn from reference 11.)

Steroid Modulation of FSH Action

Experiments in vivo and in vitro on nonprimate ovarian tissues have shown that locally produced steroids, androgens and estrogens modulate gonadotropin action on developing granulosa cells (2-5). Work with cultured granulosa cells has shown that the action of FSH in inducing granulosa cell differentiation is amplified by the presence of steroid, androgens being more active than estrogens (4,5). The follicular fluid from immature human follicles contains high levels of androgens (22), raising the question if androgens also influence FSH action at early stages of primate granulosa cell differentiation. Affirmative evidence comes from work with cultured granulosa cells from reproductively sup-

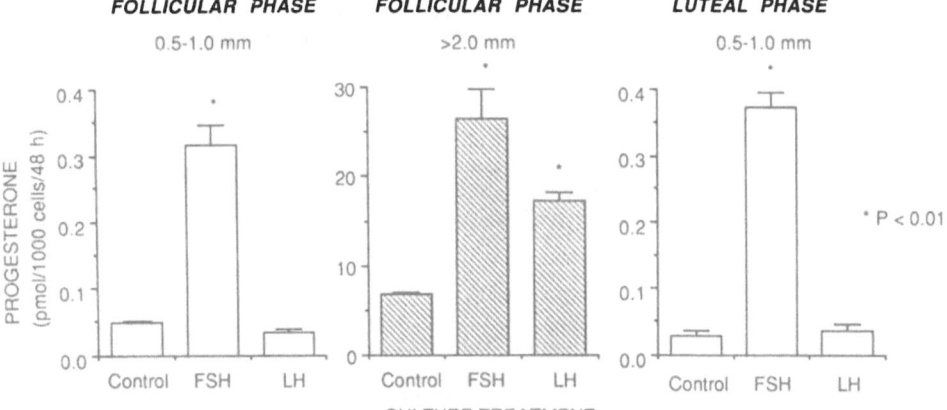

FOLLICULAR PHASE
0.5-1.0 mm

FOLLICULAR PHASE
>2.0 mm

LUTEAL PHASE
0.5-1.0 mm

* P < 0.01

PROGESTERONE (pmol/1000 cells/48 h)

CULTURE TREATMENT

Fig. 6. Effects of FSH and LH on progesterone production by marmoset granulosa cell cultures. Immature follicles (0.5-1.0 mm diameter) in the follicular phase (<u>left panel</u>) and luteal phase (<u>right panel</u>) yield granulosa cells which do not respond to LH, whereas cells from preovulatory (>2.0-mm diameter) follicles do (<u>center panel</u>). Culture was for 48 h in medium containing no gonadotropin ("control"), FSH (human FSH LER 8/116, 10 ng/ml) or LH (human LH LER 1972, 10 ng/ml). Progesterone accumulation was measured in culture medium. Data are mean ± SE from incubations in triplicate. Asterisk denotes significant stimulation (P<0.01) compared with the corresponding control value. (Unpublished results.)

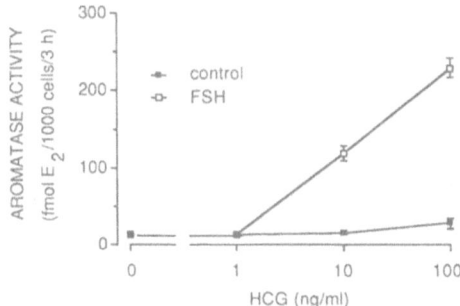

AROMATASE ACTIVITY (fmol E$_2$/1000 cells/3 h)

control
FSH

HCG (ng/ml)

Fig. 7. FSH induction of hCG–responsive aromatase activity in marmoset granulosa cell cultures. Cells obtained from "small" (0.5-1.0 mm diameter) follicles 7 days after prostaglandin-induced luteolysis were cultured for 48 h in medium without ("control") or with FSH (human FSH LER 8/116, 30 ng/ml). The medium was replaced with fresh medium containing no hormone or hCG (CR-119) at the concentrations indicated. Incubation was continued for a further 48 h. Aromatase activity was determined at 96 h in washed cell monolayers, as described in the legend to Figure 5. Data are mean ± SE from incubations in triplicate. (Unpublished results.)

pressed acyclic marmoset ovaries (13): androgens (5α–dihydrotestosterone
and testosterone) but not estradiol dramatically enhance the action of FSH
in inducing granulosa cell aromatase activity and progesterone biosynthesis (Fig. 8). Similar effects are observed using granulosa cells from
immature follicles in cyclic animals (11), as illustrated in Figures 9 and
10. These results afford the first clear–cut evidence with primate tissue
that androgens can promote FSH–induced steroidogenesis during granulosa
cell differentiation in vitro. The data also show how androgen action
varies with preovulatory granulosa cell maturity. Thus, testosterone and
5α–dihydrotestosterone act directly to enhance the sensitivity of immature
granulosa cells to the differentiation–inducing action of FSH. However,
these androgens have no consistent effect on FSH–stimulated progesterone
production by granulosa cells from preovulatory follicles (Fig. 9).
Moreover, testosterone serves to inhibit the FSH stimulation of aromatase
activity in mature granulosa cells (Fig. 10). This suggests that
granulosa cell responsiveness to androgen undergoes a shift during preovulatory follicular development. The mechanism and physiological significance of the inhibitory action of androgen on the aromatase system in
preovulatory primate granulosa cells remain to be established.

The finding that estradiol does not enhance the differentiation-
inducing action of FSH on immature marmoset granulosa cells is at variance
with much of the data from nonprimates (1–5). It remains to be determined
whether estrogen acts directly to affect gonadotropin responsiveness
during preovulatory stages of granulosa cell development, as is generally
believed to be the case in nonprimate ovaries (1–5).

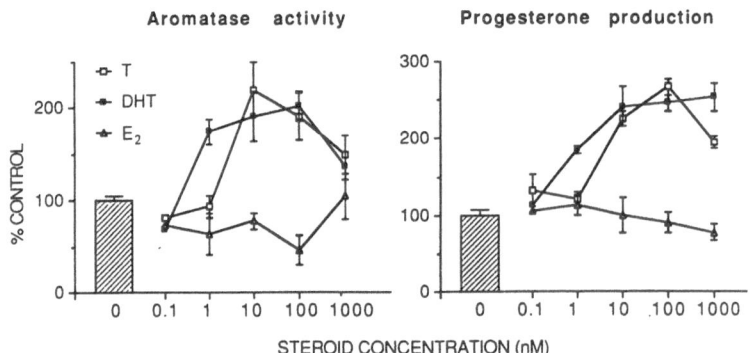

Fig. 8. Augmentation of FSH–induced steroidogenesis by testosterone and 5α–dihydrotestosterone
(DHT) but not estradiol (E₂) in cultured marmoset
granulosa cells. Granulosa cells from follicles
≤1.0–mm diameter in reproductively suppressed
marmoset ovaries were cultured for 48 h in medium
containing FSH (human FSH LER 8/116, 3 ng/ml)
alone and in the presence of steroid at the
concentrations indicated. Aromatase activity
(left panel) was measured in washed cell monolayers, as described in the legend to Figure 5;
progesterone accumulation (right panel) was
measured in the medium. Data are expressed as a
percentage of the response to FSH alone and are
mean ± SE from incubations in quadruplicate.
(Redrawn from reference 13.)

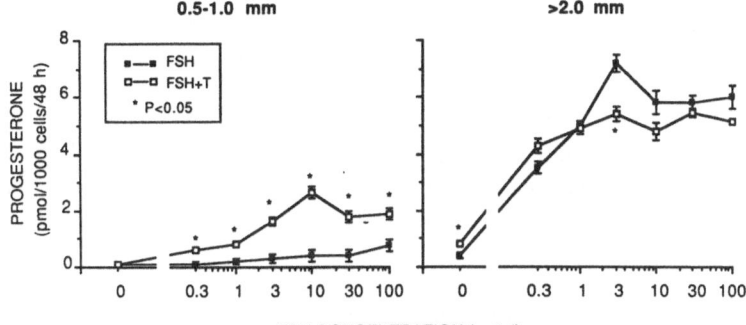

Fig. 9. Effect of testosterone on FSH-responsive progesterone production in marmoset granulosa cell cultures from "small" (0.5-1.0 mm diameter, <u>left panel</u>) and "large" (>2.0 mm diameter, <u>right panel</u>) follicles 7 days after prostaglandin-induced luteolysis. The cells were cultured in medium containing increasing doses of FSH (human FSH LER 8/116) in the absence and presence of 0.1 μM testosterone (T), as indicated. Progesterone accumulation was measured in the culture medium collected at 48 h. Data are mean ± SE from incubations in quadruplicate. Asterisk denotes statistically significant (P<0.05) levels of stimulation or inhibition due to the presence of testosterone. (Redrawn from reference 11.)

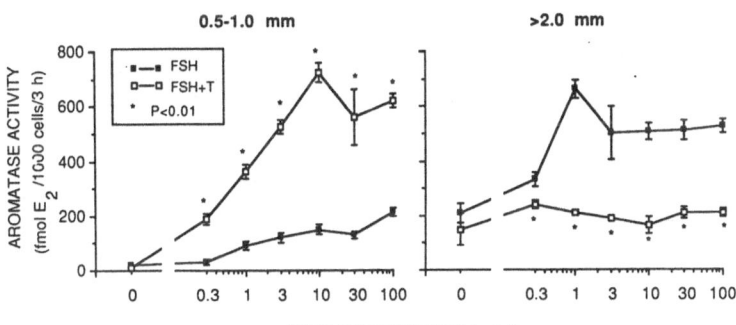

Fig. 10. Effect of testosterone on FSH-responsive aromatase activity in marmoset granulosa cell cultures from "small" (0.5-1.0 mm diameter, <u>left panel</u>) and "large" (>2.0 mm diameter, <u>right panel</u>) follicles 7 days after prostaglandin-induced luteolysis. The cells were cultured in medium containing increasing doses of FSH (human FSH LER 8/116) in the absence and presence of 0.1 μM testosterone (T). Aromatase activity was measured in washed cell monolayers at 48 h, as described in the legend to Figure 5. Data are mean ± SE from incubations in quadruplicate. Asterisk denotes significant (P<0.01) levels of stimulation or inhibition due to the presence of testosterone. (Redrawn from reference 11.)

CONCLUDING REMARKS

Perspectives on folliculogenesis in nonprimates accord FSH a pivotal function as the primary endocrine stimulus for folliculogenesis via activation of specific FSH receptors on immature granulosa cells. Phenotypic expression of functional and morphological granulosa cell changes induced by FSH is subject to a second (paracrine) level of control by factors such as androgens produced locally under endocrine control by LH. FSH-induced onset of differentiated granulosa cell function (i.e., direct LH responsiveness) is associated with altered genomic expression and the biosynthesis of new proteins, including LH receptors, steroidogenic enzymes, proteases and regulatory peptides such as somatomedins and inhibins. These factors constitute a third (autocrine) level of cellular control, culminating in terminally differentiated granulosa cell function (i.e., LH-responsive progesterone biosynthesis) in the corpus luteum.

The relevance of many of these concepts to primates remains to be shown experimentally. However, the in vitro approach using marmoset granulosa cells permits systematic work towards this end and should provide more knowledge of the cellular basis of folliculogenesis in the primate ovary.

ACKNOWLEDGMENT

This work was supported by a collaborative MRC Project Grant to JKH and SGH. We are grateful to Professor Leo R. Reichert, Jr., for providing human pituitary FSH and LH.

REFERENCES

1. Channing CP, Thanki K, Lindsey AM, Ledwitz-Rigby F. Development and hormonal regulation of gonadotrophin responsiveness in granulosa cells of the mammalian ovary. In: Birnbaumer L, O'Malley BW, eds. Receptors and hormone action. New York: Academic Press, 1978:435-55.
2. Richards JS. Maturation of ovarian follicles: actions and interactions of pituitary and ovarian hormones on follicular differentiation. Physiol Rev 1980; 60:51-89.
3. Hsueh AJW, Adashi EJ, Jones PBC, Welsh TJ Jr. Hormonal regulation of the differentiation of cultured ovarian granulosa cells. Endocr Rev 1984; 5:76-127.
4. Dorrington JH, McKeracher HL, Chan AK, Gore-Langton RE. Hormonal interactions in the control of granulosa cell differentiation. J Steroid Biochem 1983; 19:17-32.
5. Hillier SG. Sex steroid metabolism and follicular development in the ovary. In: Clarke JR, ed. Oxford reviews of reproductive biology; vol 7. Oxford: Clarendon Press, 1985:167-222.
6. Hearn JP. Marmosets and tamarins. In: Poole T, ed. The UFAW handbook on "The care and management of laboratory animals." 6th ed. Harlow: Longman Scientific & Technical, 1987:568-81.
7. Eastman SAK, Makawiti DW, Collins WP, Hodges JK. Pattern of excretion of urinary steroid metabolites during the ovarian cycle and pregnancy in the marmoset monkey. J Endocrinol 1984; 102:19-26.
8. Harlow CR, Hearn JP, Hodges JK. Ovulation in the marmoset monkey: endocrinology, prediction and detection. J Endocrinol 1984; 103:17-24.
9. Harlow CR, Gems S, Hodges JK, Hearn JP. The relationship between plasma progesterone and the timing of ovulation and early embryonic

development in the marmoset monkey (<u>Callithrix jacchus</u>). J Zool Lond 1983; 201:273-82.

10. Summers PM, Wennink CJ, Hodges JK. Cloprostenol-induced luteolysis in the marmoset monkey, <u>Callithrix jacchus</u>. J Reprod Fertil 1985; 73:133-8.

11. Harlow CR, Shaw HJ, Hillier SG, Hodges JK. Factors influencing FSH-induced steroidogenesis in marmoset granulosa cells: effects of androgens and stage of follicular development. Endocrinology (submitted).

12. Abbott DH. Behavioral and physiological suppression of fertility in subordinate marmoset monkeys. Am J Primatol 1984; 6:169-86.

13. Harlow CR, Hillier SG, Hodges JK. Androgen modulation of follicle-stimulating hormone-induced granulosa cell steroidogenesis in the primate ovary. Endocrinology 1986; 119:1403-5.

14. Hillier SG, Reichert LE Jr, van Hall EV. Control of preovulatory follicular estrogen biosynthesis in the human ovary. J Clin Endocrinol Metab 1981; 52:847-56.

15. Hillier SG, Knazek RA, Ross GT. Androgenic stimulation of progesterone production by granulosa cells from preantral follicles: further in vitro studies using replicate cell cultures. Endocrinology 1977; 100:1539-49.

16. Erickson GF. Primary cultures of ovarian cells in serum-free medium as models of hormone-dependent differentiation. Mol Cell Endocrinol 1983; 29:21-49.

17. Hillier SG, de Zwart FA. Androgen/antiandrogen modulation of cyclic AMP-induced steroidogenesis during granulosa cell differentiation in tissue culture. Mol Cell Endocrinol 1982; 28:347-61.

18. Hsueh AJW. Paracrine mechanisms involved in granulosa cell differentiation. In: Franchimont F, ed. Clinics in endocrinology and metabolism; vol 15. London: WB Saunders, 1986:117-33.

19. Zeleznik AJ, Kubik CJ. Ovarian responses in macaques to pulsatile induction of follicle-stimulating hormone (FSH) and luteinizing hormone: increased sensitivity of the maturing follicle to FSH. Endocrinology 1986; 119:2025-32.

20. Zeleznik AJ, Schuler HM, Reichert LE Jr. Gonadotropin-binding sites in the rhesus monkey ovary: role of the vasculature in the selective distribution of human chorionic gonadotropin to the preovulatory follicle. Endocrinology 1981; 109:356-62.

21. Zeleznik AJ, Midgley AR Jr, Reichert LE Jr. Granulosa cell maturation in the rat; increased binding of human chorionic gonadotropin following treatment with follicle-stimulating hormone in vivo. Endocrinology 1974; 95:818-25.

22. McNatty KP, Hillier SG, van den Boogaard AJM, Trimbos-Kemper TCM, Reichert LE Jr, van Hall EV. Follicular development during the luteal phase of the human menstrual cycle. J Clin Endocrinol Metab 1983; 56:1022-31.

II. OVULATION AND SUPEROVULATION

FACTORS CONTROLLING MAMMALIAN OOCYTE MATURATION

John J. Eppig, Ph.D.

The Jackson Laboratory
Bar Harbor, ME 04609

INTRODUCTION

The oocytes of many mammals are arrested in prophase of the first meiotic division from about the time of birth. Throughout most of their growth phase, the oocytes are incompetent of resuming the meiotic division. However, as the growth phase nears completion, the oocytes become competent of undergoing germinal vesicle breakdown (GVB) and reinitiating meiosis spontaneously when isolated from their follicles and cultured in an appropriate medium without gonadotropins or steroid hormones (1,2). These immature oocytes are said to have acquired GVB-competence. Oocytes in graafian follicles (Fig. 1) are usually GVB-competent. Accordingly, isolation and culture of these oocytes results in spontaneous maturation (Fig. 2). This observation of spontaneous GVB in oocytes liberated from the environment of the graafian follicle led to the hypothesis that some follicular components maintain the competent oocytes in meiotic arrest (3). Atretic antral follicles frequently contain mature oocytes presumably because the follicular system for maintaining meiotic arrest has degenerated. Meiosis is reinitiated in graafian follicles as a result of the preovulatory surge of gonadotropins. I will emphasize recent results that address the following problems: (a) the control of the acquisition of GVB-competence by immature oocytes, (b) the maintenance of meiotic arrest; and, (c) the initiation of GVB. Several reviews of earlier studies have been published (4-6).

THE ACQUISITION OF GVB-COMPETENCE

Growing mouse oocytes normally acquire GVB-competence when they achieve a diameter of 60-65 µm. However, the developmental program governing the acquisition of GVB-competence is independent of oocyte growth (7). Oocyte growth is dependent upon gap junction-mediated communication between the oocyte and its companion granulosa cells (8-11). But when the oocytes were co-cultured with fibroblasts with which they did not communicate via gap junctions, the oocytes acquired GVB-competence, without significant growth, within about the same time period as growing oocytes (7).

Oocytes isolated from 10-11-day-old mice are in mid-growth phase and, without further development, are GVB-incompetent. When oocyte-granulosa cell complexes were isolated from these mice and cultured for 12 days in defined medium without gonadotropins or steroid hormones, about 70% of them acquired GVB-competence (12). These results show that once the oocytes reach mid-growth phase in normal mice with circulating gonadotropin, further exposure to gonadotropins or steroid hormones is not required for the acquisition of GVB-competence. However, it is possible that the program governing the acquisition of competence could have been initiated

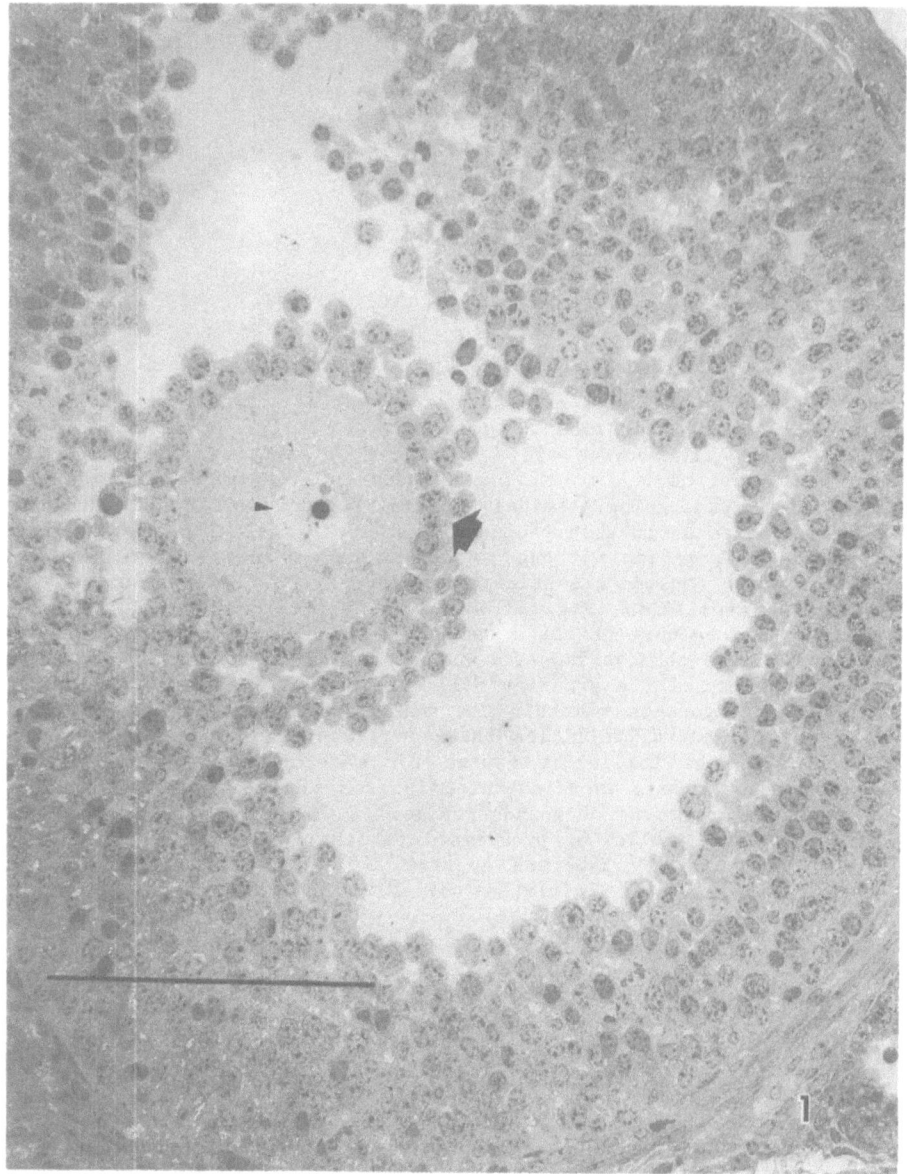

Fig. 1. Transmission electron micrograph of a graafian follicle from a 22-day-old BALB/cByJ mouse that had been injected with 5 IU of pregnant mare's serum gonadotropin (PMSG) at 20 days of age. The oocyte has intact germinal vesicle (arrowhead) containing prominent nucleoli. The oocyte is enclosed by 1-3 layers of cumulus cells (arrow). Bar indicates 100 μm.

by gonadotropins or steroid hormones before isolation of the oocyte-granulosa cell complexes.

Mice homozygous for the autosomal recessive mutation called hypogonadal (hpg) do not produce gonadotropin releasing hormone. Although the pituitary glands of these mice contain gonadotropins, there is no detectable follicle-stimulating hormone (FSH) in circulation (13). Therefore, oocytes develop in hpg/hpg females without or with extremely low levels of gonadotropin stimulation. The number of developing follicles is reduced in hpg/hpg mice, but some follicles develop to the early antral stage (13). The oocytes in these follicles are fully grown and GVB-competent (14). Apparently, the acquisition of GVB-competence by mouse oocytes can occur with little or no stimulation by gonadotropin. We have found that the kinetics of GVB by oocytes from hpg/hpg females is retarded compared to littermate controls and that injection of the hpg/hpg females with gonadotropin renders the kinetics of GVB identical to that of normal mice. Moreover, the ability of hpg/hpg oocytes matured in culture to be fertilized and undergo preimplantation development in vitro was very low compared to littermate controls. Studies in progress show that treatment of the hpg/hpg females with gonadotropin increased the frequency at which the ova can be fertilized and undergo preimplantation development. Although gonadotropins may not be required for the acquisition of GVB competence by mouse oocytes, gonadotropins have a beneficial effect on the development of maturational processes that relate to the kinetics of oocyte maturation and the developmental capacity of the ova.

Hypophysectomy reduced the percent of GVB-competent oocytes isolated from rat follicles (15). Injection of the hypophysectomized rats with either FSH or 17β-estradiol increased the percent of GVB-competent oocytes. These results suggest that FSH may play a role in the acquisition of GVB-competence by rat oocytes and that this effect is mediated by estrogen. In contrast, 95% of the oocytes isolated from mice 17 weeks after hypophysectomy underwent GVB in culture and 75% of them produced a polar body (16). Since the growth phase of mouse oocytes requires only

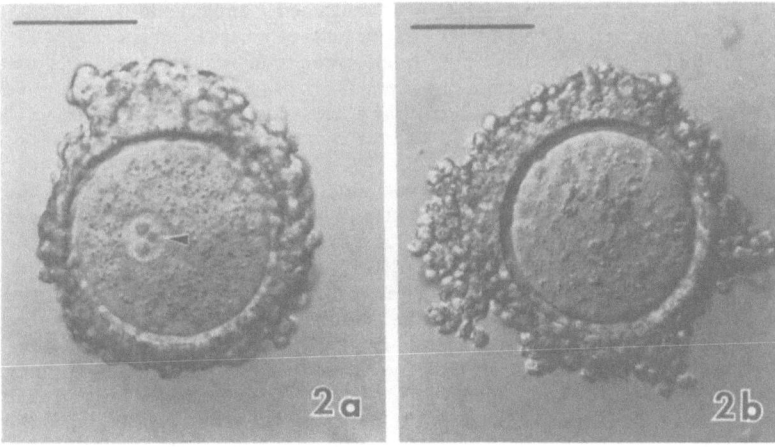

Fig. 2. Photomicrographs of cumulus cell-enclosed oocytes isolated from a 22-day-old mouse that had been injected with PMSG 2 days before isolation of the oocytes. (2a) Freshly isolated oocyte containing an intact germinal vesicle (arrowhead) with prominent nucleoli. (2b) Oocyte that has undergone spontaneous GVB during a 5-hour culture period. Nomarski interference optics; bar indicates 50 μm.

15-20 days, the entire growth of the oocytes in the hypophysectomized mice occurred in the complete absence of gonadotropin. This confirms that in mice the acquisition of GVB competence does not require gonadotropin, and may indicate a species difference in this regard between mice and rats. Polar body production by oocytes from hypophysectomized mice was increased by injection with either gonadotropin or 17β-estradiol (16). Gonadotropins, therefore, have a beneficial effect on the development of maturational processes in mice and the effect may be mediated by estrogen.

MAINTENANCE OF MEIOTIC ARREST

Cyclic adenosine monophosphate (cAMP) within the oocyte is important for maintaining meiotic arrest. Supporting evidence includes the following observations: (a) membrane-permeable analogs of cAMP and cAMP phosphodiesterase inhibitors maintain meiotic arrest in vitro (17-20); (b) levels of cAMP in mouse and rat oocytes that have undergone GVB are lower than in GV-intact oocytes (21-23); (c) injection of an inhibitor of the catalytic subunit of cAMP-dependent protein kinase induced maturation in oocytes that had been maintained in arrest by cAMP analogs or phosphodiesterase inhibitors (24); and, (d) injection into oocytes of the catalytic subunit of cAMP-dependent protein kinase maintained meiotic arrest (24). Therefore, given that elevated levels of cAMP within the oocyte are important for maintaining meiotic arrest, how are these levels of cAMP maintained within the oocyte? This may require a constant supply of cAMP because of the potentially high levels of phosphodiesterase activity in the oocytes (25).

Cyclic AMP produced in the mass of granulosa cells may be transferred to the oocytes via the gap junctions that metabolically couple granulosa cells, cumulus cells and the oocyte (20) (Fig. 3 and 4). Some evidence suggests that this is possible. Treatment of isolated oocyte-cumulus cell complexes with FSH, cholera toxin, or forskolin, and in some cases the phosphodiesterase inhibitor 3-isobutyl-1-methylxanthine (IBMX), results in an increase in the oocyte cAMP over that found in cumulus cell-denuded oocytes (23,26-28). Apparently, cAMP may be transferred from cumulus cells to oocytes under these highly stimulated conditions in vitro, but it is not clear that this occurs in vivo under normal physiological conditions. In addition, it has not been resolved whether the increase in oocyte cAMP is actually due to the transfer of cAMP from cumulus cells or to the transfer of factors that promote the generation of cAMP within the oocyte such as cAMP precursors or stimulators of oocyte adenylate cyclase.

Cyclic AMP generated within the oocyte may participate in the maintenance of meiotic arrest. Forskolin, a stimulator of the catalytic subunit of adenylate cyclase (29), increased the cAMP content of cumulus cell-denuded oocytes from mice (30,31), hamsters (28), and pigs (27). Evidence that forskolin elevates cAMP of rat oocytes is not consistent. This agent was reported to retard the kinetics of GVB by rat oocytes (32), though others reported no increase in cAMP levels in the oocytes (23). Possibly, an increase would have been detected in the denuded oocytes if cAMP degradation had been prevented with phosphodiesterase inhibitors, since forskolin did maintain meiotic arrest in the cumulus cell-denuded oocytes (23). Overall, the evidence suggests that the oocytes of several species can produce their own cAMP. Whether they can produce it in sufficient quantities to maintain oocytes in meiotic arrest under physiological conditions is unresolved. Perhaps cAMP synthesized by the oocyte is supplemented by cAMP transferred to the oocyte from granulosa cells. The relative contributions to the pool of cAMP within the oocyte made by transferred cAMP and cAMP synthesized by the oocyte itself may vary from species to species.

80

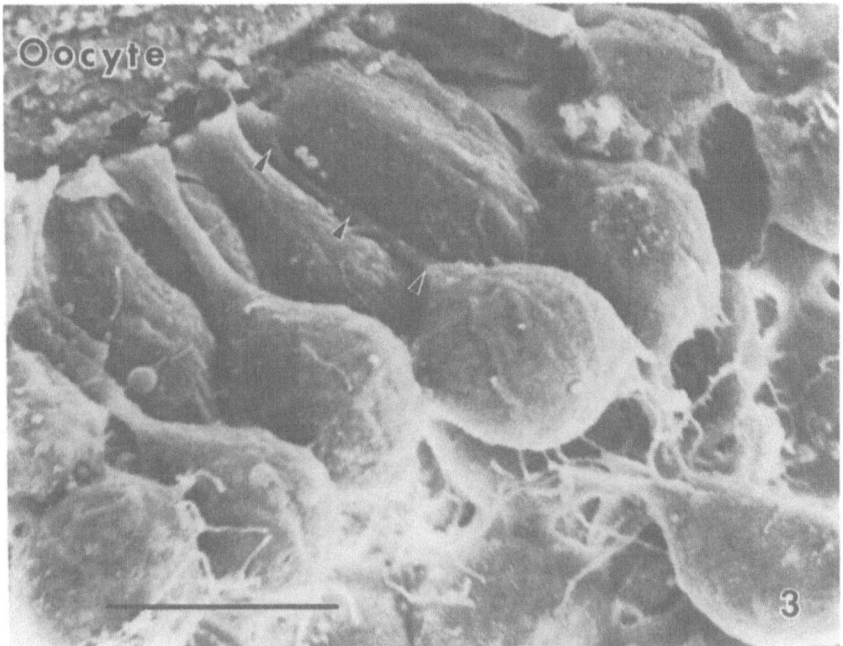

Fig. 3. Scanning electron micrograph of cumulus cells 2 days after injecting a 20-day-old mouse with PMSG. Notice that cumulus cells even in the second and third rank away from the oocyte contact the oocyte with long cytoplasmic processes (arrowheads). Apparently, most cumulus cells, even those that are not immediately adjacent to the oocyte, can communicate regulatory signals directly to the oocyte. The cytoplasmic process from the distal cumulus cells broaden where it contacts the zona pellucida (solid arrows). Bar indicates 10 μm.

Preparations of mouse and pig follicular fluid contain high concentrations of purines which maintain mouse oocytes in meiotic arrest in vitro. Mouse oocytes were reversibly maintained in meiotic arrest for 24 h by hypoxanthine and adenosine at concentrations of these purines measured in preparations of mouse follicular fluid (33). Oocytes first maintained in meiotic arrest by these purines and then allowed to mature in medium without the purines were found to be competent of undergoing fertilization and embryonic development (34). This observation supports the idea that the meiosis-arresting action of these purines in vitro is not a result of toxicity.

Three approaches were used to assess potential mechanisms for the maintenance of meiotic arrest by purines: (a) metabolism of hypoxanthine and adenosine by isolated oocyte-cumulus cell complexes and cumulus cell-denuded oocytes; (b) the effect of inhibitors of inosine monophosphate (IMP) dehydrogenase activity on meiotic arrest mediated by purines; and, (c) the role of adenosine metabolism in augmenting the meiosis-arresting action of hypoxanthine.

Both oocyte-cumulus cell complexes and denuded oocytes were able to take up radiolabeled hypoxanthine, although much more radiolabel was found in cumulus cell-enclosed oocytes than in denuded ones (35). Also, hypoxanthine was more effective in maintaining meiotic arrest in cumulus cell-enclosed than denuded oocytes (33). Most radiolabeled hypoxanthine taken up by oocyte-cumulus cell complexes or denuded oocytes was converted to uric acid, and a small amount of the hypoxanthine taken up by cumulus cells was converted to inosine and transferred to the oocyte. Radiolabeled adenosine, and/or its metabolites, was also incorporated into both cumulus cell-enclosed and denuded oocytes, but the efficiency of uptake of adenosine by denuded oocytes was much greater than the uptake of hypoxanthine. Most of the adenosine taken up was converted to phosphorylated

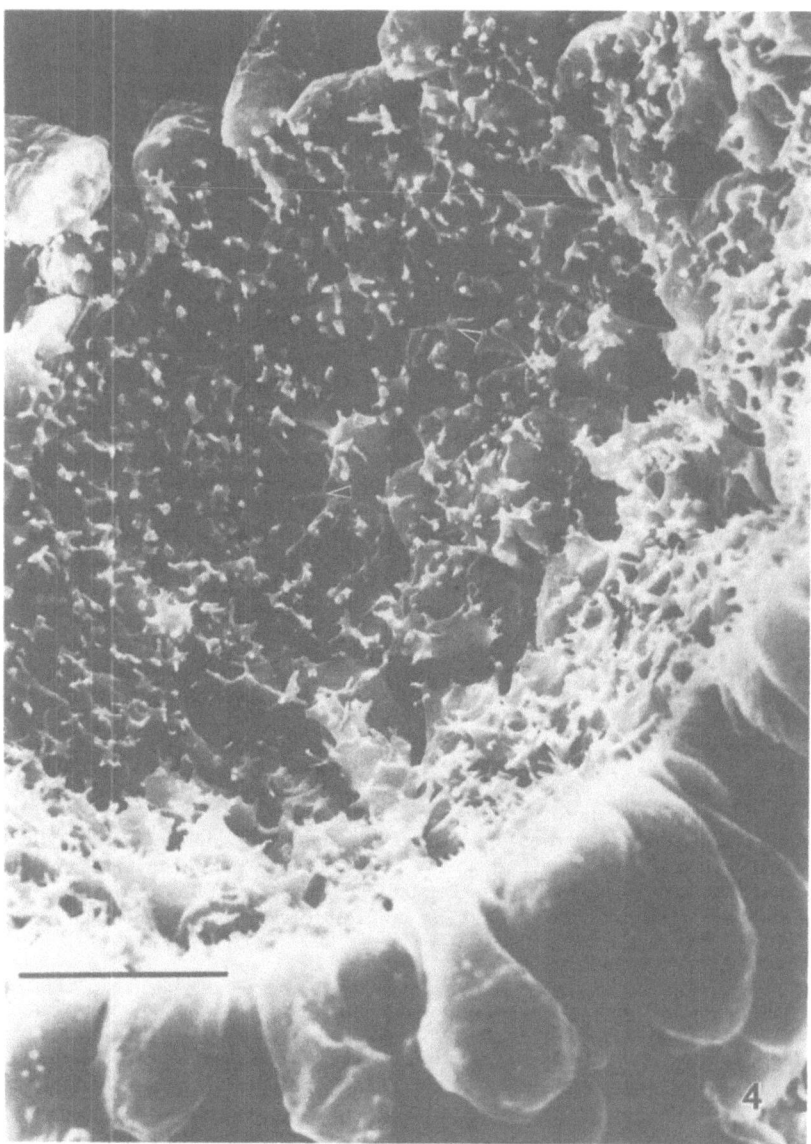

Fig. 4. Scanning electron micrograph of cumulus cells from a 22-day-old mouse that had been injected with PMSG 2 days before fixation. This is the oocyte's view of the cumulus cells. There are numerous branching processes (arrowheads) from the cumulus cells available for communication of meiosis-regulating factors to the oocyte. Bar indicates 10 μm.

derivatives, although some inosine was produced by cumulus cells and transferred to the oocytes (35).

The meiosis-arresting action of hypoxanthine could be mediated by conversion to other purines or by promoting the production of other purines. Guanosine was the most active purine tested for maintaining meiotic arrest in vitro (36), but no guanosine was detected in follicular fluid. Therefore, the effect of inhibiting a critical enzyme for the production of guanyl compounds, IMP dehydrogenase, on hypoxanthine-mediated meiotic arrest was assessed (Fig. 5). Two specific inhibitors of IMP dehydrogenase, mycophenolic acid and bredinin, induced GVB when meiotic arrest was maintained by hypoxanthine, but not by guanosine in vitro (35). The IMP dehydrogenase inhibitors also had no effect on meiotic arrest maintained by dbcAMP or IBMX (37). These results indicate that the meiosis-arresting activity of hypoxanthine in vitro is mediated by the production of guanyl compounds via the IMP dehydrogenase pathway and that these meiosis-arresting mechanisms are upstream from the arresting action of cAMP within the oocyte.

To determine whether the production of guanyl compounds is critical for the maintenance of meiotic arrest in vivo, bredinin and mycophenolic acid were injected into juvenile mice 24 h after injecting them with pregnant mare's serum gonadotropin. Both inhibitors induced maturation in vivo, but bredinin was the most active inducer (38). Injection of 6.0 μmoles bredinin induced the maturation of almost all of the cumulus cell-enclosed oocytes within 6 h. This is very strong evidence that purines, specifically guanyl compounds, participate in the maintenance of meiotic arrest in vivo. Whether production of these compounds in vivo involves hypoxanthine remains to be demonstrated.

There are several ways in which hypoxanthine could promote the production of guanyl compounds (see Fig. 5). For example, hypoxanthine

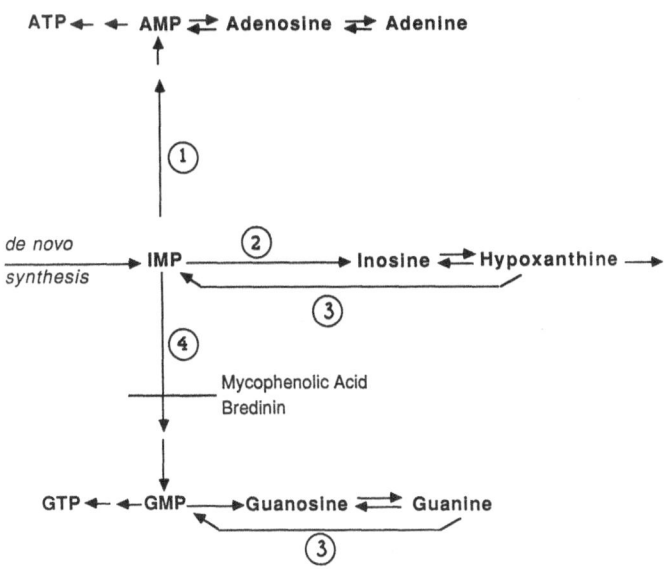

Fig. 5. Possible pathways of purine metabolism.
(1) Adenylosuccinate synthetase; (2) 5'-nucleotidase; (3) hypoxanthine guanine phosphoribosyl transferase; (4) IMP dehydrogenase.

could be metabolized to IMP via the activity of hypoxanthine guanine phosphoribosyl transferase, and then converted to guanosine monophosphate (GMP) by IMP dehydrogenase. Alternatively, hypoxanthine could inhibit 5'-nucleotidase activity and, by suppressing metabolism of IMP to inosine, promote conversion of IMP to GMP via IMP dehydrogenase.

Guanyl compounds, specifically guanosine triphosphate (GTP), are known to be important in the regulation of some biological processes (39). These actions often require the binding of GTP to specific effector molecules referred to as G-proteins. Two pathways of potential importance in maintaining meiotic arrest may be regulated by G-proteins in oocytes. First, adenylate cyclase activity is stimulated by binding of GTP to the G_s subunit and, therefore, oocyte cAMP levels may be regulated by GTP. Second, G-proteins have been implicated in the regulation of the activity of phospholipase C and the production of inositol triphosphate and 1,2-diacylglycerol (40). Protein kinase C is activated by diacylglycerol (41), and phorbol esters, which also stimulate protein kinase C, have been shown to maintain mouse oocytes in meiotic arrest (42,43).

The maintenance of meiotic arrest by hypoxanthine in vitro was continuous for 24 h (33). In contrast, adenosine had only a transient activity in maintaining meiotic arrest. However, adenosine augmented the meiosis-arresting activity of hypoxanthine, and this augmentation effect was continuous for 24 h (33). There are several potential mechanisms for this augmentation action of adenosine. The most obvious involve the generation of cAMP. Adenosine is rapidly metabolized to phosphorylated derivatives (35) and adenosine triphosphate (ATP) is the substrate for adenylate cyclase. However, the metabolism of adenosine does not appear necessary for the augmentation of the action of hypoxanthine because the poorly metabolized analog of adenosine, 2-chloroadenosine, augments the action of hypoxanthine to the same extent as adenosine itself (35). FSH suppresses GVB in mouse, pig, and rat cumulus cell-enclosed oocytes (44-47). Kinetic analysis of this effect on mouse oocytes has shown that suppression of GVB by FSH is transient, but the effect of FSH on the kinetics of maturation in rat oocytes has not been reported. Adenosine augmented the GVB-suppressing effect of FSH on rat cumulus cell-enclosed oocytes and 2-chloroadenosine mimicked the action of adenosine (47). Therefore, since adenosine need not be metabolized to augment the action of either hypoxanthine or FSH, adenosine may act primarily by stimulating adenylate cyclase activity by a receptor-mediated mechanism and thereby help to maintain elevated levels of cAMP within the oocyte. Accordingly, adenosine has been reported to increase the levels of cAMP in rat oocyte-cumulus cell complexes stimulated with FSH (48).

Other molecules may also participate in the maintenance of meiotic arrest in vivo. A small peptide has been detected in follicular fluid that can suppress GVB in the oocytes of several species in vitro (6). Additionally, some steroid hormones could participate in the maintenance of meiotic arrest (44-46). The maintenance of cAMP concentrations above certain threshold levels within the oocyte appears to be essential for the maintenance of meiotic arrest and levels above this threshold could be achieved via the participation and interaction of several follicular factors. Moreover, pathways that are not components of the cAMP-initiated cascade could also participate in the maintenance of meiotic arrest. The proportional contributions of these factors could vary between species. Therefore, it is critically important to correlate the findings of experiments in vitro with the intact follicular environment in vivo and not assume that the proportion of participation of a specific factor in the maintenance of arrest in one species is equivalent to that in another species.

Since follicular factors maintain mammalian oocytes in meiotic arrest, the preovulatory gonadotropins that initiate oocyte maturation may act to deprive the oocyte of the maturation-arresting factors. One way to isolate the oocyte from these factors would be to disrupt the pathway that delivers arresting factors to the oocyte. Gap junctions probably mediate the transfer of putative arresting factors to oocytes (20,23,32,33,45). However, studies that have utilized intercellular markers that quantify metabolic cooperativity mediated by gap junctions between cumulus cells and oocytes indicate that GVB occurs before significant reduction in transport of these markers when maturation was induced in vivo or in intact follicles in vitro (6,49-51). Nevertheless, the transfer of GVB-arresting substances may be selectively regulated by the gap junctions.

There is a massive loss in gap junctional area between cumulus cells that occurs at about the same time as gonadotropin-induced GVB in the rat (52). Although this loss may not affect communication between the cumulus cells and the oocyte since most cumulus cells appear to communicate directly with the oocyte (Fig. 3), the loss of communication between cumulus cells may indicate a decreased communication between the follicle wall and the cumulus cells and, consequently, between the follicle wall and the oocyte. This decrease could reduce the amount of putative GVB-arresting factors produced by mural granulosa cells and transferred to the oocyte via cumulus cells. However, the decrease in gap junctional area only coincides with and does not appear to precede GVB. It will be important to correlate the loss of gap junctional area with a decrease in the amount of specific inhibitory substances in the cumulus cell-oocyte complex and the time of commitment by the oocyte to undergo GVB.

Although meiosis-arresting substances may be necessary for maintaining the GV stage in vivo, a decrease in the concentration of these substances may not be a necessary requirement for GVB. There was no decrease in oocyte cAMP levels seen before GVB in sheep (53), pig (27), or hamster (28,54) oocytes, although an undetected transient decrease in cAMP may have occurred before GVB or factors other than cAMP could be responsible for the maintenance of meiotic arrest in these cases. A decrease in oocyte cAMP was reported to precede gonadotropin-induced maturation in mice (21). However, it is not known whether or not this decrease preceded commitment to undergo GVB. That is, the oocytes in vivo may have been stimulated to undergo GVB before the decline in cAMP levels. In this case, after commitment to undergo GVB was stimulated in vivo, blocking the decline in oocyte cAMP in vitro with agents that maintain cAMP levels would not have prevented GVB.

When mouse oocyte-cumulus cell complexes were incubated in medium containing FSH plus either hypoxanthine, dbcAMP, or IBMX, there was first an increase in the maturation-arresting action of these substances and then a decrease in the frequency of oocytes maintained in the GV stage (55). Cumulus cell-enclosed oocytes are more sensitive to the GVB-arresting action of hypoxanthine, dbcAMP, or IBMX than denuded oocytes (33,44,55), therefore the cumulus cells mediate some of the arresting action of these substances. If FSH induces maturation of cumulus cell-enclosed oocytes incubated in medium containing one of the inhibitors by uncoupling the cumulus cells from the oocytes, then the frequency of maturation in medium containing the inhibitor should be equal when the oocytes are denuded of cumulus cells or the cumulus cell-enclosed oocytes are stimulated with FSH. However, when this experiment was conducted in defined medium, FSH stimulated a significantly greater percent of the oocytes to undergo GVB than did mechanically denuding them (12,55). FSH had no effect on the frequency of GVB by denuded oocytes incubated in maturation-arresting substances. These results suggest that oocyte maturation is induced by a positive signal generated by cumulus cells in response to gonadotropin and not simply by deprivation of maturation-arresting substances. The same hypothesis was derived from the observation that LH induced GVB in hamster oocytes within intact follicles in vitro without a detected decrease in oocyte cAMP (54).

There are two other lines of evidence indicative of a positive effect of gonadotropin-stimulated cumulus cells on oocyte maturational processes. First, oocytes that have undergone GVB express much greater tissue plasminogen activator (tPA) activity than GV stage oocytes (56). Cumulus cells express urokinase (uPA) activity, but not tPA activity (56). Stimulation of isolated oocyte-cumulus cell complexes with FSH results in greater tPA activity in the oocyte (56). FSH may induce the cumulus cells to generate some factor(s) that stimulate(s) the oocyte to increase tPA activity, an activity that is associated with the maturing oocytes. Second, mouse oocytes that mature spontaneously in culture are often competent of undergoing fertilization and embryonic development (57). FSH treatment of the maturing oocytes increased both the frequency of fertilization and frequency of fertilized eggs developed to blastocysts (34). The increased frequency of fertilization could be due to the stimulation of cumulus expansion which might allow more easy access of the sperm to the egg, but this is not likely to account for the increased frequency of development of the eggs from the 2-cell stage to blastocysts. This increased frequency of embryonic development could be the result of a positive stimulation of an oocyte maturational process by the FSH-stimulated cumulus cells.

Maturation may be induced by a coordinated series of events that include both a reduction in the production or transfer of GVB-arresting factors and the generation of positive signals by granulosa cells that promote maturational processes. Positive signaling could provide a more precise control of maturational processes than a simple withdrawal of maturation-arresting factors. In addition, positive maturation-inducing signals have been identified in other species. For example, a progesterone-like steroid produced by follicle cells induces maturation in amphibians (58,59) and fish (60), and 1-methyladenine produced by follicle cells induces maturation in starfish (61). Identification of putative mammalian maturation-promoting signals and resolution of their mode of action is critical not only for understanding the mechanisms regulating the initiation of maturation but also the processes that promote the acquisition of potential for fertilization and embryogenesis.

STUDIES ON THE MECHANISMS CONTROLLING PRIMATE OOCYTE MATURATION IN VITRO

Pincus and Sauders (62) were the first to report the spontaneous maturation in culture of primate (human) oocytes. This observation was extended by Edwards (63) who also described the spontaneous maturation of rhesus monkey oocytes. However, primate oocytes have not been utilized to resolve the mechanisms that govern oocyte maturation because they are not so readily available as oocytes of other species. Nevertheless, it is essential that studies be conducted with primate oocytes for understanding potential differences between primate oocytes and those of other species, and for the benefit of practical applications such as the propagation of rare primates and human clinical in vitro fertilization protocols.

REFERENCES

1. Szybec K. In vitro maturation of oocytes from sexually immature mice. J Endocrinol 1972; 54:527-8.
2. Sorensen RA, Wassarman PM. Relationship between growth and meiotic maturation of the mouse oocyte. Dev Biol 1976; 50:531-6.
3. Pincus G, Enzmann EV. The comparative behavior of mammalian eggs in vivo and in vitro. I. The activation of ovarian eggs. J Exp Med 1935; 62:665-75.
4. Lindner HR, Tsafriri A, Lieberman ME, Zor U, Koch Y. Gonadotropin action on cultured Graafian follicles: induction of maturation division of the mammalian oocyte and differentiation of the luteal cell. Recent Prog Horm Res 1974; 30:79-138.
5. Moor RM, Osborn JC, Crosby IM. Cell interactions and oocyte regulation in mammals. In: Rolland R, Van Hall EV, Hillier SG, McNatty KP, Schoemaker J, eds. Follicular maturation and ovulation. Elsevier/North Holland, 1981:249-64.
6. Tsafriri A, Dekel N, Bar-Ami S. The role of oocyte maturation inhibitor in follicular regulation of oocyte maturation. J Reprod Fertil 1982; 64:541-51.
7. Canipari R, Palombi F, Riminucci M, Mangia F. Early programming of maturation competence in mouse oogenesis. Dev Biol 1984; 102:519.
8. Eppig JJ. Mouse oocyte development in vitro with various culture systems. Dev Biol 1977; 60:371-88.
9. Eppig JJ. A comparison between oocyte growth in coculture with granulosa cells and oocytes with granulosa cell-oocyte junctional contact maintained in vitro. J Exp Zool 1979; 209:345-53.
10. Brower PT, Schultz RM. Intercellular communication between granulosa cells and mouse oocytes: existence and possible nutritional role during oocyte growth. Dev Biol 1982; 90:144-53.
11. Herlands RL, Schultz RM. Regulation of mouse oocyte growth: probable nutritional role for intercellular communication between follicle cells and oocytes in oocyte growth. J Exp Zool 1984; 229:317-25.
12. Eppig JJ, Downs SM. The effect of hypoxanthine on mouse oocyte growth and development in vitro: maintenance of meiotic arrest and gonadotropin-induced oocyte maturation. Dev Biol 1987; 119:313-21.
13. Halpin DMG, Jones A, Fink G, Charlton HM. Postnatal ovarian follicle development in hypogonadal (hpg) and normal mice and associated changes in the hypothalamic-pituitary ovarian axis. J Reprod Fertil 1986; 77:287-96.
14. Eppig JJ, Downs SM. Chemical signals that regulate mammalian oocyte maturation. Biol Reprod 1984; 30:1-11.
15. Bar-Ami S, Nimrod A, Brodie AMH, Tsafriri A. Role of FSH and oestradiol-17β in the development of meiotic competence in rat oocytes. J Steroid Biochem 1983; 19:965-71.
16. Smith DM, Tenney DY. Effect of hypophysectomy on mouse oocyte maturation in vitro. J Reprod Fertil 1979; 55:415-22.
17. Cho WK, Stern JS, Biggers JD. Inhibitory effect of dibutyryl cAMP on mouse oocyte maturation in vitro. J Exp Zool 1974; 187:183-6.
18. Wassarman PM, Josefowicz WJ, Letourneau GE. Meiotic maturation of mouse oocytes in vitro; inhibition of maturation at specific stages of nuclear progression. J Cell Sci 1976; 22:531-45.
19. Magnusson C, Hillensjo T. Inhibition of maturation and metabolism of rat oocytes by cyclic AMP. J Exp Zool 1977; 201:138-47.
20. Dekel N, Beers WH. Rat oocyte maturation in vitro: relief of cyclic AMP inhibition by gonadotropins. Proc Natl Acad Sci USA 1978; 75:4369-73.
21. Schultz RM, Montgomery R, Bellanoff J. Regulation of mouse oocyte meiotic maturation; implication of a decrease in oocyte cAMP and protein phosphorylation in commitment to resume meiosis. Dev Biol 1983; 97:264-73.

22. Vivarelli E, Conti M, De Felici M, Siracusa G. Meiotic resumption and intracellular cAMP levels in mouse oocytes with compounds which act on cAMP metabolism. Cell Differ 1983; 12:271-6.

23. Racowsky C. Effect of forskolin on the spontaneous maturation and cyclic AMP content of rat oocyte-cumulus complexes. J Reprod Fertil 1984; 72:107-16.

24. Bornslaeger EA, Mattei P, Schultz RM. Involvement of cAMP-dependent protein kinase and protein phosphorylation in regulation of mouse oocyte maturation. Dev Biol 1986; 114:453-62.

25. Bornslaeger EA, Wilde MW, Schultz RM. Regulation of mouse oocyte maturation: involvement of cyclic AMP phosphodiesterase and calmodulin. Dev Biol 1984; 105:488-99.

26. Bornslaeger EA, Schultz RM. Regulation of mouse oocyte maturation; effect of elevating cumulus cell cAMP on oocyte cAMP levels. Biol Reprod 1985; 33:698-704.

27. Racowsky C. Effect of forskolin on maintenance of meiotic arrest and stimulation of cumulus expansion, progesterone and cyclic AMP production by pig oocyte-cumulus complexes. J Reprod Fertil 1985; 74:9-21.

28. Racowsky C. Effect of forskolin on the spontaneous maturation and cyclic AMP content of hamster oocyte-cumulus complexes. J Exp Zool 1985; 234:87-96.

29. Seamon KB, Padgett W, Daly JW. Forskolin: unique diterpene activator of adenylate cyclase in membranes and intact cells. Proc Natl Acad Sci USA 1981; 78:3363-7.

30. Urner F, Herrmann WL, Baulieu EE, Schorderet-Slatkine S. Inhibition of denuded mouse oocyte meiotic maturation by forskolin, an activator of adenylate cyclase. Endocrinology 1983; 113:1170-2.

31. Bornslaeger EA, Schultz RM. Adenylate cyclase activity in zona-free mouse oocytes. Exp Cell Res 1985; 156:277-81.

32. Ekholm C, Hillensjo T, Mangusson C, Rosberg S. Simulation and inhibition of rat oocyte meiosis by forskolin. Biol Reprod 1984; 30:537-43.

33. Eppig JJ, Ward-Bailey PF, Coleman DL. Hypoxanthine and adenosine in murine ovarian follicular fluid: concentrations and activity in maintaining oocyte meiotic arrest. Biol Reprod 1985; 33:1041-9.

34. Downs SM, Schroeder AC, Eppig JJ. Developmental capacity of mouse oocytes following maintenance of meiotic arrest in vitro. Gamete Res 1986; 15:305-16.

35. Downs SM, Coleman DL, Eppig JJ. Maintenance of murine oocyte meiotic arrest: uptake and metabolism of hypoxanthine and adenosine by cumulus cell-enclosed and denuded oocytes. Dev Biol 1986; 117:174-83.

36. Downs SM, Coleman DL, Ward-Bailey PF, Eppig JJ. Hypoxanthine is the principal inhibitor of murine oocyte maturation in a low molecular weight fraction of porcine follicular fluid. Proc Natl Acad Sci USA 1985; 82:454-8.

37. Eppig JJ, Downs SM. The role of purines in the maintenance of meiotic arrest in mammalian oocytes. In: Haseltine FP, First NL, eds. Meiotic inhibition: molecular control of meiosis. New York: Alan R. Liss, Inc., 1987 (in press).

38. Downs SM, Eppig JJ. Induction of mouse oocyte maturation in vivo by perturbants of purine metabolism. Biol Reprod 1987; 36:431-7.

39. Speigel AM. Signal transduction by guanine nucleotide binding proteins. Mol Cell Endocrinol 1987; 49:1-16.

40. Baldassare JJ, Fisher GJ. Regulation of membrane-associated and cytosolic phospholipase C activities in human platelets by guanosine triphosphate. J Biol Chem 1986; 261:11942-4.

41. Kishimoto A, Takai Y, Mori T, Kikkawa U, Nishizuka Y. Activation of calcium and phospholipid-dependent protein kinase by diacyglycerol, its possible relation to phosphatidylinositol turnover. J Biol Chem 1980; 255:2273-6.

42. Urner F, Schorderet-Slatkine S. Inhibition of denuded mouse oocyte meiotic maturation by tumor-promoting phorbol esters and its reversal by retinoids. Exp Cell Res 1984; 154:600-5.

43. Bornslaeger EA, Poueymirou WT, Mattei P, Schultz RM. Effects of protein kinase C activators on germinal vesicle breakdown and polar body emission of mouse oocytes. Exp Cell Res 1986; 165:507-17.

44. Eppig JJ, Freter RR, Ward-Bailey PF, Schultz RM. Inhibition of oocyte maturation in the mouse: participation of cAMP, steroid hormones, and a putative maturation-inhibitory factor. Dev Biol 1983; 100:39-49.

45. Schultz RM, Montgomery RR, Ward-Bailey PF, Eppig JJ. Regulation of oocyte maturation in the mouse; possible roles of intercellular communication, cAMP, and testosterone. Dev Biol 1983; 95:294-304.

46. Racowsky C. Androgenic modulation of cyclic adenosine monophosphate (cAMP)-dependent meiotic arrest. Biol Reprod 1983; 28:774-87.

47. Miller JGO, Behrman HR. Oocyte maturation is inhibited by adenosine in the presence of follicle-stimulating hormone. Biol Reprod 1987; 35:833-7.

48. Laufer N, Polan ML, DeCherney AH, Haseltine FP, Behrman HR. Characteristics of pre- and postovulatory oocyte cumulus complex (OCC) responses to gonadotropins and adenosine. Proceedings of the 65th Endocrine Society Meetings, 1983:300.

49. Eppig JJ. The relationship between cumulus cell-oocyte coupling, oocyte meiotic maturation, and cumulus expansion. Dev Biol 1982; 89:268-72.

50. Salustri A, Siracusa G. Metabolic coupling, cumulus expansion and meiotic resumption in mouse cumuli oophori cultured in vitro in the presence of FSH or dbcAMP, or stimulated in vivo by hCG. J Reprod Fertil 1983; 68:335-41.

51. Moor RM, Osborn JC, Cran DG, Walters DE. Selective effect of gonadotropins on cell coupling, nuclear maturation and protein synthesis in mammalian oocytes. J Embryol Exp Morphol 1981; 61:347-65.

52. Larsen WJ, Wert SE, Brunner GD. A dramatic loss of cumulus cell gap junctions is correlated with germinal vesicle breakdown in rat oocytes. Dev Biol 1986; 113:517-21.

53. Moor RM, Heslop JB. cAMP in mammalian follicle cells and oocytes during maturation. J Exp Zool 1981; 216:205-9.

54. Hubbard CJ. Cyclic AMP changes in the component cells of Graafian follicles: possible influences on maturation in the follicle-enclosed oocytes of hamsters. Dev Biol 1986; 118:343-51.

55. Downs SM, Daniel SAJ, Eppig JJ. Induction of maturation in cumulus cell-enclosed oocytes by follicle-stimulating hormone and epidermal growth factor: evidence for a positive stimulus of somatic cell origin (submitted for publication).

56. Liu YX, Ny T, Sarkar D, Loskutoff D, Hsueh AJW. Identification and regulation of tissue plasminogen activator activity in rat cumulus-oocyte complexes. Endocrinology 1986; 119:1578-87.

57. Schroeder AC, Eppig JJ. The developmental capacity of mouse oocytes that matured spontaneously in vitro is normal. Dev Biol 1984; 102:493-7.

58. Schuetz AW. Effect of steroids on germinal vesicle of oocytes of the frog (Rana pipiens) in vitro. Proc Soc Exp Biol Med 1967; 124:1307-10.

59. Masui Y. Relative roles of the pituitary, follicle cells, and progesterone in the induction of oocyte maturation in Rana pipiens. J Exp Zool 1967; 166:365-76.

60. Nagahama Y, Hirose K, Young G, Adachi S, Suzuki K, Tamaoki BI. Relative in vitro effectiveness of 17,20-dihydroxy-4-pregnen-3-one and other pregnene derivatives on germinal vesicle breakdown in

oocytes of ayu (Plecoglossus altivelis), amago salmon (Oncorhynchus rhodurus), rainbow trout (Salmo gairdneri), and goldfish (Carassius auratus). Gen Comp Endocrinol 1983; 51:15-23.

61. Kanatani H, Shirai H, Nakanishi K, Kurokawa T. Isolation and identification of meiosis inducing substance in starfish. Nature 1969; 221:273-4.

62. Pincus G, Saunders B. The comparative behavior of mammalian eggs in vivo and in vitro. IV. The maturation of human ovarian ova. Anat Rec 1939; 75:537-45.

63. Edwards RG. Maturation in vitro of mouse, sheep, cow, pig, rhesus monkey and human ovarian oocytes. Nature 1965; 208:349-51.

REGULATION OF OVULATORY PROCESSES

William J. LeMaire, M.D., Thomas E. Curry, Jr., Ph.D.,[1]
Nobuyuki Morioka, M.D., Mats Brannstrom, M.D.,[2]
Martin R. Clark, Ph.D.,[3] J.F. Woessner, Ph.D.,
and Robert D. Koos, Ph.D.[4]

The Reproductive Sciences and Endocrinology Laboratories,
and Departments of Obstetrics and Gynecology, and Biochemistry, University of Miami School of Medicine, Miami, FL
33101; [1]Center for Reproductive Medicine, Department of
Obstetrics and Gynecology, University of Kentucky, Lexing-
ton, KY 40536; [2]Department of Physiology, University of
Goteborg, S-400 33 Goteborg, Sweden; [3]Department of Obstetrics and Gynecology, University of North Carolina, Chapel
Hill, NC 27514; [4]Department of Physiology, University of
Maryland, Baltimore, MD 21201

INTRODUCTION

In all mammalian species studied to date, the process of ovulation is
initiated by a discharge from the pituitary gland of luteinizing hormone
(LH), the normal physiological trigger for ovulation (1). The ovulatory
surge of LH acts upon the mature preovulatory follicles and sets in motion
a series of biochemical and morphological events which eventually lead to
ovulation. The interval between LH stimulation and ovulation varies from
species to species. While many of the biochemical and morphological
changes within the follicle during that interval are still not known or
are controversial, we will discuss recent information from our laboratory
and others which may shed light on the key events during that period. In
addition to LH, follicle stimulating hormone (FSH) and gonadotropin
releasing hormone (GnRH) have also been shown to have direct actions on
the rat ovary sufficient to cause follicular rupture. The relevance of
these latter observations to our understanding of the ovulatory process
will also be discussed.

HORMONES CAPABLE OF INDUCING OVULATION BY DIRECT ACTION ON THE OVARY

Luteinizing Hormone

LH is considered to be the normal physiological trigger which initiates the process of ovulation by a direct action on the ovarian follicle
(1). The study of the direct ovulation-inducing effect of LH and other
substances has benefited greatly from the introduction of methods for in
vitro perfusion of rabbit ovaries (2,3), later adapted for the rat (4).
These models lend themselves well to the study of various substances
thought to stimulate or inhibit ovulation. In these methods, surgically-

isolated ovaries are placed in a perfusion chamber and continuously perfused through the ovarian artery with chemically-defined, oxygenated medium. The addition to this medium of human chorionic gonadotropin (hCG) (2) or LH (3,4) consistently causes ovulation, while in control perfusions with medium alone, ovulations seldom occur (Table 1, columns 1 and 2).

Follicle Stimulating Hormone

There is considerable evidence to suggest that FSH alone can also induce ovulation (1), but may not be required under physiological conditions (1,5). Using the in vitro perfusion system with rat ovaries, we have recently confirmed that purified heterologous and homologous FSH alone can trigger the ovulatory process (6) (Table 1). Whether this is also true for other mammalian species remains to be determined.

These in vitro observations clearly support the proposal that FSH in the absence of LH, can initiate the biochemical changes leading to follicular rupture, but do not shed light on the role of FSH under physiological in vivo conditions. These in vitro studies, however, provide an important tool to compare the mechanism of the effects of FSH to those of LH.

Gonadotropin Releasing Hormone

Classically, the role of GnRH is one of action at the pituitary level but evidence from many laboratories has established a direct extra-pituitary effect of GnRH on the gonads (7). While most of these effects have been inhibitory (7), GnRH agonists have also been shown to have stimulatory effects on the ovary, including the induction of ovulation in hypophysectomized rats (8,9). However, GnRH does not appear to be part of the biochemical mechanism by which LH causes ovulation, as LH-induced ovulation is not inhibited by a GnRH antagonist (10). Using the ovarian perfusion system, we recently demonstrated that a GnRH agonist can induce ovulation by a direct action on the rat ovary and that this action can be inhibited by simultaneous treatment with a GnRH antagonist (11) (Table 2). While it is doubtful that GnRH plays a normal physiological role in the initiation of ovulation in the rat, the studies mentioned above may help

Table 1. Ovulations in rat ovaries perfused in vitro with LH or FSH.[1]

	Control[2]	oLH-23[3] (100 ng/ml)	oFSH-211B[4] (100 ng/ml)	rFSH-I-6[5] (150 ng/ml)
No. of ovaries perfused	9	9	3	5
No. of ovaries ovulating	1	9	3	5
No. of ovulations/ovulating ovary (mean ± SEM)	1	7.9 ± 1.2	11.3 ± 2.6	13.8 ± 2.2

[1] Immature female rats were primed with 20 IU of PMSG on day 26-29 and the ovaries removed for in vitro perfusion 48 h later (prior to the endogenous LH surge). Various treatments were added after 1 h of perfusion and the medium collected and examined for oocytes 20 h later.
[2] Control ovaries were perfused with medium alone and the appropriate vehicle for the hormone treatments.
[3] NIH oLH-23 and other hormones were added directly to the perfusion medium.
[4] Papkoff oFSH G4-211B (FSH biopotency: 50-60 U/mg).
[5] NIADDK rat FSH (FSH biopotency: 100 U/mg).
Adapted from references 4 and 6.

to clarify the mechanism of ovulation. It must be pointed out that GnRH was ineffective in inducing ovulations in the perfused rabbit ovary (11). Likewise, it is doubtful that GnRH would have any direct ovarian action in primates as the majority of evidence indicates an absence of GnRH receptors and no demonstrated actions in the primate ovary (12).

ROLE FOR CYCLIC NUCLEOTIDES

Many of the actions of LH on ovarian tissue involve the activation of adenylate cyclase resulting in increased concentrations of cyclic AMP (cAMP). This increased cAMP is the principal intracellular messenger of LH's actions. This role of cAMP has been reviewed extensively elsewhere (13,14).

Given the second messenger role of cAMP in many of the actions of LH, it is logical to consider that this nucleotide might mediate the ovulatory action of LH. Direct evidence of this, however, was lacking until Holmes et al. (15) and Brannstrom et al. (16) demonstrated a direct ovulation-inducing effect for cAMP in the rabbit and rat, respectively. With in vitro perfused rabbit ovaries, these investigators demonstrated that forskolin, a nonreceptor mediated activator of adenylate cyclase, was able to induce ovulation (15). Furthermore, ovaries of immature PMSG-treated rats ovulated in response to either forskolin or dibutyryl cAMP + 3-isobutyl-1-methylxanthine (IBMX; an inhibitor of phosphodiesterase) added to the perfusion medium (16) (Table 3).

The latter investigators (16) also found that both forskolin and dibutyryl cAMP resulted in marked increases in prostaglandin E (PGE) levels in the ovary. Furthermore, the induction of ovulation by these 2 treatments was inhibited by indomethacin and this inhibition was reversed by the addition of PGE_2 (1 µg/ml) (16). LH-induced ovulation was also inhibited by indomethacin in this model and the inhibition was reversed by the addition of prostaglandins (17). These observations lend support to the idea that cAMP is the physiological mediator for LH-induced ovulation.

However, cAMP may not be the only messenger for the induction of ovulation, as another direct stimulator of ovulation in the rat, namely GnRH (11), has not been shown to increase cAMP in vitro in isolated rat

Table 2. Ovulations in rat ovaries perfused in vitro with GnRHa.[1]

	Control[2]	GnRHa[3] (100 ng/ml)	GnRHa + GnRHi[4] (100 ng/ml + 1 µg/ml)
No. of ovaries perfused	5	7	6
No. of ovaries ovulating	3	6	2
No. of ovulations/ovulating ovary (mean ± SE)	1.3	13.0 ± 2.9	1.5

[1] Same as in Table 1.
[2] Same as in Table 1.
[3] The GnRH agonist (D-ala[6], des-gly-NH$_2$[10]) LHRH-ethylamide was added directly to the perfusion medium.
[4] The GnRH antagonist [Ac-[3]-Pro[1], p-F-DPhe[2], D-Trp[3,6]] GnRH was added directly to the perfusion medium.
Adapted from reference 11.

Table 3. Ovulations in rat ovaries perfused in vitro with forskolin and dibutyryl cAMP.[1]

	Control[2]	Forskolin[3] (30 μM)	dbcAMP + IBMX[4] (1 mM + 0.2 mM)
No. of ovaries perfused	5	5	5
No. of ovaries ovulating	0	5	5
No. of ovulations/ovulating ovary (mean + SEM)	-	11.8 ± 1.8	18.6 ± 4.4

[1] Same as Table 1.
[2] Same as Table 1.
[3] Forskolin (7β-acetoxy-8, 3-epoxy-1, 6β, 9-trihydroxy-14-ene-11-one) was added directly to the perfusion medium dissolved in 42 μl of 99.5% ethanol. Controls received the same amount of ethanol.
[4] dbcAMP (N[6], 2'-O-dibutyryladenosine 3':5'-cyclic monophosphate) + IBMX (3-isobutyl-1-methylxanthine) was added directly to the perfusion medium. From reference 16.

granulosa cells (18). Whether LH, in addition to stimulating cAMP-dependent protein kinase during the induction of ovulation, also stimulates Ca^{++}-dependent phospholipid sensitive protein kinase (PKC), and whether the activation of PKC can act as an ovulatory stimulus remains to be determined. We attempted to induce ovulation during in vitro perfusion of rat ovaries by the addition to the medium of phorbol ester, which is known to activate PKC in granulosa cells (19). These experiments were unsuccessful, possibly because the addition of this agent caused a rapid and marked reduction of the flow of medium through the ovary (Brannstrom, unpublished observation). Other approaches will be required to answer this question.

ROLE FOR STEROIDS

One of the early effects of the ovulatory LH surge on the ovary is a marked stimulation of steroidogenesis, followed by a period of refractoriness during which steroidogenesis is turned off. An important role for this initial increase and/or the subsequent decrease of steroidogenesis in the ovulatory process has been postulated (20). Indeed, based on studies using inhibitors of steroidogenesis, earlier workers concluded that steroid production was essential for ovulation (21,22). However, the effect of these inhibitors could have been via an action other than inhibition of steroidogenesis (23). More recently the drug epostane, an inhibitor of the enzyme 3-β-hydroxysteroid dehydrogenase was shown to inhibit ovulation in the rat and this inhibition could be reversed by progesterone (24). The arguments in favor of a role of steroids in ovulation and their possible involvement in the LH stimulation of plasminogen activator (an important step in the ovulatory process as discussed later), was recently reviewed (25). A number of studies using various inhibitors of steroidogenesis administered in vivo either systemically or into the ovarian bursa have demonstrated an inhibition of ovulation which in many cases could be reversed by the administration of the appropriate steroid (25).

Ovarian perfusion in vitro has been used to study the role of steroids in ovulation. Using such an approach, Koos et al. (26) showed that the marked increase in estrogen production following LH stimulation in the perfused rat ovary could be inhibited by 4-OH-androstenedione, an aromatase inhibitor, without ovulation being inhibited. Because of a recent report on the possible estrogenic effect of phenol red, a common pH indicator used in the perfusion medium (27), we have repeated these studies in phenol red-free medium with similar results (Morioka et al., unpublished observations) (Fig. 1).

Kitai et al. (28) and Holmes et al. (29) have also shown in perfused rabbit ovaries that an inhibitor of cholesterol side-chain cleavage or an inhibitor of 3-β-hydroxysteroid dehydrogenase added to the perfusion media did not inhibit hCG- or LH-induced ovulation while completely abolishing the LH-induced increase in follicular progesterone levels.

A further argument against a vital role for increased steroidogenesis in ovulation comes from the observation that FSH as well as GnRH analogs are capable of inducing ovulation by themselves in the perfused rat ovary, while causing only minimal increases in steroidogenesis (6,11). Furthermore, PGF$_{2\alpha}$ added alone to the medium of perfused rabbit ovaries induces ovulation without a concomitant increase in estrogen or progesterone secretion (17). Thus, while the in vivo data seem to support an important local role for the increase in steroidogenesis prior to ovulation, recent data using the in vitro perfused ovary model do not support such a role.

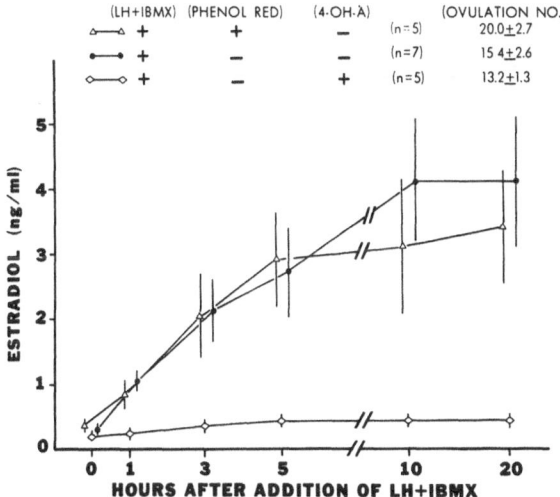

Fig. 1. Estradiol levels in the perfusion medium (mean ± SE) of ovaries from immature PMSG (20 IU) treated rats. All ovaries were perfused with LH (0.1 μg/ml of NIH-oLH-23) and IBMX (0.2 mM), added at time 0. Medium containing phenol red was first compared to medium without phenol red. Perfusion was then carried out in phenol red-free medium in the presence of an inhibitor of aromatase, 4-OH-androstenedione (5 μM). The number (mean ± SE) of oocytes recovered in the medium at the end of the perfusion is indicated as well. From Morioka et al., unpublished observations.

It has been proposed that the decline in the production of estradiol, which is seen sometime after the LH surge, may in fact play a role in follicular rupture, possibly by allowing the activation of ovarian collagenase (20). Again using the in vitro perfused rabbit ovary, we have found that sustained levels of ovarian estrogen did not prevent LH-induced ovulation (30). Similar studies in the rabbit have demonstrated, however, that the addition of progesterone to the medium markedly reduced LH-induced ovulation (29).

ROLE FOR PROSTAGLANDINS

The evidence in favor of an important role of prostaglandins in the ovulatory process at the local ovarian level is very strong (reviewed in 31). First, it was demonstrated that either systemic or local administration of cyclooxygenase inhibitors, which inhibit prostaglandin synthesis (indomethacin, aspirin), inhibits LH-induced ovulation in the rat and rabbit and that this inhibition could be reversed by the administration of exogenous prostaglandins (31). Such an inhibition of gonadotropin-induced ovulation has also been demonstrated for the rhesus monkey (32) and the marmoset (33). In the latter case, inhibition of ovulation by indomethacin was accompanied by entrapment of oocytes within the luteinized follicle and by normal luteal progesterone levels. A similar finding has been reported for the rabbit (34). While these studies support the role for prostaglandins in ovulation, it should be noted that in both monkey experiments the follicular development was induced by exogenous FSH (human menopausal gonadotropin) and ovulation was induced by exogenous hCG. In a subsequent experiment using normal cycling rhesus monkeys, Wright et al. demonstrated that indomethacin was incapable of inhibiting spontaneous ovulation (35). Similarly, the administration of aspirin failed to block spontaneous ovulation in women (36). In the latter study, however, the dose of aspirin used (600 mg, 3 times/day) may not have been sufficient to block prostaglandin synthesis in the ovarian follicles, a parameter which was not assessed in that study nor in the study with rhesus monkeys discussed above (35).

Additional arguments in favor of a role for prostaglandins in ovulation derive from in vitro perfusion experiments. Ovulations induced in in vitro perfused rabbit ovaries by hCG or LH can be prevented by indomethacin added to the perfusion medium (17,37) without interfering with oocyte maturation (38). The addition of exogenous $PGF_{2\alpha}$ to the perfusion medium reversed this inhibition (17,39). In fact, the addition of $PGF_{2\alpha}$ alone to the medium without LH or hCG was capable of inducing ovulation (17,39). In perfused rat ovaries, forskolin- or FSH-induced ovulation was also inhibited by indomethacin and this block could be overcome by adding prostaglandins to the medium (16,40) (Table 4 for FSH). Furthermore, GnRH-induced ovulation in hypophysectomized rats in vivo could be inhibited by indomethacin administration (41).

During the process of ovulation, the endogenous levels of prostaglandins in the rat and rabbit follicle increase markedly and this increase can be inhibited by indomethacin (reviewed in 31). Furthermore, Koos et al. (42) found a marked preovulatory increase in follicular levels of prostaglandins (PGE and PGF) during in vitro perfusion of rabbit ovaries. Abundant evidence exists to demonstrate that prostaglandins are produced locally within the ovarian tissues and that their synthesis is under gonadotropic control (31).

The above discussion has dealt with the possible role of the classical prostaglandin products of the cyclooxygenase pathway, namely $PGF_{2\alpha}$ and PGE_2. Recent evidence from Reich et al. (43) has also implicated

Table 4. Ovulations in rat ovaries perfused in vitro[1] with FSH: inhibition by Indomethacin.

	rFSH[2]	rFSH[2] Indo[3]	rFSH[2] Indo[3] PGF[4]$_{2\alpha}$	rFSH[2] Indo[3] PGE[5]$_2$
No. of ovaries perfused	5	5	4	3
No. of ovaries ovulating	5	1	2	3
No. of ovulations/ovulating ovary (mean/SE)	6.4 ± 2.0	1	5.0 ± 1.0	4.7 ± 1.7

[1] Same as in Table 1.
[2] NIADDK rat FSH (FSH biopotency: 100 U/mg) added after 1 h of perfusion at a final concentration of 100 ng/ml.
[3] Indomethacin was dissolved in 50 μl of ethanol and added at the beginning of the perfusion at a concentration of 5 μg/ml.
[4] PGF$_{2\alpha}$ was added after 1 h of perfusion at a final concentration of 1 μg/ml.
[5] PGE$_2$ was added after 1 h of perfusion at a final concentration of 0.5 μg/ml.
Adapted from reference 40.

products of the lipoxygenase pathway in ovulation. Furthermore, Koos and Clark (44) demonstrated that isolated rat granulosa cells synthesize prostacyclin (PGI$_2$) and that this synthesis could be stimulated by LH as well as a GnRH agonist, suggesting a possible role for PGI$_2$ in ovarian function. Indeed, Yoshimura et al. recently provided preliminary evidence that PGI$_2$ added to the perfusion medium in the absence of gonadotropin can induce ovulation (45). At this time it is unclear which prostaglandin or prostaglandin-like compounds are involved in follicular rupture, but as a group they undoubtedly play an important role in the induction of ovulation by gonadotropin.

What is the mechanism by which prostaglandins are involved in follicular rupture? Since a crucial event in follicular rupture appears to be a weakening of the wall of the follicle by proteolytic enzymes (see below), it is plausible to propose a role for prostaglandins in this process. Espey et al. (46) and Downs and Longo (47) have shown that prostaglandins may be involved in the morphological degradation of the follicular wall prior to ovulation in the rat and mouse, respectively, suggesting a role for prostaglandins in the activation of proteinases required for follicular rupture. Indeed, Reich et al. (48) showed that inhibition of prostaglandin synthesis by intrabursal administration of indomethacin in the rat inhibited collagenolysis as measured by the release of ^{3}H-hydroxyproline from endogenously labeled collagen. Kawamura et al. (49), using a synthetic substrate as an index of collagenase activity, obtained similar results. Furthermore, Murdoch et al. (50) recently showed that intrafollicular injection of indomethacin in the sheep inhibited the preovulatory increase of follicular collagenase activity. Curry et al. (51), on the other hand, found no inhibition by indomethacin of LH-stimulated follicular collagenase utilizing a specific assay which measures true latent collagenase production (Fig. 2).

These seemingly contradictory findings can be reconciled. LH may act, directly or indirectly depending on the cell type, to increase tissue collagenase production in fibroblasts, germinal epithelium, granulosa

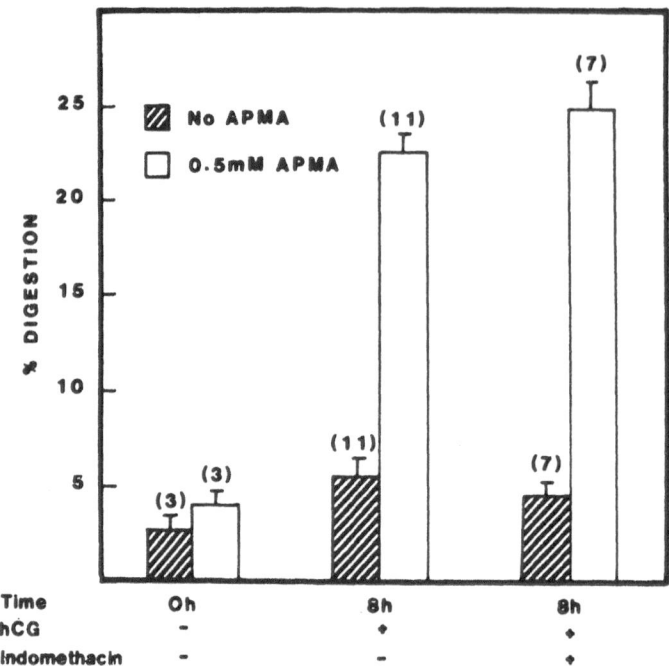

Fig. 2. Collagenase activity in ovarian extracts from
immature rat ovaries collected at 0 h (52 h after 20
IU of PMSG) and 8 h post-hCG (10 IU) with or without
pretreatment with indomethacin. Ovarian extracts (100
μl aliquots) were incubated with 17.6 μg ^{3}H-labeled
collagen for 44-46 h with or without p-aminophenylmercuric acetate (APMA). Each value represents the
mean ± SEM. The number of experiments is in parentheses, and in each experiment the measurements were
carried out in triplicate. APMA activates latent
collagenase. From reference 51.

cells, or macrophages. This action of LH appears independent of
prostaglandins (51). LH also may stimulate the release and/or activation
of this collagenase prior to follicular rupture. This latter process of
activation or release of the enzyme may be prostaglandin dependent (48).
The preovulatory LH surge also stimulates plasminogen activator activity
and this enzyme may be an important step in the activation of collagenase
(see below). However, products of either the cyclooxygenase or the
lipoxygenase pathway seem not to be involved in the increase of plasminogen activator activity (52-54).

Another possible mechanism by which prostaglandins may be involved in
ovulation is by stimulation of smooth muscle contraction in the ovary.
Such contractions have been implicated in the process of ovulation in a
number of species including the human (55), the rhesus monkey (55), and
the hamster (56). However, the role of such contractions remains
controversial (57,58).

LH/hCG also induces marked changes in the perifollicular capillaries
including dilatation and increased permeability (59), as well as changes
in blood flow in the preovulatory period (60). These changes, which may
have important implications for follicular rupture, can be prevented to a

large extent, by treatment with indomethacin, suggesting another possible mechanism by which prostaglandins may be involved in the ovulatory process (59,60).

While all the evidence discussed above points to an important role for prostaglandins in ovulation, Espey et al. (61) recently introduced a note of caution in the interpretation of this body of data. They found in the rabbit that they could demonstrate a dissociation between the ovulation inhibiting effect of indomethacin and its capability to inhibit follicular PGF and PGE levels, i.e., that ovulation could take place even when prostaglandin levels were kept low by the administration of indomethacin. These observations have been confirmed in the rat (Espey, personal communication). The explanation of these findings is not clear at this time, but they may indicate that prostaglandins are not the sole mediators of the ovulation-inducing action of LH.

ROLE FOR PROTEASES IN FOLLICULAR RUPTURE

Collagenase

In the final hours prior to follicular rupture, there is a remarkable thinning of the follicular wall at the apex (reviewed in 62) with an eventual breakthrough at the area of the stigma (63). Cinematographic and photographic observations of the rabbit graafian follicle in an in vitro perfusion model clearly show this process (64) (Fig. 3).

This thinning of the follicular wall is accompanied by a dissociation and fragmentation of the collagen fibrils (63,65-68). Martin and Miller-

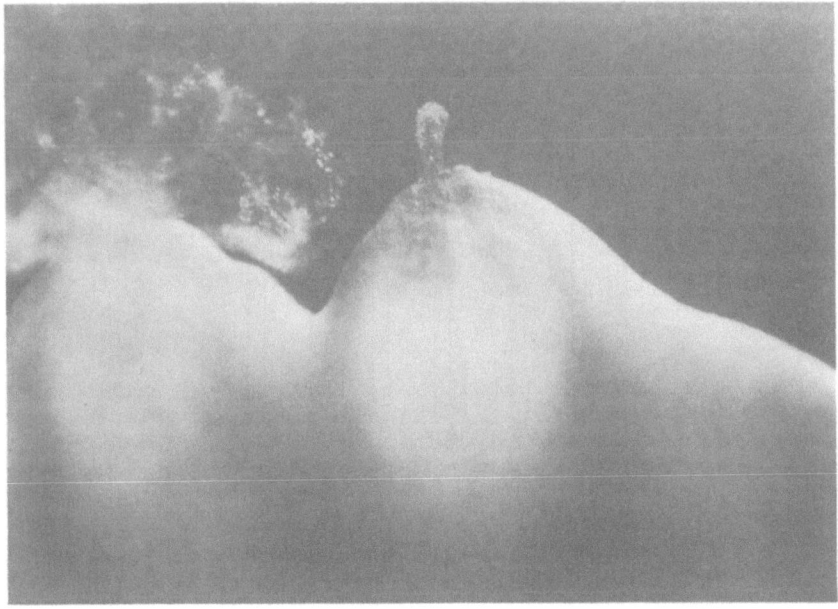

Fig. 3. Photograph of a rabbit ovary in ovarian perfusion just at the moment of follicular rupture, with an initial release of granulosa cells escaping from the ruptured follicular wall on the right. The follicle on the left ovulated some minutes earlier and a mass of dispersed granulosa cells can be seen attached to its surface. From reference 64.

Walker (68) concluded from their scanning electron microscopic observations in the hamster that this fragmentation is due to a breakdown of the intermolecular bonds that hold the collagen fibers together, thereby allowing them to separate and give way to form the stigma. Biochemically, however, this process is also associated with a decrease in ovarian and follicular collagen content (48,69). While collagen breakdown in the follicle wall can be demonstrated prior to ovulation, the measurement of an increase in true collagenase in ovarian tissue has met with considerable difficulty (69-71). This difficulty can probably be attributed to the presence of tissue and serum-borne inhibitors of collagenase which are released at the time of homogenization of the tissue prior to measurement of the enzyme (69,72).

Reich et al. (48) showed a modest preovulatory increase in the digestion of endogenously-labeled collagen in the rat. The specificity of their assay for collagenase is open to question, however, as endogenously-labeled collagen could yield radioactive fragments from telopeptide ends, cleaved by noncollagen-specific proteases (73).

Using a telopeptide-free collagen as substrate, Curry et al. (74) overcame to a substantial degree the problem of collagenase inhibitors by introducing a step of reduction and alkylation (dithiothreitol and iodoacetamide) prior to the assay of collagenase. This step appears to eliminate most of the inhibitors. With this method we found that the ovarian collagenase is present in the homogenates in an inactive form and requires activation by substances such as p-aminophenylmercuric acetate (APMA) prior to assay of the enzyme activity (74). It is likely that in vivo such an activation is also required, perhaps by proteases such as the serine protease plasmin (see below). Using this specific assay, we have recently demonstrated a marked increase in true collagenase in rat ovaries prior to ovulation (74) (Fig. 4).

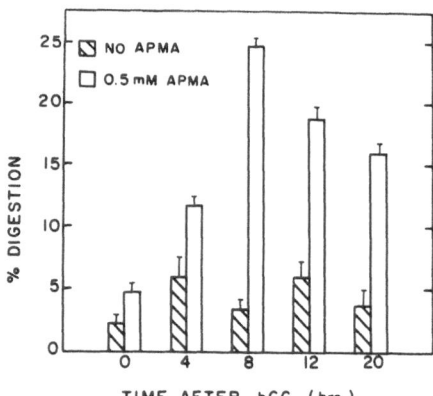

Fig. 4. Collagenase activity in ovarian supernatants treated with dithiothreitol and iodoacetamide. The ovaries were collected from immature PMSG (20 IU) treated rats at various times after administration of an ovulatory dose of hCG (10 IU). Ovarian extracts (100 µl aliquots) were incubated with 17.6 µg of telopeptide-free ^{3}H-collagen for 48 h with or without APMA to examine the latent and active forms of the enzyme respectively. Each value represents the mean ± SEM of 5 experiments in triplicate. From reference 74.

100

Interestingly, we have also recently found that homogenates of rat ovaries contain inhibitors of metalloproteases (the group of enzymes to which collagenase belongs) which also appear to increase as ovulation approaches (Fig. 5). This inhibitory activity is markedly reduced by reduction and alkylation (75). Tissue inhibitors of metalloprotease (TIMP) have been proposed as major regulators of collagenase activity in cartilage, bone, and skin (76), and it is possible that such a TIMP-like inhibitor may also play an important role in regulation of collagenase during ovulation.

The concomitant increase of collagenase activity and TIMP-like inhibitor in ovarian homogenates prior to ovulation probably represents an additional control over the collagenolytic process. While collagenase levels increase about fivefold, inhibitor levels increase only about threefold, so that collagenase may escape inhibition around the time of ovulation, at least in localized areas. A concomitant increase in collagenase and collagenase inhibitors has also been reported for fibroblasts (78) and osteoblast-like cells (79). We have recently found that rat granulosa cells in vitro produce a TIMP-like inhibitor which is stimulated by the addition of LH (80) (Table 5).

Although granulosa cells in the rat (81) and human (82) have been reported to produce collagenolytic activity, we have not been able to demonstrate the production of true collagenase in cultures of rat granulosa cells (Slackman et al., unpublished observations).

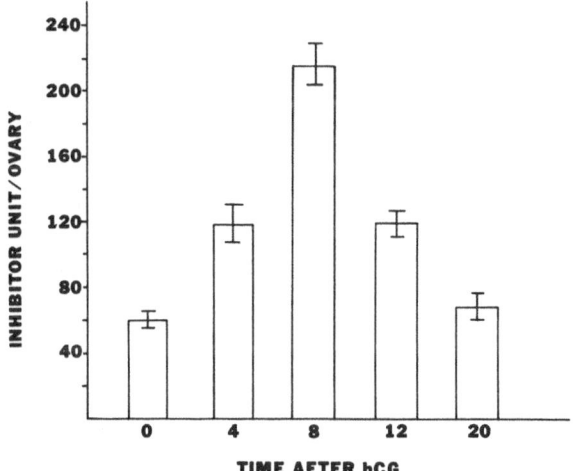

Fig. 5. Metalloprotease inhibitor in rat ovaries. Ovaries were collected from immature rats treated with PMSG (20 IU) at various times after an ovulatory dose of hCG (10 IU). The ovarian homogenate was tested for inhibitor activity using a spectrophotometric assay based on the degradation of a general proteolytic substrate (Azocoll) by uterine metalloprotease (77). The inhibitory activity is expressed as units/ovary, where 1 U represents a decrease of 77 ng of Azocoll digested/min at 37 C. From reference 75 and Curry et al., unpublished observations.

Table 5. Inhibitor activity of a neutral metalloprotease
in medium of rat granulosa cells cultured in vitro.

Hours of Incubation[2]	LH[3]	Inhibitor Activity[1]	
		Without R/A[4]	With R/A[4]
0	none	15.6 ± 10.1	-
20	none	29.3 ± 17.3	14.7 ± 9.9
20	10 ng/ml	51.4 ± 20.3	8.4 ± 7.8

[1]Inhibitor activity was measured by determining the ability of aliquots of the media to inhibit a uterine neutral metalloprotease, using a spectrophotometric assay based on the degradation of a general proteinase substrate Azocoll (77). The activity is expressed as percent inhibition of the total metalloprotease activity in the absence of any inhibitor.
[2]Granulosa cells were obtained from immature rats 48 h after treatment with PMSG (20 IU) and cultured in medium 199.
[3]NIH oLH-23.
[4]R/A = reduction and alkylation by sequential incubation with dithiothreitol and iodoacetamide (74).
From reference 80 and Slackman et al., unpublished observations.

Clearly, the hormonal regulation of collagenase and its local control by inhibitors and activators requires further study. A very intricate mechanism may emerge which operates to limit the greatest collagen breakdown to a local area within the follicle wall where rupture will occur. It appears that activation of ovarian collagenase prior to ovulation plays an important role in this process, as putative collagenase inhibitors block follicular rupture when added to the explanted hamster ovary in vitro (83) and when injected into the bursa of the rat ovary in vivo (48). Using the in vitro perfused rat ovary, our laboratory has recently demonstrated that both phenanthroline, an inhibitor of metalloproteases, and a specific synthetic peptide inhibitor of mammalian collagenase (CI-1) can inhibit LH-induced ovulation (84) (Table 6).

While the majority of morphological and biochemical studies have focused on the collagen network surrounding the follicle (Type I collagen), the basement membranes (Type IV collagen), which separate the granulosa cells from the theca cells and the germinal epithelium from the tunica albuginea, must also be broken down for ovulation to occur. Such a breakdown has indeed been observed with the use of histochemical techniques (86). The enzymes responsible for the breakdown of these basement membranes remain, however, to be determined.

The data discussed above support overwhelmingly a role for collagen breakdown and collagenase activity in ovulation. While considerable progress has been made, much further work is needed to determine the nature, the cellular origin, and the control of the collagenolytic enzyme(s) in the ovary as they relate to the process of follicular rupture.

Plasminogen Activator

Substantial evidence has linked the activity of plasminogen activator (PA) and plasmin to ovulation. This has included the demonstration that

Table 6. Ovulations in rat ovaries perfused in vitro with collagenase inhibitors.[1]

Treatment (n)	Ovulations/Ovulating Ovary[1] mean ± SE (ovulating ovaries)
Control (4)	0 (0)
LH + IBMX (4)	17.2 ± 0.5 (4)
LH + IBMX + pht 10^{-3} (4)[2]	1 (1)
LH + IBMX + pht 10^{-4} (4)[2]	2.0 ± 0.8 (4)
LH + IBMX + pht 10^{-5} (4)[2]	12.5 ± 3.5 (4)
LH + IBMX + CI-1 (25 µM) (6)[3]	7.6 ± 2.5 (5)
LH + IBMX + CI-2 (25 µM) (6)[4]	24.0 ± 3.4 (5)

[1] Same as in Table 1. LH (0.1 µg/ml of NIH-oLH-24) and IBMX (0.2 mM) were added at 0 time to all perfusions, except the control.
[2] After 1 h, 1,10-phenanthroline was added at the concentration indicated.
[3] After 1 h, CI-1, a specific inhibitor of collagenase (85), was added.
[4] After 1 h CI-2, the inactive stereoisomer of CI-1 was added.
From reference 84 and Brannstrom et al., unpublished observations.

PA activity increases in the rat ovary as ovulation approaches (87) and that granulosa cells in vitro produce PA and increase this production under stimulation by gonadotropin (87). At first it was thought that FSH was the most potent stimulator of PA in granulosa cells (53,88), but recent evidence has demonstrated that both LH and FSH are equally effective in stimulating PA production by isolated preovulatory rat follicles (52) and isolated preovulatory granulosa cells (89-91). While this difference is not clearly understood, it may be due to the stage of maturity of the granulosa cells, with more mature cells responding to both gonadotropins.

Furthermore, evidence of the involvement of PA in the ovulatory process was provided by Reich et al. (52). These investigators injected inhibitors of either PA or plasmin into the bursa of the rat ovary and blocked LH-induced ovulation in a dose-dependent manner. Preliminary evidence from our laboratory indicates that addition of a potent inhibitor of PA (tranexamic acid) to the perfused rat ovary causes a dose-dependent inhibition of ovulation (Morioka et al., unpublished observations).

The ovary produces both the tissue type of PA (tPA) and a urokinase type of PA (uPA) (90,91). The cellular origin and the gonadotropic control of these two enzymes is complex. While thecal tissue produces some PA, the granulosa cells account for the majority of the total follicular PA activity. Gonadotropins stimulate tPA production by granulosa cells while uPA is not increased (90,91). Furthermore, most of the gonadotropin-stimulated PA activity produced by GC is found in the culture medium or follicular fluid (90). Interestingly, Ny et al. (91) found that granulosa cells in culture also secrete an inhibitor of fibrinolysis and that this secretion is suppressed by gonadotropin addition to the medium.

The substrate for PA is apparently blood-borne plasminogen which is present in the follicular fluid (92). The resulting plasmin could act within the follicle antrum itself or in the follicle wall and surrounding tissue. Plasmin itself is not capable of digesting collagen, but has been shown in other tissues to activate collagenase (93). Furthermore, Reich et al. (48) have shown that plasmin is able to activate ovarian collagenase and that the time course of stimulation by gonadotropin of both enzymes (PA and collagenase) within the ovary is such that PA via plasmin may function as the physiological activator of ovarian collagenase necessary to digest the follicular wall (see above). It is possible, of course, that PA and plasmin may have other functions in the ovulatory process such as dissociation of the ground substance between collagen fibrils or dissociation of oocyte-cumulus complexes. In this regard, it is of interest that oocyte-cumulus complexes produce tPA and that this production can be stimulated in vitro by gonadotropin (94).

All this evidence indicates an important role for PA and the fibrinolytic system in ovulation. Further studies to elucidate their control and action are necessary.

BIOCHEMICAL MODEL FOR OVULATION

We have limited the above discussion to investigations of five distinct aspects of the ovulatory process in which our laboratory is involved, namely the role of (1) the various hormones capable of initiating the process; (2) cyclic nucleotides; (3) steroids; (4) prostaglandins; and, (5) proteolytic enzymes. There are undoubtedly many more factors, such as histamine, catecholamines, serotonin, kinins, and Ca^{++}, which may be involved but have not been discussed. The complexity of the entire process of ovulation and the similarity of many components of this process to an inflammatory reaction have lead Espey to propose that ovulation is a type of inflammatory process within the follicle (95). There is much merit to this proposal, but an in-depth discussion of the multitude of factors which support this comparison is clearly not within the scope of this review and the reader is referred to the review by Espey (95).

Some years ago we proposed a simplified model for the biochemical mechanism of ovulation based on the then available information from our laboratory and others (20). Much new information is now available and we propose the following sequence of events schematized in Figure 6. Although most of the information on which this model is based is derived from studies of the rabbit and the rat, there is good reason to believe that the basic mechanisms of ovulation may be similar in other species as well. All of these events are probably not encompassed in any single cell type. It is probable that several cell types—granulosa cells, theca cells, fibroblasts, smooth muscle cells, and possibly also macrophages and other leukocytes—interact during the biochemical process leading to ovulation. The exact cell types in which each biochemical event occurs remains to be determined.

It is obvious that LH, perhaps with some contribution from FSH, is the normal physiological trigger for the ovulatory sequence of events and it appears from the available information that LH's effects are mainly mediated via adenylate cyclase and increased cAMP. The cAMP in turn, via cAMP-dependent protein kinase, influences at least two distinct steps in the ovulatory process which seem to be of crucial importance, namely: (1) the stimulation of cyclooxygenase/lipoxygenase leading to increased prostaglandin/leukotriene synthesis; and, (2) the stimulation of plasminogen activator which catalyzes the conversion of plasminogen in plasmin.

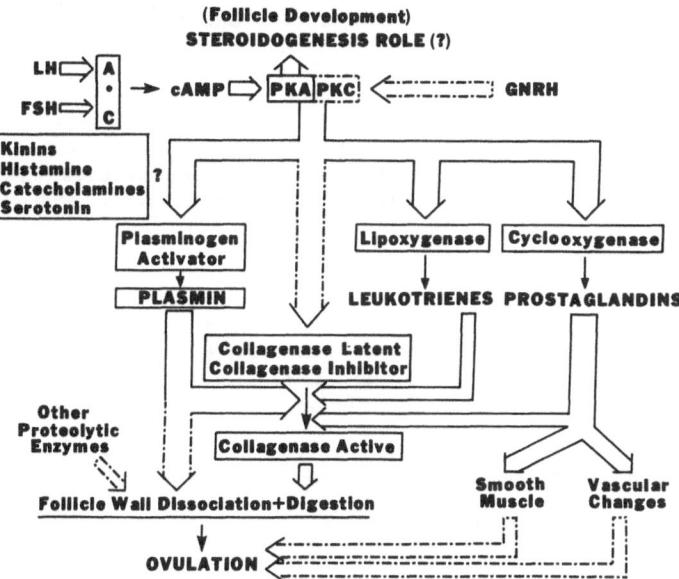

Fig. 6. Hypothetical model of some of the biochemical events occurring during the ovulatory process. LH = luteinizing hormone; FSH = follicle stimulating hormone; AC = adenylate cyclase; cAMP = cAMP; PKA = cAMP-dependent protein kinase; PKC = protein kinase C; GnRH = gonadotropin releasing hormone. Rectangular boxes are for enzymes involved. Open arrows ($\Rightarrow$) indicate stimulation, while closed arrows ($\longrightarrow$) indicate conversions. Solid lines indicate proven stimulation, while dashed lines indicate that the stimulation remains unproven.

A third crucial step in the ovulatory mechanism is the LH-induced increase in latent collagenase, but it remains to be determined if this step is mediated via cAMP. Concomitant with the increase in latent collagenase, there also appears to be an LH-dependent increase in collagenase inhibitors. The latent collagenase is then activated and it appears that leukotrienes and prostaglandins as well as plasmin may be involved in this process. The active collagenase causes a digestion of the collagen in the follicle wall. Plasmin as well as possibly other proteolytic enzymes such as proteoglycanase (81) may cause a further dissociation of the follicular wall. These processes of digestion of collagen and dissociation of the collagen fibers result in an opening in the follicular wall with the formation of the stigma and rupture. While the weakening of the follicular wall takes place throughout the entire wall, rupture remains for the most part a localized process at the apex of the follicle. This localization of the rupture may be explained on the basis of mechanical factors operating when the follicle wall thins and weakens (96).

FSH by itself can also cause ovulation, but its physiological role in this regard has not been demonstrated. Its mechanism is most likely also via cAMP-dependent protein kinase (97). GnRH's ability to trigger ovulation in the rat does not involve cAMP (18), but may instead involve activation of PKC (98). However, there is no evidence at present that GnRH plays a physiologic role in ovulation.

While it is clear that prostaglandins and leukotrienes can influence smooth muscle by causing contractions and that these compounds can cause vascular changes such as increased permeability, vasodilatation and vasoconstriction, it is not clear what the exact role of these latter processes are in ovulation. There is controversy as well regarding the obligatory role for the increase in steroids in the ovulatory process. Most in vivo data seem to point to a role for steroids while in vitro perfusion data suggest that the increase in estrogen and progesterone, seen in the preovulatory follicle after LH stimulation, is not required for follicular rupture.

We realize that our model is not complete and most certainly does not include all the factors that may play a role in the mechanism by which LH triggers ovulation. It presents, however, a working model upon which further experimentation can be designed. While progress has not been rapid, a great deal of new information has emerged since our previous review (20). Little information is available on the primate, but many of the mechanisms discussed here and derived from studies on other mammalian species may apply to the primate as well. Arriving at a clear understanding of the ovarian mechanisms leading to ovulation is of major importance, as ovulation is a central event in the female reproductive process. From this understanding new methods for the control of ovulation may emerge, whether they be for induction of ovulation in cases of anovulatory infertility, or in vitro fertilization, or for inhibition of ovulation for contraceptive purposes.

ACKNOWLEDGMENTS

This manuscript was supported in part by NIH grants HD-08747, HD-06773, HD-07129. We thank Maria A. Sanchez for the very careful preparation of the manuscript. We wish to thank Drs. P. O. Janson and K. E. B. Ahren for their continuing interest and collaboration with our studies and Dr. L. L. Espey for many fruitful discussions and helpful suggestions. Dr. M. Brannstrom received support from the Swedish Medical Research Council (Grant No. 27).

REFERENCES

1. Schwartz NB. The role of FSH and LH and their antibodies on follicle growth and on ovulation. Biol Reprod 1974; 10:236-72.
2. Wallach EE, Wright KH, Hamada Y. Investigation of mammalian ovulation with an in vitro perfused rabbit ovary preparation. Am J Obstet Gynecol 1978; 132:728-38.
3. Janson PO, LeMaire WJ, Kallfelt B, et al. The study of ovulation in the isolated perfused rabbit ovary. I. Methodology and patterns of steroidogenesis. Biol Reprod 1982; 26:456-65.
4. Koos RD, Jaccarino FJ, Magaril RA, LeMaire WJ. Perfusion of the rat ovary in vitro: methodology, induction of ovulation, and patterns of steroidogenesis. Biol Reprod 1984; 30:1135-41.
5. Sheela-Rani GS, Moudgal NR. Examination of the role of FSH in periovulatory events in the hamster. J Reprod Fertil 1977; 50:37-45.
6. Shaykh M, LeMaire WJ, Papkoff H, Curry TE, Sogn JH, Koos RD. Ovulations in rat ovaries perfused in vitro with follicle stimulating hormone. Biol Reprod 1985; 33:629-36.
7. Hsueh AJW, Jones PBC. Extrapituitary actions of gonadotropin releasing hormone. Endocr Rev 1981; 2:437-61.
8. Ekholm C, Hillensjo I, Isaksson O. Gonadotropin releasing hormone agonists stimulate oocyte meiosis and ovulation in hypophysectomized rats. Endocrinology 1981; 108:2022-4.

9. Corbin A, Bex FJ. Luteinizing hormone releasing hormone agonists induce ovulation in hypophysectomized proestrus rats: direct ovarian effect. Life Sci 1981; 29:185-92.

10. Dekel N, Sherizly A, Tsafriri A, Noar Z. A comparative study of the mechanism of action of luteinizing hormone releasing hormone analog on the ovary. Biol Reprod 1983; 28:161-92.

11. Koos RD, LeMaire WJ. The effect of a gonadotropin-releasing hormone agonist on ovulation and steroidogenesis during perfusion of rabbit and rat ovaries in vitro. Endocrinology 1985; 116:628-32.

12. Fraser HM, Bramley TA, Miller WR, Sharpe RM. Extrapituitary actions of LHRH analogues in tissues of the human female and investigation of the existence and function of LHRH like peptides. In: Rolland R, Chadha DR, Willemsen WNP, eds. Gonadotropin down regulation in gynecologic practice. New York: Alan R. Liss Inc., 1986:29-54.

13. Marsh JM. The role of cyclic AMP in gonadal function. Adv Cyclic Nucleotide Res 1975; 6:137-99.

14. Birnbaumer L, Kirchick HJ. Regulation of gonadotropin action: the molecular mechanisms of gonadotropin induced activation of ovarian adenylyl cyclases. In: Greenwald GS, Terranova P, eds. Factors regulating ovarian function. New York: Raven Press, 1983:287-310.

15. Holmes PV, Hedin L, Janson PO. The role of cyclic AMP in the ovulatory process of the in vitro perfused rabbit ovary. Endocrinology 1986; 118:2195-202.

16. Brannstrom M, Koos RD, LeMaire WJ, Janson PO. Cyclic AMP induced ovulation in the perfused rat ovary and its mediation by prostaglandins. Biol Reprod 1987 (in press).

17. Holmes PV, Janson PO, Sogn J, et al. Effects of $PGF_{2\alpha}$ and indomethacin on ovulation and steroid production in the isolated rabbit ovary. Acta Endocrinol (Copenh) 1983; 104:233-9.

18. Clark MR, Thibier C, Marsh JM, LeMaire WJ. Stimulation of prostaglandin accumulation by luteinizing hormone-releasing hormone (LHRH) and LHRH analogs in rat granulosa cells in vitro. Endocrinology 1980; 107:17-23.

19. Kawai Y, Clark MR. Phorbol ester regulation of rat granulosa cell prostaglandin and progesterone accumulation. Endocrinology 1985; 116:2320-6.

20. LeMaire WJ, Clark MR, Marsh JM. Biochemical mechanism of ovulation. In: Hafez ESE, ed. Human ovulation. Amsterdam: Elsevier/North Holland Biochemical Press, 1979:159-75.

21. Lipner H, Greep RO. Inhibition of steroidogenesis at various sites in the biosynthesis pathway in relation to induced ovulation. Endocrinology 1971; 88:602-7.

22. Lipner H, Wendelken L. Inhibition of ovulation by inhibition of steroidogenesis in immature rats. Proc Soc Exp Biol Med 1971; 136:1141-5.

23. Bullock DW, Kappauf BH. Dissociation of gonadotropin induced ovulation and steroidogenesis in immature rats. Endocrinology 1975; 92:1625-8.

24. Snyder BW, Beechan GD, Schane HP. Inhibition of ovulation in rats with Epostane, an inhibition of 3-beta-hydroxysteroid dehydrogenase (418G5). Proc Soc Exp Biol Med 1984; 176:238-42.

25. Tsafriri A, Abisogun AO, Reich R. Steroids and follicular rupture at ovulation. Proceedings VII International Congress on Hormonal Steroids, Madrid, 1986 (in press).

26. Koos RD, Feiertag M, Brodie A, LeMaire WJ. Inhibition of estrogen synthesis does not inhibit LH-induced ovulations. Am J Obstet Gynecol 1984; 148:939-45.

27. Berthois Y, Katzenellenbogen JA, Katzenellenbogen BS. Phenol red in tissue culture media is a weak estrogen: implications concerning the study of estrogen-responsive cells in culture. Proc Nat Acad Sci 1986; 83:2496-500.

28. Kitai H, Bongiovanni A, Santulli R, Wallach EE. The effect of ovarian steroidogenesis on ovulation in the rabbit [Abstract]. Fertil Steril 1983; 39:397.

29. Holmes PV, Sogn J, Schillinger E, Janson PO. Effects of high and low preovulatory concentrations of progesterone on ovulation from the isolated perfused rabbit ovary. J Reprod Fertil 1985; 75:393-9.

30. LeMaire WJ, Janson PO, Kallfelt BJ, et al. The preovulatory decline in follicular estradiol is not required for ovulation in the rabbit. Acta Endocrinol (Copenh) 1982; 101:452-7.

31. LeMaire WJ, Clark MR, Chainy GBN, Marsh JM. The role of prostaglandins in the mechanism of ovulation. In: Tozzini RI, Reaves G, Pineda RL, eds. International symposium on the endocrine physiopathology of the ovary. Amsterdam: Elsevier/North Holland, 1980; 207-17.

32. Wallach EE, de la Cruz A, Hunt J, Wright KH, Stevens VC. The effect of indomethacin on hMG-hCG induced ovulation in the Rhesus monkey. Prostaglandins 1975; 9:654-8.

33. Maia H, Barbosa I, Coutinho EM. Inhibition of ovulation in marmoset monkeys by indomethacin. Fertil Steril 1978; 29:565-70.

34. O'Grady JP, Caldwell BV, Auletta FJ, Speroff L. The effects of an inhibitor of prostaglandin synthesis (indomethacin) on ovulation, pregnancy and pseudopregnancy in the rabbit. Prostaglandins 1972; 1:97-106.

35. Wright KH, Stevens VC, Hamada Y, Wallach EE. The effect of indomethacin on spontaneous ovulation in Rhesus monkeys [Abstract]. Fertil Steril 1977; 29:239.

36. Chaudhuri G, Elder MG. Lack of evidence for inhibition of ovulation by aspirin in women. Prostaglandins 1976; 11:727-32.

37. Hamada Y, Bronson RA, Wright KH, Wallach EE. Ovulation in the perfused rabbit ovary: the influence of prostaglandin inhibitors. Biol Reprod 1977; 17:58-63.

38. Kobayashi Y, Santulli R, Wright KH, Wallach EE. The effect of prostaglandin synthesis inhibition by indomethacin on ovulation and ovum maturation in the in vitro perfused rabbit ovary. Am J Obstet Gynecol 1981; 141:53-7.

39. Hamada Y, Wright KH, Wallach EE. In vitro reversal of indomethacin blocked ovulation by prostaglandin F_2. Fertil Steril 1978; 30:702-6.

40. Sogn JH, Curry TE, Brannstrom M, et al. Inhibition of FSH induced ovulation by indomethacin in the perfused rat ovary. Biol Reprod (in press).

41. Ekholm C, Clark MR, Magnuson C, Isaksson O, LeMaire WJ. Ovulation induced by a gonadotropin releasing hormone analog in hypophysectomized rats involves prostaglandins. Endocrinology 1982; 110:288-90.

42. Koos RD, Clark MR, Janson PO, Ahren KEB, LeMaire WJ. Prostaglandin levels in preovulatory follicles from rabbit ovaries perfused in vitro. Prostaglandins 1983; 25:715-24.

43. Reich R, Kohen F, Naor Z, Tsafriri A. Possible involvement of lipoxygenase products of arachidonic acid pathway in ovulation. Prostaglandins 1983; 26:1011-20.

44. Koos RD, Clark MR. Production of 6-keto-prostaglandin F_1 by rat granulosa cells in vitro. Endocrinology 1982; 111:1513-8.

45. Yoshimura Y, Dharmarajan AM, Gipps S, et al. Local effects of prostacyclin on in vitro ovulation [Abstract]. Society for Gynecologic Investigation, 34th Annual Meeting, Atlanta, Georgia, 1987.

46. Espey LL, Coons PJ, Marsh JM, LeMaire WJ. Effect of indomethacin on preovulatory changes in the ultrastructure of rabbit Graafian follicles. Endocrinology 1981; 108:1040-48.

47. Downs SM, Longo FJ. Effects of indomethacin on preovulatory follicles in immature superovulated mice. Am J Anat 1982; 164:265-74.

48. Reich R, Tsafriri A, Mechanic GL. The involvement of collagenolysis

in ovulation in the rat. Endocrinology 1985; 116:522-7.

49. Kawamura N, Himeno N, Okamura H, Mori T, Fukomoto M, Midorikawa O. Effect of indomethacin on collagenolytic enzyme activities in rabbit ovary. Nippon Sanka Fiyuika, Gakkai Zasshi, 1984; 26:2099-105.

50. Murdoch WJ, Peterson TA, Van Kirk EA, Vincent DL, Inskeep EK. Interactive roles of progesterone prostaglandins and collagenase in the ovulatory mechanism of the ewe. Biol Reprod 1986; 35:1187-94.

51. Curry T, Clark MR, Dean DD, Woessner JF, LeMaire, WJ. The pre-ovulatory increase in ovarian collagenase activity in the rat is independent of prostaglandin production. Endocrinology 1986; 118:1823-8.

52. Reich R, Miskin R, Tsafriri A. Follicular plasminogen activator: involvement in ovulation. Endocrinology 1985; 116:516-21.

53. Strickland S, Beers WH. Studies on the role of plasminogen activator in ovulation. J Biol Chem 1976; 251:5694-702.

54. Shimada H, Okamura H, Noda Y, Suzuki A, Tojo S, Takada A. Plasminogen activator in rat ovary during the ovulatory process: independence of prostaglandin mediation. J Endocrinol 1983; 97:201-5.

55. Owman CH, Sjoberg NO, Wallach EE, Walles B, Wright KH. Neuromuscular mechanisms of ovulation. In: Hafez ESE, ed. Human ovulation. Amsterdam: Elsevier/North Holland, 1979:57-100.

56. Martin GG, Talbot P. The role of follicular smooth muscle cells in hamster ovulation. J Exp Zool 1981; 216:469-82.

57. Espey LL. Ovarian contractility and its relationship to ovulation: a review. Biol Reprod 1978; 19:540-51.

58. Kitai H, Santulli R, Wright KH, Wallach EE. Examination of the role of calcium in ovulation in the in vitro perfused rabbit ovary with use of ethylene glycol bis (β-aminoethyl ether)-n,n'-tetraacetic acid and verapamil. Am J Obstet Gynecol 1985; 152:705-8.

59. Okuda Y, Okamura H, Kanzaki H, Fujii S, Takenaka A, Wallach EE. An ultrastructural study of ovarian perifollicular capillaries in the indomethacin treated rabbit. Fertil Steril 1983; 39:85-92.

60. Murdoch WJ, Myers DA. Effect of treatment of estrous ewes with indomethacin on the distribution of ovarian blood flow to the peri-ovulatory follicle. Biol Reprod 1983; 29:1229-32.

61. Espey LL, Norris C, Saphire D. Effect of time and dose of indomethacin on follicular prostaglandins and ovulation in the rabbit. Endocrinology 1986; 119:746-54.

62. Espey LL. Ovulation. In: Jones RE, ed. The vertebrate ovary. New York: Plenum Press, 1978:503-32.

63. Espey LL. Ultrastructure of the apex of the rabbit Graafian follicle during the ovulatory process. Endocrinology 1962; 81:267-76.

64. Lofman CO, Janson PO, Kallfelt BJ, Ahren K, LeMaire WJ. The study of ovulation in the isolated perfused rabbit ovary. II. Photographic and cinematographic observations. Biol Reprod 1982; 26:467-73.

65. Bjersing L, Cajander S. Ovulation and the mechanism of follicular rupture. I. Light microscopic changes in rabbit ovarian follicles prior to induced ovulation. Cell Tissue Res 1974; 149:287-300.

66. Bjersing L, Cajander S. Ovulation and the mechanism of follicle rupture. III. Transmission electron microscopy of rabbit germinal epithelium prior to induced ovulation. Cell Tissue Res 1974; 149:313-27.

67. Downs SM, Longo FJ. An ultrastructural study of preovulatory apical development in mouse ovarian follicles: effect of indomethacin. Anat Rec 1983; 205:159-68.

68. Martin GG, Miller-Walker C. Visualization of the three-dimensional distribution of collagen fibrils over preovulatory follicles in the hamster. J Exp Zool 1983; 225:311-9.

69. Morales TI, Woessner JF, Marsh JM, LeMaire WJ. Collagen, collagenase and collagenolytic activity in rat Graafian follicles during follicular growth and ovulation. Biochim Biophys Acta 1983; 756:119-22.

70. Espey LL, Stacy S. Failure of an ovarian collagenolytic extract to decompose the connective tissue in the mature sow Graafian follicle [Abstract]. Fed Proc 1970; 29:833.

71. Paar EL. Absence of neutral proteinase activity in rat ovarian follicle walls at ovulation. Biol Reprod 1984; 11:509-12.

72. Espey LL. Ovarian proteolytic enzymes and ovulations. Biol Reprod 1974; 10:216-35.

73. Dean DD, Woessner JF. A sensitive, specific assay for tissue collagenase using telopeptide free [^{3}H-acetyl]-collagen. Anal Biochem 1985; 148:174-81.

74. Curry TE, Dean DD, Woessner JF, LeMaire WJ. The extraction of a tissue collagenase associated with ovulation in the rat. Biol Reprod 1985; 33:981-91.

75. Curry TE, Dean DD, Koos RD, LeMaire WJ. A metalloprotease inhibitor in the rat ovary: changes in activity during the preovulatory period [Abstract]. Proceedings of the VIth Ovarian Workshop, Ithaca, NY, 1986.

76. Sellers A, Murphy G. Collagenolytic enzymes and their naturally occurring inhibitors. Int Rev Connect Tissue Res 1981; 9:151-90.

77. Dean DD, Woessner JF. Extracts of human articular cartilage contains an inhibitor of tissue metalloproteases. Biochem J 1984; 218:277-80.

78. Murphy G, Reynolds JJ, Werb Z. Biosynthesis of tissue inhibitor of metalloproteinases by human fibroblasts in culture. J Biol Chem 1985; 260:3079-83.

79. Otsuka K, Sodek J, Limeback H. Synthesis of collagenase and collagenase inhibitors by osteoblast-like cells in culture. J Biochem 1984; 145:123-9.

80. Slackman RL, Curry TE, Koos RD, LeMaire WJ. A neutral metalloprotease inhibitor from rat granulosa cells [Abstract]. The Endocrine Society 68th Annual Meeting, Anaheim, CA, 1986.

81. Too CKL, Bryant-Greenwood GD, Greenwood FC. Relaxin increases the release of plasminogen activator, collagenase, and proteoglycanase from rat granulosa cells in vitro. Endocrinology 1984; 115:1043-50.

82. Kukumoto M, Yajima Y, Okamura H, Midorikawa O. Collagenolytic enzyme activity in human ovary: an ovulatory enzyme activity. Fertil Steril 1981; 36:746-50.

83. Ichikawa S, Morioka H, Ohta M, Oda X, Murao S. Effect of various proteinase inhibitors on ovulation of explanted hamster ovaries. J Reprod Fertil 1983; 68:407-12.

84. Brannstrom M, Woessner JF, Koos RD, Sear CKJ, LeMaire WJ. Inhibition of mammalian tissue collagenase and a general metalloproteinase inhibitor [Abstract]. First European Congress of Endocrinology, Copenhagen, 1987.

85. Delaisse JM, Eeckhout Y, Sear C, Galloway A, McCullough K, Vaes G. A new synthetic inhibitor of mammalian tissue collagenase inhibits bone resorption in culture. Biochem Biophys Res Commun 1985; 133:483-90.

86. Palotie A, Peltonen L, Foidart JM, Rajaniemi H. Immunohistochemical localization of basement membrane components and interstitial collagen types in preovulatory ovarian follicles. Coll Relat Res 1984; 4:279-87.

87. Beers WH, Strickland S, Reich E. Ovarian plasminogen activator. Relationship to ovulation and hormonal regulation. Cell 1975; 6:387-94.

88. Martinat N, Cambernous Y. The release of plasminogen activator by rat granulosa cells is highly specific for FSH activity. Endocrinology 1983; 113:433-5.

89. Wang C, Leung A. Gonadotropins regulate plasminogen activator production by rat granulosa cells. Endocrinology 1983; 112:1201-7.

90. Reich R, Miskin R, Tsafriri A. Intrafollicular distribution of plasminogen activator and their hormonal regulation in vitro. Endocrinology 1986; 119:1588-601.

91. Ny T, Bjersing L, Hsueh A, Loskutoff DJ. Cultured granulosa cells produce two plasminogen activators and an antiactivator, each regulated differently by gonadotropins. Endocrinology 1985; 116:1666-8.

92. Beers WH. Follicular plasminogen and plasminogen activator and the effect of plasmin on ovarian follicle wall. Cell 1975; 6:379-86.

93. Werb Z, Mainardi CL, Vater C, Harris ER Jr. Endogenous activation of latent collagenase by rheumatoid synovial cells. N Engl J Med 1977; 296:1017-23.

94. Lui YX, Ny T, Sarkar D, Loskutoff D, Hsueh AJW. Identification and regulation of tissue plasminogen activator activity in rat cumulus-oocyte complexes. Endocrinology 1986; 119:1578-87.

95. Espey LL. Ovulation as an inflammatory reaction—a hypothesis. Biol Reprod 1980; 22:73-106.

96. Rodbard D. Mechanism of ovulation. J Clin Endocrinol Metab 1968; 28:849-61.

97. Hsueh AJW, Adashi EY, Jones PBC, Welsh TH Jr. Hormonal regulation of the differentiation of cultured ovarian granulosa cells. Endocr Rev 1984; 5:76-127.

98. Davis JS, West JA, Farese RV. Gonadotropin releasing hormone (GnRH) rapidly stimulates the formation of inositol phosphates and diacylglycerol in rat granulosa cells: further evidence for the involvement of Ca^{2+} and protein kinase C in the action of GnRH. Endocrinology 1986; 118:2561-71.

ANGIOGENESIS IN THE OVARY

Kenneth J. Ryan, M.D., and Anastasia Makris

Laboratory of Human Reproduction and Reproductive Biology
and Department of Obstetrics, Gynecology and
Reproductive Biology
Harvard Medical School, Boston, MA 02115

ANGIOGENESIS DURING CYCLIC FOLLICLE AND CORPUS LUTEUM DEVELOPMENT

Angiogenesis associated with follicle and corpus luteum cyclicity and ovulation is an important example of recurrent capillary development in an adult physiological system. Angiogenesis is ordinarily stimulated in response to trauma, infection, inflammation or neoplasia. Such pathological conditions have offered the most common experimental models with which to study the control of capillary growth (1). Progress in our understanding of angiogenesis in general has stimulated a fresh look at this process in the ovary (2).

An independent blood supply is achieved for the follicle only after its transition from a primordial to a primary follicle, by which time it consists of several layers of granulosa cells separated from a well-defined theca interna by a basement membrane (3). Capillaries form a spherical wreath that perfuses the theca interna but blood vessels are excluded from direct contact with the granulosa cells by their failure to penetrate the basement membrane boundary. A secondary more peripheral wreath of capillaries perfuse the theca externa of the follicle. When a cohort of primary follicles are recruited for development in an ovulatory cycle, they progress through a secondary antral stage in a period of less than two weeks accompanied by extensive capillary growth in the theca of the follicles. Immediately after ovulation, the basement membrane of the follicle is breached by capillary ingrowth that then proceeds among the granulosa lutein cells of the corpus luteum. In a short period the corpus luteum consists of a dense spherical ball of intertwined capillary vessels (2,4).

Ovulation does not occur for most developing follicles and they undergo atresia with accompanying loss of their capillary vascular wreaths. When the corpus luteum regresses, it loses both its endocrine function and its anatomic structure including the well-developed capillary network (3).

This process of angiogenesis and capillary regression hence takes place recurrently over every ovulatory cycle during the reproductive life of the individual, accompanying folliculogenesis, atresia, ovulation and corpora lutea formation and regression (3,4).

In the past, these vascular changes could be understood largely in only anatomic terms or with respect to blood flow (3). Assay systems for angiogenesis have now been developed and some angiogenic factors isolated and identified (5). It should now be possible to define which factors are responsible for angiogenesis in the ovary and to explore the role that vascular changes may play in controlling ovarian cyclicity.

ASSAYS FOR ANGIOGENESIS AND STUDIES OF CAPILLARY GROWTH AND REGRESSION

Introduction of the use of the word angiogenesis to describe placental capillary formation is attributed to Hertig in 1935, but the bulk of subsequent study of angiogenesis has been related to its putative role in tumor growth and spread (5-7). Folkman has described his early observations that tumors would not grow when implanted into isolated perfused organs but could grow extensively and rapidly if implanted into host animals. When it was recognized that isolated perfused organs did not support tumor growth because they could not sustain neovascularization due to degeneration of capillaries, a theory of tumor dependence on angiogenesis evolved. This was followed by observations that a diffusible factor extracted from tumors or conditioned media could induce angiogenesis (5). The challenge was next to develop assay methods to assist in the isolation of angiogenic factors and to study the details of capillary growth and regression (8). The hope was that if we knew what made tumors grow, it might be feasible to block or reverse the process.

Assays for Angiogenic Factors

In vivo assays. In vivo assays are the reference standards for attributing angiogenic activity to a test substance. The chorioallantoic membrane (CAM) of the chick embryo and the cornea of the rabbit eye are two in vivo assays that are used most extensively by those studying angiogenesis (8).

In the chorioallantoic membrane assay, a window is made in the shell of fertilized eggs on day 9 or 10. The test substance is ordinarily dried on a small plastic coverslip and placed face down on the membrane. A positive response is the formation of a halo or spoke wheel pattern of newly formed capillaries oriented toward the test spot. Unfortunately, the CAM assay also responds to nonspecific stimuli like mechanical injury or egg dust. Folkman has used heparin on the covetslip along with an angiogenic factor to induce angiogenesis earlier than is seen with nonspecific stimuli. In some laboratories CAM is used predominantly as a negative screen (1,6-8).

A second in vivo assay is one based on use of a corneal pocket in the rabbit eye and polymer pellets for controlled release of angiogenic factors (7). A small incision is made in the cornea, 1.5 mm from the limbal edge to a depth half the thickness of the cornea. A small pocket 1.5 mm x 4 mm is fashioned with a spatula and test substances of size 1 mm^3 are inserted into the pocket. The advantage of the corneal assay is that the cornea is normally avascular; thus, new vessel growth can be measured and studied more easily. In addition, the assay has proved useful in studies of angiogenesis inhibitors (1,6,8).

In vitro assays. The basis of in vitro assays are the effects of putative angiogenic substances on endothelial cells in culture. Endothelial cells were originally obtained from the umbilical vein and aorta, but subsequently have been obtained from calf adrenal capillaries. Endothelial cells have been tested with angiogenic factors with respect to stimulation of mitogenic activity protein and DNA synthesis and migration.

In one elaborate test, not widely used, capillary and endothelial cells are plated on a coverslip covered with gold particles. Under stimulation of angiogenic factors, the cells ingest gold and migrate leaving a bare track which can be measured (7).

Endothelial cells grown in culture will form tubes when they reach confluence and it is believed that the information needed to construct a capillary tube resides in the endothelial cell itself (1). In a recently developed in vitro model of angiogenesis, endothelial cells are grown in a collagen matrix which allows three-dimensional growth. Under such circumstances, the cells form tubular structures consisting of endothelial cells folded on themselves (9).

Studies of Capillary Growth and Regression

The morphological events involved in capillary formation under angiogenic stimulus have been described by Folkman (1). Within a day of the application of an angiogenic stimulus, the endothelial cells on the side of the venule facing the stimulus thicken and increase endoplasmic reticulum, ribosomes and display a prominent Golgi apparatus. They resemble regenerating endothelium. Next, the basement membrane fragments with cell processes protruding through the area where the basal lamina is lost. This is believed due to the proteases, plasminogen activator and collagenase contained in the endothelial cells that are activated by angiogenic factors. Within 2 days, DNA synthesis is increased and continues in waves at intervals of 2 or 3 days. The endothelial cells next migrate out in the form of a sprout following one another. There is surprisingly little leakage of blood and the parent vessel seems to maintain the integrity of the basement membrane. The advance cells migrate toward the angiogenic stimulus followed by cells which are dividing. The sprouts finally form a lumen and join together to assemble into loops. The mechanism for forming arteriolar connections, however, remain to be established.

Regression of capillaries is equally intriguing and in many instances simply follows withdrawal of an angiogenic signal. It has also been established that protamine that binds heparin, inhibits angiogenesis. When heparin, usually a facilitator of angiogenesis is present with certain adrenal steroids, capillary growth is inhibited, possibly the basis of the effectiveness of corticoids in certain collagen vascular disease states. In addition, cartilage contains an angiogenesis inhibitor that is believed to be a positively charged protein (1,7,8).

ANGIOGENIC FACTORS

Angiogenic activity has been attributed to a wide variety of substances from many tissue sources (5). Some factors stimulate angiogenesis in vivo but will not induce mitosis or migration of endothelial cells in vitro. It has been postulated that there are two general types of angiogenic activity: (1) a direct angiogenesis activity that elicits all of the biological activities necessary for an endothelial cell to respond; and, (2) an indirect angiogenesis activity that mobilizes macrophages and activates them to secrete the necessary factors, or that releases extracellular mitogenic factors, or that induces endothelial cells to release the factors themselves (1). From the Walker 256 carcinoma, many protein angiogenic fractions were isolated that suggested molecular weights from a low of 200 to a high of 100,000 (2). One characteristic many of the angiogenic factors had in common was the ability to bind to heparin and this facilitated purification of one class of compounds with a molecular weight close to 18,000 (1). It is reported that one of the low molecular weight angiogenic factors in the Walker 256 carcinoma may be simply nicotinamide (10).

Fibroblast Growth Factors

Fibroblast Growth Factor (FGF) has direct angiogenic activity in addition to stimulating mitogenesis and differentiation of mesoderm and neuroectoderm derived cells (11,12). Fibroblast Growth Factor (FGF) has been isolated from a wide variety of normal cells and probably accounts for most of the diverse angiogenic and growth factors identified in neoplastic cells. The tissues with the highest concentrations of FGF are the pituitary and adrenal glands, although the brain has been a major starting material.

FGF was isolated in two closely related forms with 55% homology. A polypeptide of 140 amino acids with an acidic isoelectric point was isolated from brain, eye and retina and designated acidic FGF. The other FGF was designated basic with an amino acid content of 146 and an isoelectric point of 8 to 10. Basic FGF has been isolated from a wider range of tissue than acidic FGH including the corpus luteum (12).

Other angiogenic substances designated endothelial cell growth factors were shown to be identical to the FGFs. All these factors bound to heparin which facilitated their isolation. The gene sequence for both forms of FGF have been identified and the native amino acid composition set at 155. The shorter polypeptides isolated may be artifacts of the extraction process. Acidic FGF has been assigned to human Chromosome 5 and basic FGF to Chromosome 4. They are believed to be derived from a common ancestral protein. Basic FGF is said to be thirty- to one hundredfold more active than acidic FGF but the difference can be overcome by testing acidic FGF with heparin (12). Basic FGF has been isolated from the corpus luteum and induces angiogenesis in both the chorioallantoic membrane (CAM) assay and the rabbit cornea and also stimulates endothelial cell proliferation in vitro (13).

It is intriguing that the FGFs have no signal peptide sequence and are not ordinarily secreted by cultured cells (11,12). Its role in ovarian angiogenesis must remain speculative until FGF can be shown to control cyclic vascular events in the follicle and corpus luteum.

Other Angiogenic Factors

Angiogenin is a polypeptide isolated from tumor cells that stimulates angiogenesis in vivo. This substance has a molecular weight of 14,400, does not bind to heparin and has no homology to FGFs. Angiogenin does have a 35% homology with pancreatic ribonucleases. In contrast to FGF, angiogenin has a signal peptide and does not stimulate endothelial cells in vitro. Thus far angiogenin has not been found in the ovary (1).

Transforming Growth Factor α (TGFα), a polypeptide first isolated from viral-transformed cells, has been shown to stimulate angiogenesis in vivo and to stimulate mitoses in endothelial cells (1). There is a 35% homology between Epidermal Growth Factor (EGF) and TGFα. EGF and TGFα have been shown to be active in ovarian systems especially with effects on granulosa cells.

ANGIOGENIC FACTORS IN THE OVARY

The presence of angiogenic activity in the bovine corpus luteum was first described utilizing the CAM assay and the rabbit cornea (14,15).

Subsequently, porcine corpora lutea extracts were shown to stimulate proliferation of cultured endothelial cells (16). Although angiogenic activity was not observed in follicular extract when first tested, studies in another laboratory using the CAM assay revealed the presence of an angiogenic stimulus in follicles of PMSG-stimulated rats (2,15). Using the corneal assay, angiogenic activity has been detected in human and porcine follicular fluid (17,19). Rat granulosa cell-conditioned media was also shown to contain a stimulus for endothelial cell proliferation (19). In our own laboratory, nonluteal extracts and thecal extracts of porcine ovaries stimulated angiogenesis in the CAM assay and to stimulate proliferation and migration of bovine capillary endothelial cells (20).

Gospodarowicz and colleagues have isolated a truncated form of basic fibroblast growth factor from bovine corpora lutea and believes it is the luteal angiogenic factor (13). Utilizing heparin affinity chromatography, ion exchange chromatology and affinity dye columns and high pressure liquid chromatography, we have separated angiogenic activity into several fractions which seem to be related to each other by amino acid analysis and peptide mapping. There also seems to be a relatedness to both basic and acidic fibroblast growth factors (unpublished).

In a very preliminary study using an immunoblot technique and a cDNA probe, we have been able to observe evidence for acidic FGF mRNA in porcine corpus luteum but not in the follicle or remaining ovary (unpublished). While FGF is angiogenic and can be isolated from the ovary, its role in normal physiology is far from resolved. There is still doubt that FGF is normally secreted from the ovarian cells, and there is no evidence yet that the angiogenic factor in follicular fluid is FGF. On the other hand, FGF is a well-known mitogen for granulosa cells and affects gonadotropin action on receptor formation and steroid production.

ANGIOGENESIS AND OVARIAN FUNCTION

It is not known whether angiogenesis drives ovarian function by favoring follicle selection or is a secondary phenomenon facilitating follicle development, ovulation and corpus luteum formation. It remains to be determined if the angiogenic signal for the follicle resides in the theca, the granulosa cell, the extracellular matrix or within the endothelial cell itself. Now that angiogenic factors have been identified in the ovary itself, progress should be made in relating other ovarian cyclic activities to the remarkable cyclic formation and regression of capillaries in the follicle and corpus luteum.

REFERENCES

1. Folkman J. Angiogenesis. In: Jaffe EA, ed. Biology of endothelial cells. Boston: Martinus Nijhoff Publishers, 1984:412-28.
2. Koos RD, Lemaire WJ. Factors that may regulate the growth and regression of the blood vessels in the ovary. Seminars in Reproduc Endocrinol, 1983; 1:295-307.
3. Reynolds SRM. Blood and lymph systems of the ovary. In: Greep RO, ed. Handbook of physiology, endocrinology, female reproductive system, part I. Washington, DC: American Physiological Society, 1973:261-316.
4. Lipner H. Mechanism of mammalian ovulation. In: Greep RO, ed. Handbook of physiology, endocrinology, female reproductive system, part I. Washington, DC: American Physiological Society, 1973:409-37.
5. Folkman J, Klagsbrun M. Angiogenic factors. Science 1987; 442-7.

6. Folkman J, Cotran R. Relation of vascular proliferation to tumor growth. Int Rev Exp Pathol 1976; 16:207-48

7. Folkman J. Angiogenesis: initiation and control. Ann NY Acad Sci 1982; 401:212-27.

8. Gullino PM. Angiogenesis factor(s). In: Baserga R, ed. Tissue growth factors. Berlin: Springer-Verlag, 1981:427-49.

9. Montesano R, Vassali JD, Baird A, Guillemin R, Orci L. Basic fibroblast growth factor induces angiogenesis in vitro. Proc Natl Acad Sci USA 1986; 83:7279-301.

10. Kull FC Jr, Brent DA, Parikh I, Cuatrecasas P. Chemical identification of a tumor-derived angiogenic factor. Science 1987; 236:843-5.

11. Gospodarowicz D, Ferrara N, Schweigerer L, Neufeld G. Structural characterization and biological functions of fibroblast growth factor. Endocr Rev 1987; 8:95-114.

12. Gospodarowicz D, Neufeld G, Schweigerer L. Fibroblast growth factor. Mol Cell Endocrinol 1986; 46:187-204.

13. Gospodarowicz D, Cheng J, Lui GM, Baird A, Esch F, Bohlen P. Corpus luteum angiogenic factor is related to fibroblast growth factor. Endocrinology 1985; 117:2283-391.

14. Jacob W, Jentzsch KD, Mauresberger B, Oehme P. Demonstration of angiogenesis activity in corpus luteum of cattle. Exp Pathol 1977; 13:231-6.

15. Gospodarowicz D, Thrakal KK. Production of a corpus luteum angiogenic factor responsible for proliferation of capillaries and neovascularization of the corpus luteum. Proc Natl Acad Sci USA 1978; 75:847-51.

16. Heder G, Jacob W, Halle W, et al. Influence of porcine corpus luteum extract on DNA synthesis and proliferation of cultured fibroblasts and endothelial cells. Exp Pathol 1979; 17:493-7.

17. Frederick J, Shimanuki T, diZerega GS. Initiation of angiogenesis by human follicular fluid. Science 1984; 224:389-90.

18. Frederick JL, Hoa N, Preston DS, et al. Initiation of angiogenesis by porcine follicular fluid. Am J Obstet Gynecol 1985; 152:1073-8.

19. Koos RD. Stimulation of endothelial cell proliferation by rat granulosa cell-conditioned medium. Endocrinology 1986; 119:481-9.

20. Makris A, Ryan K, Yashumizu T, Hill CL, Zetter BR. The nonluteal porcine ovary as a source of angiogenic activity. Endocrinology 1984; 15:1672-7.

OOCYTE MATURATION AND IN VITRO FERTILIZATION

IN THE RHESUS MONKEY

Barry D. Bavister

University of Wisconsin Regional Primate Research Center
1223 Capitol Court, Madison, Wisconsin 53715

INTRODUCTION

Follicular Regulation of Oocyte Maturation

Normal embryonic development can only take place after fertilization of a normal oocyte. Assuming that there are no inherent defects in an oocyte, the milieu provided by the ovarian follicle determines whether or not a viable oocyte is produced. At present, we know very little about how oocyte maturation is regulated within the preovulatory follicle. Lack of information restricts our ability to obtain normal maturation of oocytes under controlled in vitro conditions. There are practical consequences of this situation. Incomplete or otherwise abnormal oocyte maturation may contribute to embryonic losses during pregnancy, and to failure of pregnancy following transfer of embryos produced by in vitro fertilization (IVF). The practice of IVF, whether for research or for treatment of infertility, is compromised by inadequate knowledge about the control of oocyte maturation. Both in primates and in domesticated species, ovarian stimulation with exogenous gonadotropins is likely to result in the recovery of at least a few immature oocytes. Unless these can be brought to full maturity in vitro, they represent a loss of efficiency in the treatment cycle. In our research with gonadotropin-stimulated monkeys, substantial numbers of immature but potentially viable oocytes are frequently recovered. Excised ovaries represent a potential windfall of oocytes, but these are of limited value in the absence of protocols for achieving full maturity in vitro.

The limited availability of mature oocytes is the most important rate-limiting factor for research into fertilization mechanisms using nonhuman primates. If oocytes harvested from ovaries, either in vivo or in vitro, could be brought to full maturity under controlled experimental conditions, then the supply of fertilizable eggs would be greatly increased. In addition, increasing the supply of viable cleavage stage embryos by this means would have a dramatic effect on our ability to study the regulatory mechanisms involved in early stages of preimplantation embryo development. Superovulation (i.e., multiple ovulation of gonadotropin-stimulated follicles) has been difficult to achieve in nonhuman primates, and current protocols do not consistently provide large numbers of ovulated ova. Because of this difficulty, we have placed our emphasis on IVF as a means for obtaining substantial numbers of early cleavage stage primate embryos, which in turn underscores the need to

119

obtain mature, viable oocytes. Increasing the efficiency of successful oocyte maturation in vitro would thus improve our ability to study fertilization mechanisms, which in turn would provide information on the quality of oocyte maturation. This positive feedback cycle has considerable potential for accelerating basic research into early primate development.

Understanding the regulation of oocyte maturation in primates has implications for treatment of human infertility as well as for basic embryological research. Although the majority of oocytes in human IVF programs can usually undergo fertilization followed by 1 or 2 cleavage divisions, the subsequent developmental fate of most embryos is unknown. The predicted success rate (clinical pregnancies) with transfer of 3 IVF embryos per patient is about 19% (1). This means that at least 80% of embryo transfer attempts, and 90% of all embryos transferred, fail to establish clinical pregnancy (1). Primate blastocysts secrete substantial amounts of chorionic gonadotropin (2,3). If most of the transferred embryos were able to reach the blastocyst stage in vivo, even if implantation was unsuccessful, detection of hCG secretion would be expected. In other words, if most transferred embryos are viable, the majority of embryo transfer attempts should be associated with a so-called "biochemical" pregnancy. Since this is not the case, one suspects that defects in IVF embryos, possibly originating in the oocyte, are a substantial contributing factor to the low overall efficiency of human IVF.

Since production of a normal oocyte is one of the two primary functions of the follicle, evaluation of oocyte maturation could have important implications for understanding the regulation of folliculogenesis. If the oocyte produced by a follicle is shown to be capable of undergoing fertilization and subsequent embryo development is normal, then steroid or other data obtained for that follicle can be considered as normal. By eliminating from consideration follicular data associated with incompetent oocytes, a clearer picture of the regulation of normal follicular development might begin to emerge.

Some investigators have begun to rigorously examine the fertilizability of oocytes matured under experimental conditions and the ability of the resulting embryos to produce offspring. The reason why this approach has not been pursued more vigorously until now is the technical difficulty of confirming oocyte viability by IVF followed by embryo culture (EC) and transfer of embryos to recipients. Routine IVF-EC protocols have not been available for the majority of species until recently. At least one group of investigators has avoided these technical problems by transferring in vitro matured (sheep) oocytes to recipients' oviducts for fertilization and development (4). It is unlikely that significant breakthroughs in the understanding of oocyte maturation will come from human IVF studies because these do not involve experimental procedures and the requirements of clinical IVF are usually incompatible with the needs of research. As discussed later, nonhuman primates are the most appropriate models for experimental studies on the control of oocyte maturation.

Endpoints for Oocyte Maturation

There is an enormous literature on the regulation of oocyte maturation. However, the great majority of studies have used only superficial morphological criteria of oocyte maturity, nearly always considering the breakdown of the so-called "germinal vesicle" and extrusion of the first polar body (PB1) as definitive endpoints for completion of maturation. However, by themselves, these are quite inadequate indicators of the completion of oocyte maturation, because they are primarily signs of nuclear maturation. It is crucial to examine, in addition, the question of cytoplasmic maturation, which is frequently abnormal in oocytes that are matured in vitro. Cytoplasmic maturation defects associated with subsequent developmental anomalies have been reported in a number of studies in humans and in animals. These defects range from: (i) failure to decondense the nuclei of penetrating sperm, resulting in inability to complete fertilization (5,6); (ii) errors in cortical granule distribution and/or response, resulting in either polyspermy (leading to embryonic death) or premature zona block (leading to failure of sperm penetration) (7,8); and, (iii) decreased viability and/or retarded development of embryos subsequent to apparently normal fertilization, resulting in embryonic death, or asynchrony between the embryos and the mother which compromises pregnancy (9,10). Thus, it is essential to study the developmental competence of oocytes before any statement can be made concerning their maturation status or normality (see Figure 1).

Studies on the developmental competence of oocytes following fertilization, as a means of providing feedback about the control of maturation, have been conducted primarily in the human, mouse and sheep. These studies comprise two different approaches to the analysis of regulatory events involved in oocyte maturation. In the in vivo or "indirect" approach, hormone concentrations in follicular fluid are retrospectively correlated with the known developmental capacity of oocytes, including their ability to develop into viable fetuses and term offspring. In a study of this kind in the human, it was concluded that the follicular fluid ratio of progesterone to estradiol was an important correlate of normal oocyte maturation (11). A later study indicated that

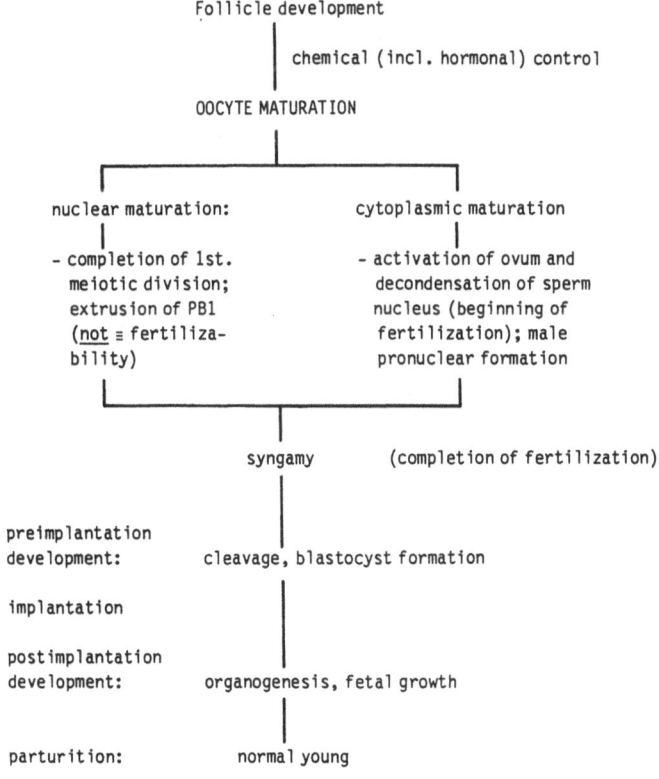

Fig. 1. Sequence of events influenced by follicular control of oocyte maturation.

the absolute estradiol concentration, and that of other follicular steroids, correlates with oocyte viability (12). An alternative, the in vitro or "direct" experimental approach, is to subject normal-looking immature oocytes to different treatments in culture, then to test their developmental capacity. In one recent study, germinal vesicle stage oocytes from inbred mice were matured and fertilized in vitro, then grown to the morula stage before transfer to recipients. About 30% of these embryos produced offspring (13). This is a remarkable achievement, especially compared to results obtained with most other species in which obtaining normal oocyte maturation in vitro has been much less successful. In the mouse, serum in the culture environment was required to support oocyte maturation, apparently functioning to prevent zona hardening; co-culture with cumulus cells was helpful but not essential (14). In another study, sheep oocytes were matured in vitro, then transferred to oviducts of ewes for in vivo fertilization and development (4). Contrary to the results of the mouse experiments, maturation of sheep oocytes in vitro required the presence of an intact corona cell layer and supplementary follicle (granulosa) cells. In these experiments with sheep oocytes, serum, gonadotropins and estradiol were routinely included in the culture medium.

Although these studies with nonprimates can give valuable suggestions about the experimental approach to be used, we cannot extrapolate these findings directly to oocyte maturation in primates. For one thing, experiments with mice and sheep have shown species variations in the factors required for supporting oocyte maturation in vitro. Moreover, the time course of oocyte maturation in these species is quite different. In the mouse, about 3 days elapse between the start of the rise in FSH and the LH surge that induces final oocyte maturation. In the sheep, this period lasts only about 2 days, although antral follicles are found during the luteal phase. In contrast, in primates such as rhesus monkeys, the time course of follicle maturation from the initiation of the rise in FSH to the LH surge is approximately 10 days. During this time period, substantial changes occur in the follicular granulosa cells and in the cumulus oophorus cells surrounding the oocyte; moreover, the degree of follicular development during the luteal phase needs to be considered. The interval between the LH surge and ovulation, when the process of oocyte maturation is completed, occupies only about 11 h in mice and 26 h in sheep, but closer to 36 h in nonhuman primates and in women. Furthermore, there are probably considerable differences in the patterns of follicular control between animals that usually ovulate only one ovum per cycle, such as the higher primates, and those that produce several ova. These differences suggest that, although the basic pattern of events taking place during folliculogenesis and oocyte maturation may be similar, the details of the regulatory mechanisms probably vary substantially.

Virtually nothing is known about the intraovarian regulation of oocyte maturation in primates. We do not know what similarities and differences exist in this respect between primates and animal models such as the mouse and sheep. Recent evidence shows that meiotic arrest in mouse oocytes is associated with elevated intracellular cyclic AMP levels, which may be maintained by hypoxanthine or other factors (15). Not only is this information of fundamental importance for understanding the regulation of oocyte maturation, but it has potential practical applications, especially for primate and domesticated animal IVF. If immature oocytes could be prevented from continuing meiosis by using hypoxanthine or other compounds, they could be stored for one or more days in vitro until it became convenient to perform IVF. This would be particularly important if, for example, oocytes became available at short notice and there was insufficient time to prepare for IVF. Once oocytes complete maturation, however, their fertile life is quite short. Unfortunately, we have no information at present on the effects of phosphodiesterase inhibitors on primate oocytes, nor on the relationship between cyclic AMP levels and oocyte maturation.

Because of the practical and ethical difficulties of using human embryos in experimental situations, there is clearly a need to develop a nonhuman primate model for the study of oocyte maturation and its regulation. We have made a start towards this objective using the rhesus monkey, as discussed in the following sections.

AN EXPERIMENTAL APPROACH FOR STUDYING CONTROL OF OOCYTE MATURATION IN NONHUMAN PRIMATES

We are using the rhesus monkey because of its similarity to humans and because it is a reasonably available nonhuman primate. During the past 6 years, we have developed techniques for routinely accomplishing in vitro fertilization of rhesus monkey oocytes in vitro and for culturing the resulting embryos up to peri-implantation stages of development. Details of our procedures for follicular stimulation, sperm preparation and capacitation, IVF, embryo culture and transfer have all been published (16-22). These procedures are useful for evaluating sperm fertilizing ability, oocyte maturation and the control of embryo development. With respect to the study of oocyte maturation, our recent experiments have followed two main approaches (see Figure 2). In one approach (Fig. 2A), oocytes that undergo partial or complete maturation in vivo are recovered by aspiration of follicles at laparoscopy. Maturation of oocytes is completed in vitro if necessary before testing their developmental competence by IVF. In the majority of these experiments to date, we stimulated monkeys with gonadotropins in order to obtain as many oocytes as possible for IVF studies (Fig. 2A1). In some cases, the maturation of oocytes was correlated with follicular fluid steroids in matched samples (23). Most recently, we have started to recover single oocytes from unstimulated animals (Fig. 2A2; ref 24). This is extremely tedious and data collection is slow. However, examination of oocytes obtained from unstimulated cycles is essential to provide normal baseline data against which to compare results from stimulated cycles and from studies on in vitro matured oocytes.

The second major approach has been to recover immature oocytes from excised ovaries of unstimulated rhesus monkeys and to mature the oocytes completely in vitro (Fig. 2B; ref 25). The major advantage of this approach is that the relative importance of different factors for oocyte maturation (e.g., gonadotropins, granulosa cells) can be studied under controlled, reproducible conditions. In a variation of these two approaches, oocytes are recovered from monkeys that have been superstimulated with gonadotropin (usually PMSG) but no hCG is given; instead, maturation of the oocytes is carried out in vitro (Fig. 2C). The idea here is to produce substantial numbers of oocytes for factorial experimental designs and to study the major part of the total maturation control process, including maturation and development of cumulus oophorus, under well-defined culture conditions. As we become more successful in accomplishing oocyte maturation in vitro, oocytes will be recovered earlier in the menstrual cycle to increase the proportion of the total maturation process that takes place under in vitro conditions.

In all cases, the endpoint of the experiments was the ability of oocytes to undergo normal fertilization in vitro and for the resulting embryos to undergo apparently normal cleavage in vitro in a timely manner, at least as far as the 6- to 8-cell stage (16,23). The competence of each oocyte to undergo normal maturation was correlated with its environmental conditions in vitro and/or in vivo. The data obtained from these experiments will be used to design improved in vitro oocyte maturation conditions, to design more critical experiments and to increase knowledge of maturation control mechanisms. The following sections provide more details about these experimental approaches and the results that we have obtained to date.

In Vitro Fertilization of Rhesus Monkey Oocytes

In the absence of reliable protocols for superovulation of monkeys, we have relied on superstimulation with gonadotropins to recruit the growth of multiple follicles, which we aspirate at laparoscopy at a set time (usually 30 h) after the injection of hCG. Oocytes collected in this way are cultured in vitro for at least 6 h to complete maturation prior to insemination with capacitated sperm (16). Washed ejaculated sperm are capacitated by incubation in a defined culture medium and are stimulated with cyclic nucleotide mediators just before (1.5 h) insemination of eggs (17). Following sperm/egg co-incubation (about 18 h), embryos are cultured for varying periods of time in a complex medium containing blood serum (19). These procedures permit all of the different phases contributing to early embryogenesis, i.e., oocyte maturation, sperm capacitation, fertilization and regulation of embryo development, to be examined (22). Accurate measurements can be made of the cleavage timing of embryos

Experimental Approach and Conditions

Advantages and Disadvantages

A. In vivo
  1. Stimulated cycles (PMSG or hMG + hCG):
        Recover late preovulatory oocytes; correlate FF constituents with oocyte maturation and embryo development after fertilization.

        Substantial nos. of oocytes. Quality may be compromised by stimulation regimen; FF data not "normal"; repeatbility of regimen usually limited.

        Recover less mature ("immature") oocytes; complete maturation in vitro (>8hr).

        Higher variability of FF volume and constituents.

  2. Spontaneous (unstimulated cycles):
        As in A1, correlate FF data with oocyte maturity and viability.

        Provides normal data on FF parameters and oocytes, provided that fertilization and embryo development are normal. Very limited nos. of oocytes; difficult to recover at precise stage of maturity.

B. In vitro (unstimulated cycles):
        Recover immature ("GV") oocytes from excised ovaries (antral follicles <2mm).

        Relatively large nos. of oocytes; complete control over maturation conditions; mature in vitro. But culture conditions empirical.

C. In vivo/in vitro (partially stimulated cycles - PMSG, no hCG):
        Recover oocytes not exposed to primate LH in vivo (no LH surge); ± FF data; complete maturation in vitro; progressively advance time of recovery.

        More control over oocyte maturation than in A1. But culture conditions are empirical; stimulation regimen not repeatable.

Fig. 2. Experimental strategy for analyzing control of oocyte maturation in the rhesus monkey. In all cases, the endpoint is ability of oocytes to undergo normal fertilization in vitro and for resulting embryos to undergo apparently normal cleavage in vitro, at least to 6- to 8-cell stage, in a timely manner. Parameters of maturation environment in vitro and/or in vivo are then correlated with competence of the corresponding oocyte to undergo normal fertilization and embryonic development. The overall strategy is to use a combination of approaches A-C. Data are used to improve in vitro oocyte maturation conditions, and to design more critical experiments for increasing our basic knowledge about maturation control mechanisms.

because the time of insemination is known with certainty. Stimulation of rhesus monkeys with gonadotropins usually provides substantial numbers of oocytes (sometimes as many as 40 per treatment cycle), although their maturation status and quality can vary widely. In order to use these IVF techniques for obtaining useful information on oocyte maturation, it is necessary to ensure that at least some of the embryos produced subsequent to IVF of oocytes are capable of undergoing apparently normal development in vitro as far as the blastocyst stage and that normal offspring can be produced. We have focused primarily on growing embryos in vitro, rather than on achieving pregnancies after embryo transfer, since more information can be obtained about the regulation of embryo development in this way. However, we have produced 3 normal rhesus offspring from the transfer of IVF embryos for the purpose of validating our culture procedures (18,20 and unpublished data).

Oocyte Maturity and IVF

We have modified our published procedures (16) for evaluating the maturation status of oocytes. An initial visual assessment of the aspirated egg cumulus complex is made through a dissecting microscope at 100x magnification, and the appearance of the cumulus and corona cells layers is recorded. This is followed by a more detailed evaluation with an inverted microscope using Nomarski optics at 200x or 400x magnification. If the details of the oocyte are not obscured by tightly condensed cumulus cells, then information is recorded concerning the shape of the oocyte, the presence or absence of a perivitelline space (PVS), the presence of the first polar body (PB1), the appearance of the oocyte cytoplasm (color, granularity) and the visibility and integrity of the zona pellucida (Fig. 3A). If necessary, the cumulus cells are stretched out with sterile needles and attached to the bottom of the culture dish to enhance visualization of the oocyte. Oocytes are protected from changes in temperature (26) and pH during this examination period by using an environmental chamber that maintains a constant temperature of 37°C on the stage of the inverted microscope. The drops of culture medium containing oocytes (or embryos) are gassed continuously with humidified 5% CO_2 in air during examination on the microscope so that pH is maintained at about 7.4 (27). Oocytes are classified as either immature, nearly mature, mature or atretic. If PB1 is not observed and there is no PVS suggestive of PB1, then oocytes are returned to culture for several hours before reexamination. If oocytes are classified as mature (on the basis of cumulus appearance and presence of PVS) but PB1 was not visible due to optical interference from overlying cumulus or corona cells, then insemination may be performed, but the presence of PB1 is always confirmed following removal of cumulus cells, usually 12 to 18 h after insemination.

Assessment of Fertilization

Following co-incubation with sperm, usually for 12 to 18 h, eggs are reexamined for the occurrence of fertilization. Since the tail remnants of the fertilizing sperm cannot be seen with the light microscope in primate eggs (16,28), normal fertilization is defined as the presence of 2 well-developed pronuclei and 2 polar bodies (16,22). At this time, it is important to detect if polyspermy has occurred, as shown by the presence of more than 2 pronuclei. Polyspermy may occur either because of excessive sperm numbers in the insemination medium, or because of some defect in the block to polyspermy response (7). The latter condition would suggest a defect in oocyte maturation. Polypronucleate monkey and human embryos are able to develop in vitro at least up to the morula or early blastocyst stage (8,22), so that cleavage of IVF embryos in vitro is not by itself a sufficiently stringent indicator of normal fertilization without the important assessment at the presyngamy stage (22).

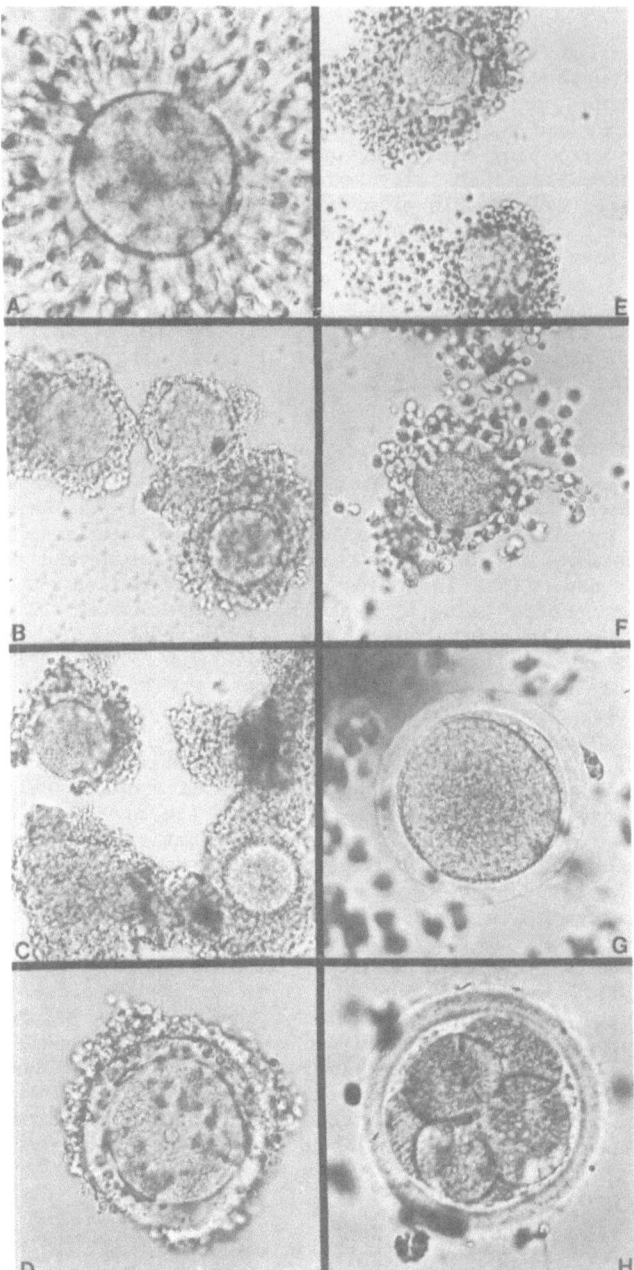

Fig. 3. Appearance of oocytes collected from unstimulated rhesus monkey and of oocytes matured in vitro. A: Mature oocyte from untreated follicle after 8-h incubation in TALP + 20% calf serum. PB1 is visible at 4 o'clock. The zona pellucida is discernible as a pale shadow surrounding the oocyte, and the corona cells show characteristic radiating pattern. B, C: Immature oocytes freshly recovered from follicles of excised ovaries. Cumulus and corona cells form a dense, compact layer around the oocytes, obscuring cytoplasmic details. D: At the time of recovery from an excised ovary, some oocytes show a prominent "germinal vesicle" nucleus, as shown here. [Legend continues on opposite page.]

Timing of Rhesus Embryo Development In Vitro

For assessing the normality of oocyte maturation, even if normal monospermic fertilization appears to have taken place, it is not sufficient to simply show that IVF embryos are capable of undergoing 1 or 2 cleavage divisions in culture. In our early work on the culture of IVF rhesus embryos (16), we found that cleavage beyond the 4-cell stage is necessary before substantial differences can be detected in the timing of development. After the 4-cell stage, some embryos ceased development while others developed as far as the morula stage. Therefore, we have used the timing of cleavage to the 6- or 8-cell stage as a criterion for normal fertilization ("timely" cleavage, 19,22,23). The time course for rhesus embryo development up to the morula stage is the same for embryos grown in vivo and in vitro (22).

Relationship Between Oocyte Maturity and Embryo Development

The use of IVF as a research tool to probe the normality of oocyte maturation has revealed that the normal sequence of events can be disturbed and that nuclear maturation can occur in an oocyte in which cytoplasmic maturation is incomplete or otherwise defective. Disturbances in cytoplasmic maturation are most often encountered following attempts to mature oocytes in vitro. Defects are usually manifested as an inability of the egg cytoplasm to decondense the nucleus of the penetrating sperm and/or for the fertilized egg to undergo normal embryonic development (6,10). As mentioned earlier, defective oocyte maturation may account for some of the conception failures or embryonic wastage observed in old-world primates. Such losses have been estimated as between 25 and 50% of the probable conceptions (29-32). Defective preimplantation embryos have been recovered by flushing the reproductive tract of mated rhesus monkeys (30,32). Both retarded embryo cleavage as well as abnormal morphology have been noted in such embryos. Compared with laboratory rodents, preovulatory oocytes of primates appear to have a high frequency of defects in oocyte (cytoplasmic) maturation. This difference may explain the discrepancy between the low early-pregnancy losses in rodents vs. the situation in primates. Experiments using IVF permit the relationship between oocyte maturity and embryo development (Fig. 1) to be examined more critically. Using rhesus monkeys, we observed that events occurring during folliculogenesis and oocyte maturation can have significant effects on embryo development subsequent to fertilization. Animals were stimulated with gonadotropins (PMSG and hCG). Oocytes were aspirated from preovulatory follicles a few hours before the anticipated time of ovulation (which was estimated to be 36 h post-hCG). The oocytes were classified according to whether they required less than or more than 8 h in culture for extrusion of PB1 (mature [M], and initially immature, matured in vitro [MIV], respectively). As shown in Table 1, there was no significant difference in the percentage of ova from these two categories that

---

[Figure 3 legend continued from preceding page.] E: Immature oocytes after 23-h culture in CMRL (control medium) showing partial loosening of cumulus/corona cell layers. F: Same as E except that CMRL + FSH was used to culture oocyte. G: Oocyte completely matured in vitro (CMRL control). PB1 is visible at 2 o'clock. Cumulus and corona cells are absent from this oocyte. H: Seven-cell embryo derived from IVF of an oocyte that was matured in vitro with CMRL + FSH-P + hCG. This embryo was cultured for 50-h post-insemination in TALP + 20% calf serum. Magnifications (optical): A, D, G and H, 40x; B, C, E and F, 10x.

were fertilized in vitro. However, there was a significant difference in the percentage of fertilized ova that were able to develop to the 6- to 8-cell stage. When the development of IVF embryos was expressed as ability to cleave in a timely manner to the 6- to 8-cell stage, we found that only 3/14 embryos derived from MIV oocytes had normal cleavage timing vs. 11/14 of those from M oocytes (23). Clearly, embryo development is a critical endpoint for classification of oocyte maturity. Our finding that the timing of embryo cleavage in vitro is retarded subsequent to disturbed oocyte maturation may be relevant to the etiology of embryo losses in vivo.

Development of Embryos After Transfer

In order to verify that embryos obtained by in vitro fertilization were capable of undergoing normal postimplantation development, we transferred embryos to surrogate recipient monkeys. Although there are some problems in establishing the timing of ovulation in rhesus monkeys and in finding synchronous recipients when needed (22), the use of normal surrogates does have the advantage that their cycles have not been disturbed by exogenous gonadotropins. Following transfer of IVF embryos nonsurgically (via the uterine cervix), we obtained two normal male rhesus offspring, the oldest of which ("Petri," 20) is almost 4 years old. Using a laparoscopic oviductal transfer technique (33), we obtained a third offspring, also a male. Although our embryo transfer success rates need to be improved by better synchronization of embryos and recipients, results to date show that at least some of the IVF embryos are normal.

CORRELATION OF FOLLICULAR FLUID PARAMETERS WITH OOCYTE MATURATION

Gonadotropin-Stimulated Cycles

During some of our oocyte collections from stimulated rhesus monkeys, we also recovered matched follicular fluid samples to study the relationships between follicular steroids and oocyte maturation (Fig. 2A1; ref 23). While follicle stimulation produces substantial numbers of oocytes (18), the quality of oocytes is likely to be compromised to some extent by the gonadotropin stimulation treatment. We have often found that some of the oocytes obtained from gonadotropin-stimulated animals look abnormal at the time of recovery, although the numbers of defective oocytes are nearly always in the minority. No doubt the follicular fluid data are not normal; in fact, mean steroid concentrations per follicle of estradiol and progesterone are significantly less in stimulated cycles than in spontaneous cycles (see section on Unstimulated Cycles). Another disadvantage of using gonadotropin stimulation in monkeys is the limited repeatability of the treatment protocol with nonhuman primates. We have mainly used pregnant mare serum gonadotropin (PMSG) for stimulation of rhesus monkeys because this preparation usually produces a large number of good quality oocytes (18). However, animals rapidly develop immunity to PMSG and cannot be stimulated more than once (34). The response of rhesus monkeys stimulated with Pergonal® is inconsistent; in our experience, the average number of oocytes recovered per treatment cycle is significantly less than with PMSG (18). In addition, Pergonal® also seems to stimulate an immune response after a few cycles of treatment.

We have usually recovered oocytes from stimulated animals 30 h after hCG injection. This time interval was selected as the optimum for obtaining oocytes that are close to completion of maturation without risk of losing oocytes due to ovulation. In practice, we recovered a variety of oocytes which we classified as: mature (M) or matured in vitro (MIV), as defined above, or as nonmature or atretic, i.e., oocytes that failed to

Table 1. Maturation status of oocytes aspirated from follicles of gonadotropin-stimulated rhesus monkeys and their developmental competence following in vitro fertilization.

Class	No. ova fertilized/ no. inseminated (%)	No. ≥6- to 8-cells in vitro (% ova fertilized)
Mature (M)[a]	40/61 (65.6)	35/37[c,d] (94.6)
Maturation completed in vitro (MIV)[b]	35/49 (71.4)	21/35[d] (60.0)

[a] Incubated <8 h prior to insemination, first polar body (PB1) confirmed after cumulus dispersal.
[b] Incubated >8 h prior to insemination, PB1 confirmed after cumulus dispersal.
[c] Excludes 2 embryos transferred (1 live birth [ref. 18] and 1 lost prior to 6- to 8-cell stage).
[d] χ^2, $P \leq 0.001$.

produce a polar body after extensive culture or that were clearly atretic at the time of recovery. Figure 4 shows the hormonal data associated with oocytes from 5 gonadotropin-stimulated monkeys (3 with PMSG + hCG, 2 with hMG + hCG). Follicular fluid samples were analyzed for estradiol, progesterone, testosterone, and dihydrotestosterone and grouped according to the maturation status of their corresponding oocytes. A significant difference between the three categories of oocyte was found only for progesterone (Fig. 4). The oocytes in the first two categories (mature and matured in vitro) were inseminated in vitro. When the follicular fluid data were reanalyzed according to whether oocytes were or were not fertilized in vitro, there were no significant differences between the two groups for any of the 4 steroids tested (Fig. 5). Viability of IVF oocytes was then expressed as timely development of embryos to the 6- to 8-cell stage by 50 h postinsemination. This analysis (Fig. 6) showed a significant difference ($P < 0.01$) between the embryos derived from fertilized M oocytes (8 out of 13 [61.5%]) vs. embryos from MIV oocytes (5 out of 22 [23%]).

In summary, our preliminary data indicate that follicular fluid steroid concentrations of estradiol, testosterone and dihydrotestosterone do not correlate significantly with oocyte maturity at the time of recovery. The concentrations of all 4 steroids measured did not correlate significantly with the ability of oocytes to undergo IVF. Nevertheless, there was a significant difference in the ability of M vs. MIV oocytes to undergo timely embryo development in vitro. These results emphasize that (i) follicular steroid concentrations (in our experience) are not adequate indicators of the true maturity of aspirated oocytes; (ii) the ability of oocytes to undergo morphologically normal-looking fertilization in vitro is also not an adequate indicator; and, (iii) it is important to examine the time course of embryo development in vitro in addition to the morphological appearance at fertilization. The results that we have obtained to date are not consistent with reports that the ratio of follicular fluid progesterone to estradiol (11) or the absolute concentration of estradiol (12) was significantly correlated with oocyte maturity and viability. Our data also differ from another study which reported a negative correlation between testosterone in follicular fluid and oocyte fertilizability (36).

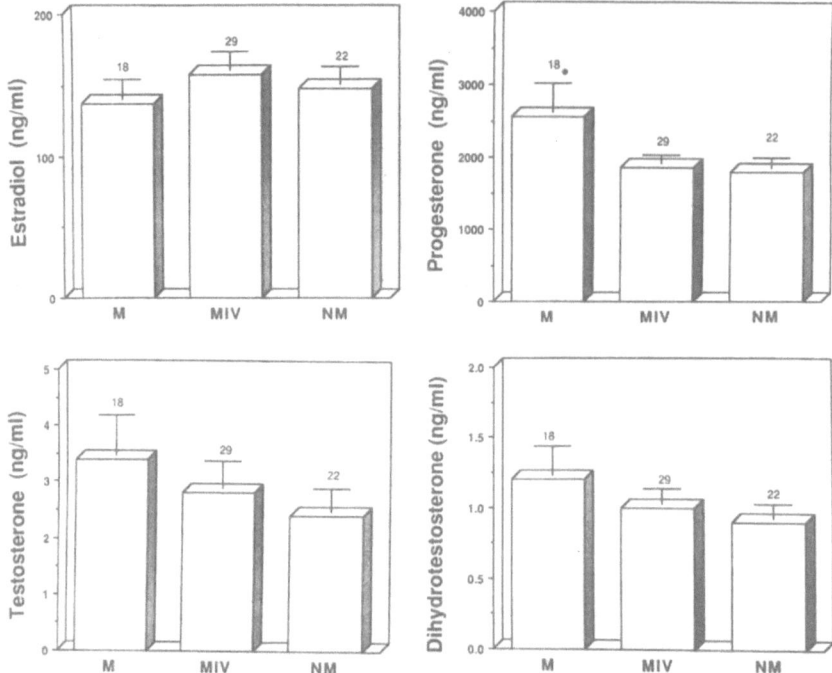

Fig. 4. Stimulated cycles: comparison of follicular fluid concentrations of estradiol, progesterone, testosterone and dihydrotestosterone associated with oocyte maturation status. M (mature) = oocytes requiring <8 h in culture for PB1 to appear; MIV (matured in vitro) = oocytes requiring >8 h for PB1 extrusion; NM = nonmaturable/atretic oocytes. Numbers above each bar show number of oocytes and matched follicular fluid samples that were analyzed. No significant differences were found between oocyte maturation categories for estradiol, testosterone or dihydrotestosterone. Values for progesterone were significantly different (P<0.05) for M vs. MIV and M vs. NM. (Data from 35.)

As a by-product of the gonadotropin stimulation protocol, some immature oocytes are usually recovered (Fig. 2A1). These oocytes require longer incubation to reach maturity than preovulatory oocytes and may be treated as described later for oocytes recovered from excised ovaries that are matured completely in vitro (see Oocyte Maturation in Vitro). Because these oocytes have been subjected to follicle-stimulating gonadotropins in vivo, they may have better prospects for achieving maturation in vitro than those obtained from excised ovaries of untreated animals.

A variation on this experimental approach that we are starting to use is to aspirate oocytes from follicles of stimulated monkeys before the endogenous LH surge and without giving any hCG (Fig. 2C). The oocyte-cumulus complexes will have been subjected to the follicular environment for several days, but the completion of oocyte maturation is carried out in vitro. Using PMSG for follicular stimulation is useful for this procedure because it prevents the endogenous LH surge; however, a disadvantage is the presence of LH activity in PMSG preparations. This approach attempts to separate pre- and post-LH phases of oocyte-cumulus maturation. When normal maturation is accomplished with these oocytes, the time of oocyte aspiration will be progressively advanced so that increasing amounts of the "pre-LH surge" maturation phase are also examined in vitro.

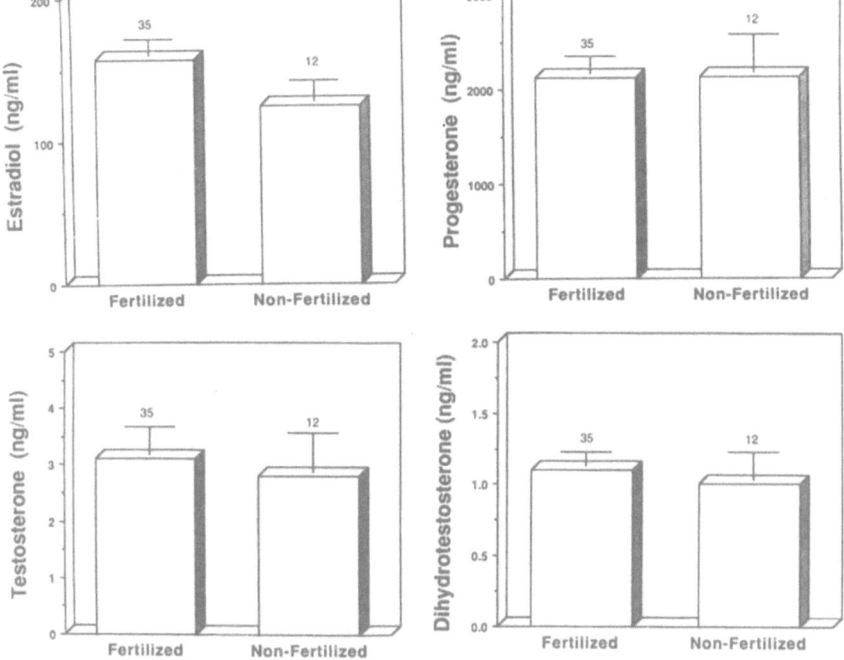

Fig. 5. Stimulated cycles: comparison of follicular fluid concentrations of estradiol, progesterone, testosterone and dihydrotestosterone associated with oocytes that were fertilized or nonfertilized in vitro. Data from same experiments represented in Figure 4 were reanalyzed (only M and MIV oocytes and their corresponding steroid values).

Unstimulated Cycles

Because of the uncertainties about interpretation of data following any experimental manipulation of the normal events involved in oocyte maturation, it becomes necessary to obtain control data on follicular fluid and oocytes from unstimulated primates (Fig. 2A2). Such data will establish the baselines for results of all experimental treatments. However, it is extremely tedious to collect single oocytes from unstimulated monkeys. Prediction of the optimum time for aspiration of the mature oocyte is difficult because no rapid RIA is available for monkey LH, so we rely on estradiol RIAs which are less accurate predictors of ovulation. Moreover, the time/cost effectiveness of this procedure is poor, since only one oocyte is collected after a substantial amount of work. Nevertheless, the information gained may be invaluable. The morphological appearance of oocytes from unstimulated monkeys provides normative data against which oocytes from treated cycles can be compared. These normal oocytes have finely granulated cytoplasm with a light brown color. There is a well-defined perivitelline space containing PB1, and the corona cells radiate out from the oocyte in a characteristic pattern (Fig. 3A). The cumulus oophorus layer is either "fluffy" with loose cells, or virtually absent with only a few cumulus cells adhering to the corona layer.

Our preliminary steroid data (Table 2) show significant differences in follicular fluid concentrations of estradiol and progesterone associated with mature oocytes (here defined as having PB1 at the time of

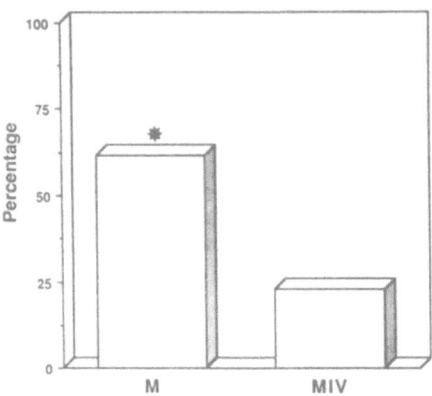

Fig. 6. Comparison of in vitro development
of embryos derived from M and MIV oocytes,
expressed as timely development to the 6- to
8-cell stage (should reach this stage by 50
h postinsemination). (Data from 35.)

aspiration) vs. initially immature oocytes (PB1 extruded within 24-h
culture). To date, we have found no difference in the fertilizability of
these two classes of oocyte. Comparison of estradiol concentrations
associated with mature oocytes from stimulated cycles (described in
preceding section) and from spontaneous cycles showed no significant
differences (137 ± 14 and 153.2 ± 31 ng/ml, respectively). Neither was
any significant difference found in progesterone values for these two
groups (2.6 ± 0.4 and 3.2 ± 0.2 μg/ml, respectively). However, when these
steroids were compared for the MIV oocytes, highly significant differences
were found (Fig. 7). The estradiol concentration in follicular fluid
associated with MIV oocytes was 158 ± 13 ng/ml from stimulated cycles, and
772.6 ± 291 ng/ml from spontaneous cycles (P<0.001). Corresponding values
for progesterone were 1.9 ± 0.1 and 4.7 ± 0.6 μg/ml, respectively
(P<0.001).

In summary, there appear to be some differences in follicular steroids associated with the maturation status of oocytes, but these differences are not yet clear-cut. Interpretation of follicular fluid
steroid data correlated with oocyte maturation/viability is difficult
because aspiration of the follicular contents interrupts a dynamic process, and single time-point determinations of follicular fluid constituents
may give an inaccurate picture of the pattern of events taking place
within the follicle. Additionally, the developmental competence of the
oocyte may be compromised to differing extents depending on when it is
aspirated from the follicle, and abnormalities of cumulus cell function
may be produced. It is possible that changes in the profiles of follicular steroids during folliculogenesis are not as significant for oocyte
maturation as they might seem. Provided that the concentration of a
particular steroid is above (or below) a threshold value, large variations
in the concentration may not be important. Since receptors determine the
responsiveness of cells, we need information about the numbers of receptors for particular steroids present in the cumulus cells (and in the
oocyte?) before we can fully assess the significance of steroid concentrations in follicular fluid for oocyte maturation.

Thus, it remains to be seen whether or not follicular fluid data are
helpful in understanding the chemical regulation of oocyte maturation.
Assessment of the value of such information is made difficult by the

Table 2. Spontaneous cycles: comparison of follicular fluid concentrations of estradiol and progesterone associated with maturation status of oocytes.[a]

	M (n = 6)	IM (n = 5)
Estradiol (ng/ml)	153.2 ± 31[b]	772.6 ± 291[b]
Progesterone (µg/ml)	3.2 ± 0.2[c]	4.7 ± 0.6[c]

[a]Data from reference 24.
M = mature (PB1) at time of aspiration from follicle.
IM = initially immature but extruded PB1 within 24-h culture.
[b,c]Significantly different, P<0.05.

uncertainties introduced by disturbing the dynamic relationship between the oocyte and follicle, and by lack of knowledge at the biochemical level about the functional role played by steroids in oocyte maturation. It may well be that the mechanisms underlying regulation of oocyte maturation can be identified more readily by studying maturation totally in vitro.

Oocyte Maturation in Vitro

In this experimental approach, immature (GV-intact) oocytes are obtained from excised ovaries and matured in vitro (Fig. 2B). This approach has been used successfully in mice and in sheep (4,13,14). Substantial numbers of oocytes can be obtained in this way. For example, a pair of rhesus monkey ovaries can yield up to 100 or more viable immature oocytes. Conditions provided for supporting oocyte maturation are empirical, being derived in part from the use of culture media which may have been devised for somatic cells, and partly from the application of knowledge gained from in vivo studies as described in the preceding two sections. Preliminary studies were done in our laboratory with ovaries from 4 unstimulated rhesus monkeys (25). Immature oocytes enclosed in several (more than 2) cell layers of tightly condensed cumulus oophorus

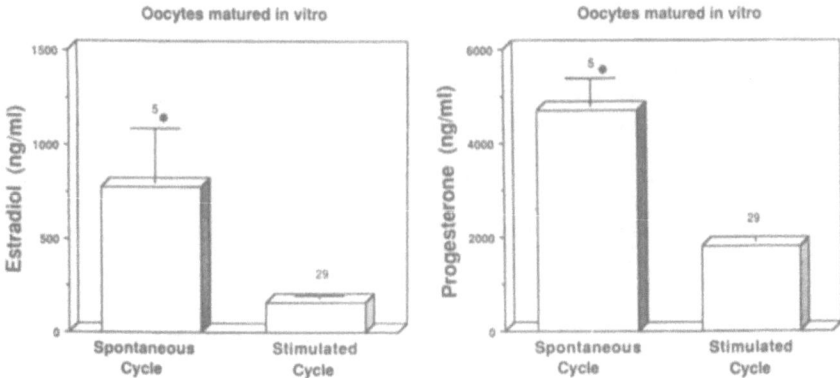

Fig. 7. Comparison of spontaneous vs. stimulated cycles for follicular fluid concentrations of estradiol and progesterone associated with oocytes that matured in vitro. Values for estradiol and for progesterone between the two categories shown here are significantly different (P<0.001).

(Fig. 3B,C) were collected in a HEPES-buffered balanced salt solution (TALP, 22) containing 5% heat-inactivated calf serum. In some oocytes with sparse cellular investments, the germinal vesicle nucleus could easily be seen (Fig. 3D). Care was taken to maintain the oocytes at 32°C during collection because of the detrimental effect of lower temperatures on oocyte viability (26). A total of 139 oocytes were assigned randomly to 6 culture groups in a 2 x 3 experimental design. Three of the groups used a complex culture medium (modified CMRL-1066, 22) and 3 groups used TALP. An animal pituitary gonadotropin preparation (FSH-P, Burns-Biotec, Omaha, Nebraska) was used in these preliminary experiments. The subtreatments were: 20% calf serum (CS); 20% calf serum + 10 µg/ml FSH-P (CS + FSH); 20% calf serum + 10 µg/ml FSH-P at 0 h + 5 IU/ml hCG after 24 h of culture (CS + FSH + hCG). Oocytes were incubated in groups of 5 in 50 µl drops of culture medium under oil. After culture for about 24 h (Fig. 3E,F), oocytes were examined for evidence of PB1 or a distinct PVS (Fig. 3G). If 3 or more oocytes per group showed one of these signs, they were all inseminated. If not, culture of oocytes was continued for additional periods of time before insemination, up to a maximum of 50 h. Oocytes were co-incubated with sperm for 16 to 20 h, then examined for evidence of fertilization. If oocytes were fertilized, they were cultured until embryo development ceased. At the end of culture, all oocytes and embryos were fixed and stained (25).

Significantly more oocytes that were incubated in TALP + CS + FSH underwent germinal vesicle breakdown compared to all other treatments (25). Approximately twice as many of the oocytes cultured in TALP + CS ± FSH extruded PB1 compared to oocytes in the three CMRL treatments. To date, the percentage of in vitro-matured oocytes able to undergo fertilization in vitro has been low. There were no significant differences in ability of oocytes to undergo IVF correlated with use of the complex or the simple culture medium, but there were significant subtreatment effects (CS + FSH + hCG > CS + FSH >> CS only (P<0.05). About half of the fertilized oocytes cleaved to the 6- to 8-cell stage in vitro (Fig. 3H) and one embryo developed as far as the morula stage (25). These preliminary results show that oocytes recovered from excised ovaries of unstimulated rhesus monkeys can undergo maturation, fertilization and cleavage in vitro. Better results should be obtained now that human FSH is available to us and as we develop improved culture procedures.

SUMMARY AND FUTURE DIRECTIONS

IVF of monkey oocytes is a powerful experimental approach for analyzing the regulation of oocyte maturation in primates. The use of reasonably stringent endpoints, such as the timely cleavage of IVF embryos at least to the 6- to 8-cell stage, appears to be mandatory for detecting subtle anomalies of cytoplasmic maturation which may not be apparent at earlier stages of development. Using nuclear maturation, evidenced by completion of the first meiotic division and extrusion of PB1, as the sole criterion of oocyte maturation is unacceptable. A large part of the early literature on oocyte maturation control is compromised because of the use of inadequate endpoints. The most rapid progress in understanding the control of primate oocyte maturation is likely to come from a combination of studies on maturation in vivo and in vitro (Fig. 2). Each of these experimental approaches, as outlined in the preceding discussion, has advantages and drawbacks. Data obtained on the follicular milieu in vivo may help us to design more suitable artificial environments for sustaining normal oocyte maturation. Examination of oocytes during and after maturation in vitro allows us to obtain dynamic information on the time course and quality of oocyte maturation.

134

Attaining the goal of complete normal oocyte maturation in vitro will benefit research on early primate embryo development by providing a convenient supply of gametes and will, in addition, improve the efficiency of primate IVF by reducing the wastage of oocytes that are unfertilizable at present. Attempts to support oocyte maturation in vitro should become more proficient as improved culture media and supplements are devised for this purpose and as more pertinent information is obtained on the natural follicular environment.

Studies on the maturation and developmental capability of oocytes will also benefit understanding of the regulation of folliculogenesis. Since the functional endpoint of follicular development is the production of a developmentally competent oocyte, then assessment of oocyte quality using IVF and embryo culture techniques can give useful feedback about the normality of the follicle from which that oocyte was derived. This information will allow attention to be directed at those follicles, and their cellular and chemical products, that are associated with normality. Our preliminary data on the relationship between follicular steroids and maturity of oocytes suggests that these chemical parameters of follicular development may not be good indicators of the "normality" of follicles from a strictly embryological viewpoint. However, there may be functionally significant relationships (such as steroid ratios) which we have not examined or which may require additional experimental data for their detection.

Much more attention should be focused on the use of nonhuman primates for studying the regulation of oocyte maturation, so that information relating directly to the human situation can be obtained. Studies in rodents or in women cannot provide the same quality of relevant experimental data. Information derived from studies with mice, for example, can provide valuable clues on the direction that research into primate oocyte maturation should take. However, there are some striking differences in the physiology of oocyte maturation regulation between rodents and primates, so that direct extrapolation of information is not appropriate. On the other hand, although a considerable amount of information has already been obtained from human IVF studies, particularly from attempts to correlate follicular fluid steroid concentrations with oocyte maturation, the human clinical IVF situation does not lend itself to critical experimental studies on oocyte maturation. In particular, it is not feasible or ethical to design experiments involving human IVF solely for the purpose of investigating the control of oocyte maturation, which would involve loss of some oocytes (e.g., those assigned to control treatments) as well as requiring prolonged culture of embryos in order to evaluate their viability. These difficulties emphasize the value of the nonhuman primate species for undertaking experiments on oocyte maturation. Now that reliable IVF procedures have been developed and the protocols are readily available, and inroads are being made into mechanisms of oocyte maturation in other species, it is to be hoped that investigators will begin to direct more attention towards the study of oocyte maturation in nonhuman primates.

ACKNOWLEDGMENTS

I am grateful to my colleagues Dorothy Boatman, Emily Kraus, Patricia Morgan, and Pradeep Warikoo for providing data described in this report. I am especially grateful to Dr. Morgan for data analysis and for providing the figures. The research described in this chapter was supported by a grant from NICHD (HD14765) and by the Wisconsin Primate Center (base operating grant number RR00167).

REFERENCES

1. Soules MR. The in vitro fertilization pregnancy rate: let's be honest with one another. Fertil Steril 1985; 43:511-3.
2. Fishel SB, Edwards RG, Evans CJ. Human chorionic gonadotropin secreted by preimplantation embryos cultured in vitro. Science 1984; 223:816-8.
3. Pope VZ, Pope CE, Beck LR. Gonadotropin production by the baboon embryo in vitro. In: Hafez ESE, Semm K, eds. In vitro fertilization and embryo transfer. Lancaster, England: MTP Press, 1982; 129-34.
4. Staigmiller RB, Moor RM. Effect of follicle cells on the maturation and developmental competence of ovine oocytes matured outside the follicle. Gamete Res 1984; 9:221-9.
5. Thibault C. Are follicular maturation and oocyte maturation independent processes? J Reprod Fertil 1977; 51:1-15.
6. Leibfried ML, Bavister BD. Fertilizability of in vitro matured oocytes from golden hamsters. J Exp Zool 1983; 226:481-5.
7. Sathananthan AH, Trounson AO. Ultrastructure of cortical granule release and zona interaction in monospermic and polyspermic human ova fertilized in vitro. Gamete Res 1982; 6:225-34.
8. Van Blerkom J, Henry G, Porreco R. Preimplantation human embryonic development from polypronuclear eggs after in vitro fertilization. Fertil Steril 1984; 41:686-96.
9. Shalgi R. Developmental capacity of rat embryos produced by in vivo or in vitro fertilization. Gamete Res 1984; 10:77-82.
10. Fleming AD, Evans G, Walton EA, Armstrong DT. Developmental capability of rat oocytes matured in vitro in defined medium. Gamete Res 1985; 12:255-63.
11. Carson RS, Trounson AO, Findlay JK. Successful fertilization of human oocytes in vitro: concentrations of estradiol-17β, progesterone and androstenedione in the antral fluid of donor follicles. J Clin Endocrinol Metab 1982; 55:798-800.
12. Botero-Ruiz W, Laufer N, DeCherney AH, Polan ML, Haseltine FP, Behrman HR. The relationship between follicular fluid steroid concentration and successful fertilization of human oocytes in vitro. Fertil Steril 1984; 41:820-6.
13. Schroeder AC, Eppig JJ. The developmental capacity of mouse oocytes that matured spontaneously in vitro is normal. Dev Biol 1984; 102:493-7.
14. Eppig JJ, Schroeder AC. Culture systems for mammalian oocyte development: progress and prospects. Theriogenology 1986; 25:97-106.
15. Downs SM, Coleman DL, Ward-Bailey PF, Eppig JJ. Hypoxanthine is the principal inhibitor of murine oocyte maturation in a low molecular weight fraction of porcine follicular fluid. Proc Natl Acad Sci USA 1985; 82:454-8.
16. Bavister BD, Boatman DE, Leibfried ML, Loose M, Vernon MW. Fertilization and cleavage of rhesus monkey oocytes in vitro. Biol Reprod 1983; 28:983-99.
17. Boatman DE, Bavister BD. Stimulation of rhesus monkey sperm capacitation by cyclic nucleotide mediators. J Reprod Fertil 1984; 77:357-66.
18. Boatman DE, Morgan PM, Bavister BD. Variables affecting the yield and developmental potential of embryos following superstimulation and in vitro fertilization in rhesus monkeys. Gamete Res 1986; 13:327-38.
19. Morgan PM, Boatman DE, Collins K, Bavister BD. Complete preimplantation development in culture of in vitro fertilized rhesus monkey oocytes. Biol Reprod 1984; 30(suppl 1):96a.
20. Bavister BD, Boatman DE, Collins K, Dierschke DJ, Eisele SG. Birth of rhesus monkey infant following in vitro fertilization and nonsur-

gical embryo transfer. Proc Natl Acad Sci USA 1984; 81:2218-22.

21. Bavister BD, Collins K, Eisele S. Non-surgical embryo transfer in the rhesus monkey. Theriogenology 1985; 23:177a.

22. Boatman DE. In vitro growth of non-human primate pre- and peri-implantation embryos. In: Bavister BD, ed. The mammalian preimplantation embryo: regulation of growth and differentiation in vitro. New York: Plenum Press, 1987; 273-308.

23. Morgan PM, Boatman DE, Kraus EM. Relationship between follicular fluid steroid hormone concentrations and in vitro development of rhesus monkey embryos. Biol Reprod 1986; 34(suppl 1):94a.

24. Morgan PM, Warikoo PK, Erwin MJ, Kraus EM. Recovery of oocytes from spontaneously cycling rhesus monkeys: timing, follicular steroids and in vitro fertilization. Biol Reprod 1987; 36(suppl 1):130a.

25. Morgan PM, Warikoo PK, Bavister, BD. In vitro maturation and fertilization of rhesus monkey oocytes [Abstract]. The primate ovary, final program and abstract book, Oregon Regional Primate Research Center, Beaverton, OR, May 16-17, 1987:28.

26. Moor RM, Crosby IM. Temperature-induced abnormalities in sheep oocytes during maturation. J Reprod Fertil 1985; 75:467-73.

27. Bavister BD. A mini-chamber device for maintaining a constant carbon dioxide atmosphere during prolonged culture of cells on the stage of an inverted microscope (in preparation).

28. Soupart P, Strong PA. Ultrastructural observations on human oocytes fertilized in vitro. Fertil Steril 1974; 25:11-44.

29. Hertig AL, Rock J, Adams EC. A description of 34 human ova within the first 17 days of development. Am J Anat 1956; 98:435-93.

30. Hurst PR, Jeffries K, Eckstein P, Wheller AG. Recovery of uterine embryos in rhesus monkeys. Biol Reprod 1976; 15:429-34.

31. Hendrickx AG, Binkerd PE. Fetal deaths in nonhuman primates. In: Porter IH, Hook EB, eds. Human embryonic and fetal death. New York: Academic Press, 1980; 45-69.

32. Enders AC, Hendrickx AG, Binkerd PA. Abnormal development of blastocysts and blastomeres in the rhesus monkey. Biol Reprod 1982; 26:353-66.

33. Bavister BD, Boatman DE, Morgan PM, Collins K, Kraus EM, Eisele S. Surgical and non-surgical transfer of in vitro fertilized embryos in the rhesus monkey (in preparation).

34. Bavister BD, Dees HC, Schultz RD. Refractoriness of rhesus monkeys to repeated gonadotropin stimulation is due to formation of nonprecipitating antibodies. Am J Reprod Immunol Microbiol 1986; 11:11-6.

35. Morgan PM, Boatman DE, Bavister BD. Relationships between follicular fluid steroid concentrations, oocyte maturation, in vitro fertilization and embryonic development in the rhesus monkey (in preparation).

36. Uehara S, Naganuma T, Tsuiki A, Kyono K, Hoshiai H, Suzuki M. Relationship between follicular fluid steroid concentrations and in vitro fertilization. Obstet Gynecol 1985; 66:19-23.

PERSPECTIVES ON OVARIAN STIMULATION AND

IN VITRO FERTILIZATION IN PRIMATE MODELS

Gary D. Hodgen, Ph.D.

Professor and Scientific Director
The Jones Institute for Reproductive Medicine, Lewis Hall
Room 2001, 700 Olney Road, Norfolk, Virginia 23507

Since the inception of in vitro fertilization and embryo transfer (IVF/ET) therapy by Edwards and Steptoe in the mid-70s, nothing has increased the pregnancy rate of this procedure as dramatically as the decision to employ enhancement of the natural ovarian/menstrual cycle in order to attempt collection of several oocytes from each patient during each treatment cycle. Here, we will review first the underlying physiological mechanisms in the natural ovarian cycle in order to serve us in the second case, where our purpose is to override selection of the dominant follicle to facilitate aspiration of several preovulatory oocytes for IVF/ET therapy (Fig. 1).

Over the past 15 years, we have studied basic mechanisms of ovarian function in the primate menstrual cycle. As previously reviewed, these investigations were directed at understanding follicular growth and atresia (1), corpus luteum function (2,3), ovum maturation (4), and the initiation of ovulatory menstrual cycles after menarche and the postpartum hiatus (5). Here, it is our challenge to convey the relevance of this research to the practitioner of reproductive medicine, especially the physicians and scientists providing IVF/ET therapy, with the expectation that these new findings may enrich existing skills and knowledge in clinical care (6).

Both human and laboratory primate data will be considered. The principal advantages in employing nonhuman primate models lie in: (1) their extensive mimicry of many fundamental properties (anatomic, functional, and temporal) of the human hypothalamic-pituitary-ovarian-uterine (HPOU) axis; (2) the freedom to pursue aggressive protocols having the capacity to resolve questions about the reproductive process, thereby accelerating and guiding the course of subsequent clinical research; and, (3) freedom from inherent moral constraints on direct clinical investigation. Prevailing ethical and legal standards restrict the design and conduct of studies on many of the foremost endocrine-infertility problems confronting the clinician; and quite appropriately, our concern for individual patient welfare supersedes the quest for new understanding.

There are obvious limitations in the use of these surrogate primates (rhesus and cynomolgus monkeys) that must be realized. Respect for these limitations is shown in their selective application in the laboratory, followed by conservative interpretation and use of the results toward the resolution of clinical problems.

Realizing that many recent advancements confirm the activity of contiguous clinical and laboratory studies, this review builds upon previous texts (1-5) in discussing the dominant ovarian follicle of the natural cycle or folliculogenesis during ovulation induction or IVF/ET therapy.

The Natural Ovarian/Menstrual Cycle

The specialized gonadal tissue of the growing preovulatory follicle and its successor, the corpus luteum, establish and maintain the changing hormonal milieu which nurtures the ovum through maturation, fertilization, and the initial stages of embryogenesis. Indeed, it is the ovarian cycle which temporally modulates hypothalamic-pituitary function through both negative and positive feedback on gonadotropin release, as well as orchestration of uterine proliferative and secretory phases of the men-strual cycle (Fig. 2). No wonder, then, the sequelae to aberrancies during folliculogenesis (spontaneous or induced) include abnormalities of the cervical mucus, the endometrium, circulating gonadotropins, the corpus luteum, and even the ovum. Accordingly, fertility in the female depends fundamentally on an underpinning of intraovarian processes that account for timely follicular growth, culminating in ovulation of a fertilizable oocyte, as well as its subsequent nurturing.

Whereas many follicles may begin this developmental course each ovarian/menstrual cycle, typically only a single follicle sustains its inherent gametogenic potential, all others succumb to atresia (Fig. 3). Of course, provision of more gonadotropins in stimulated or induced cycles

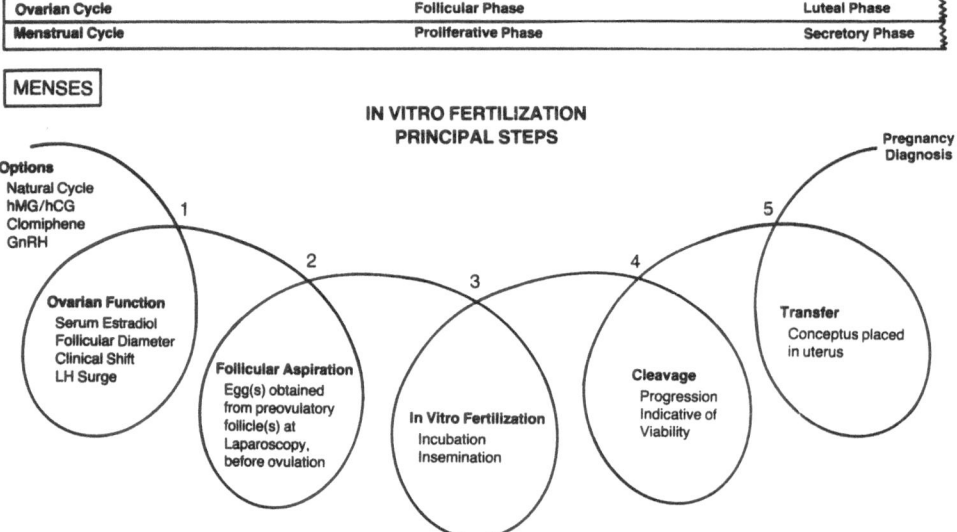

Fig. 1. The five principal steps in IVF/ET therapy. Hormonal stimulation of the ovarian cycle is of crucial importance for collection of several oocytes of high quality. The success of these first and second steps greatly influences the pregnancy rate after one or more embryos are transferred to the uterus (from Hodgen).

(clomiphene citrate [CC] and/or human menopausal gonadotropin [hMG]) will violate the normal monovular quota (Fig. 4). On a controlled basis, this may be desirable in order to facilitate IVF/ET. Even so, the attendant risk is to have impaired (qualitatively) the normality of the growing follicles and the sequelae of the ovarian/menstrual cycle, requisite for establishing a viable pregnancy. Moreover, aspiration of the preovulatory follicle to accomplish ovum collection necessarily is associated with removal of some follicular fluid and granulosa cells. These constituents of the intrafollicular milieu surely participate in ovum maturation, engendering the ovum's fertilizable status in the final hours of the preovulatory gonadotropin surge.

We have hypothesized (1) that the precise regulation of follicle growth and selection is accomplished primarily by specific ovarian factors that act directly on the ovaries; and, (2) that gonadotropins, at tonic levels, are merely permissive to folliculogenesis (7). We envisage a two-tier ovarian mechanism. At the first tier, specific ovarian factors govern the progressive winnowing of the cohort of developing follicles down to the size of the species-characteristic ovulatory quota in each cycle. Some factors may act within the ovary of origin as intraovarian regulators; other ovarian factors may be secreted and circulate to the opposite ovary, to act as extraovarian signals (but of ovarian origin). Together, they regulate the culling-out or inhibit the maturation of supernumerary-growing follicles. This first tier of the proposed ovarian mechanism which precisely regulates follicle selection is operative, however, only when circulating gonadotropins are above minimal levels and

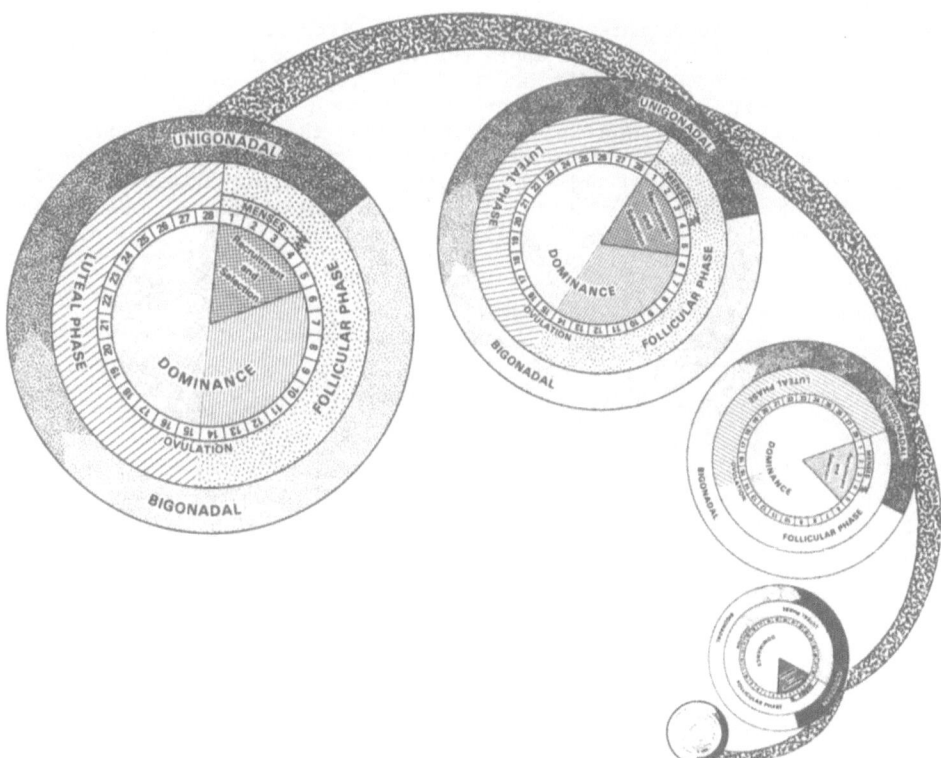

Fig. 2. Conceptualization of the primate ovarian/menstrual cycle. The dominant follicle is selected in the same cycle as it achieves ovulation (from diZerega and Hodgen).

141

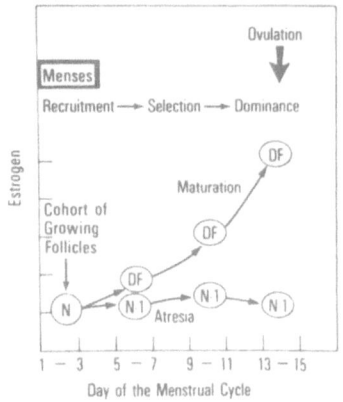

Fig. 3. Time course for recruitment, selection, and ovulation of the dominant ovarian follicle, with onset of atresia among other follicles of the cohort (from Hodgen).

near the tonic "set-point." At the second tier, ovarian hormones (steroidal and nonsteroidal) inhibit gonadotropin secretion in a negative feedback fashion to constrain circulating gonadotropin levels to an appropriate range around the tonic set-point. If gonadotropin levels are too far below this tonic set-point, then folliculogenesis will be arrested as a result of inadequate stimulation. Contrariwise, if circulating gonadotropin levels are too far above the tonic set-point, then first-tier ovarian mechanisms, ordinarily at work to regulate the size of the ovulatory quota, are impaired or inactivated; in such instances, superovulation occurs. That is, we propose that the mergence of multiple follicles on both ovaries after administration of exogenous gonadotropins to monkeys or women is not only the result of augmenting the availability of gonadotropins, per se, but is also an indirect result of overriding first-tier ovarian mechanisms of follicle selection (Fig. 5).

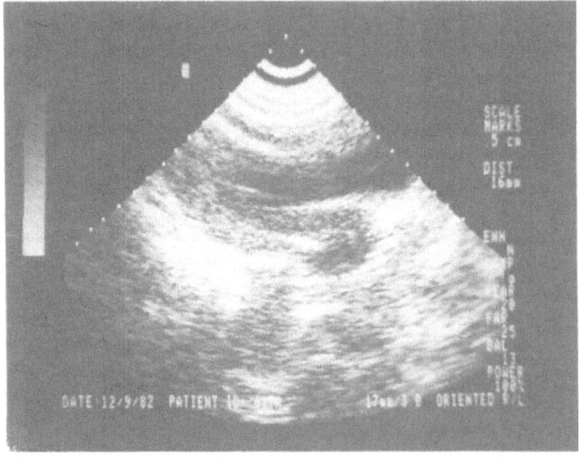

Fig. 4. Ovarian sonogram illustrating single dominant follicle on primate cycle day 13 after onset of menses.

142

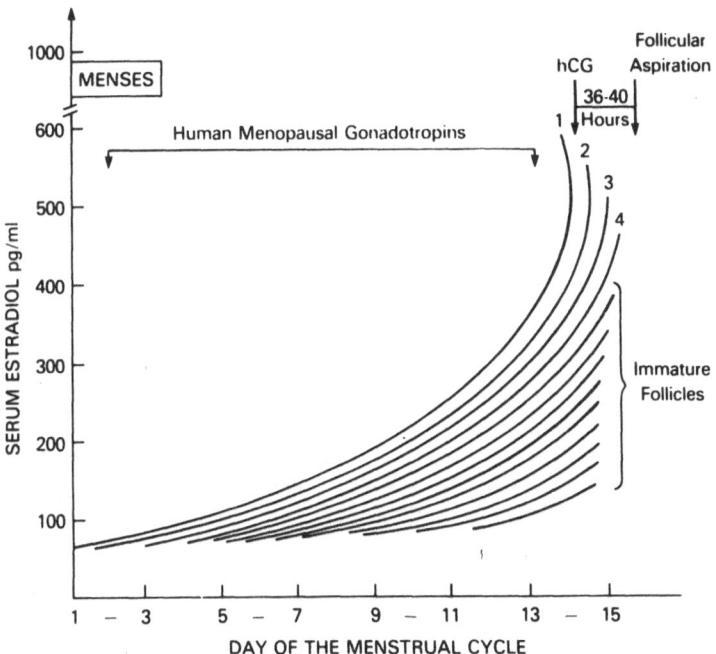

Fig. 5. Induced follicular maturation, hMG/hCG. HMG stimulates follicular maturation overriding selection of a single dominant follicle in the natural cycle. Note that only a few follicles can be regarded as developing quasi-synchronously. If hCG is given too late, the most advanced follicles may yield post-mature eggs of low viable potential (from Hodgen).

Clearly, as exploited in several well-known bioassays for gonadotropins, both FSH and LH can have graded, dose-dependent effects on the ovary. However, in the physiological setting of the menstrual cycle, we find it more useful to consider that the folliculogenic actions of gonadotropins (principally FSH) are permissive at tonic levels and that the steroidogenic actions of gonadotropins (principally LH) are graded. If FSH at tonic levels is actually permissive to folliculogenesis, then graded effects observed may be attributable to supraphysiological (supratonic) levels. Graded actions of gonadotropins on steroidogenesis [and perhaps on "inhibin" secretion(s) as well, see below] are necessary for the second tier of the ovarian mechanism to constrain circulating gonadotropins near the tonic set-point, so that first-tier mechanisms of follicle selection are effective. Evidence that these two activities (tiers) are dissociable, in some circumstances, is presented below. More direct evidence for this hypothesis must come from future studies.

Terminology

Before considering how we arrived at this hypothesis, we shall explain some important terms. These terms are now new, yet although in wide used, they have not been employed with uniform precision. While even our definitions remain lacking, they are, nonetheless, useful in drawing important distinctions.

The ovary performs dual roles as an organ of reproduction and a gland of internal secretion. To distinguish the regulation of these ovarian activities, we shall refer to the gametogenic activity as <u>folliculogenesis</u> and to the secretory activity as <u>hormonogenesis</u> (Fig. 5). Extra or intraovarian factors that directly influence the ovary's gametogenic role have a folliculogenic action or elicit a folliculogenic response. While some may balk at the introduction of a term like hormonogenesis, it is used here because we find current nomenclature inadequate. Since, in our scheme, some ovarian secretions may act locally within the ovary in a paracrine (or perhaps even autocrine) fashion, they are not, in the strictest sense, endocrine. In addition, since some ovarian hormones secreted into the circulation may be nonsteroidal ("inhibins"), steroidogenesis is too restrictive. Consequently, we will use the term hormonogenesis to encompass all nature and manner of such ovarian secretions.

During each cycle, primordial follicles depart the resting pool and begin a well-characterized pattern of growth and development (8,9). Groups of (quasi) synchronously growing follicles are called <u>cohorts</u>. In the same or some subsequent cycle, a few (or only one) members of one cohort continue to develop and escape atresia, until they become preovulatory graafian follicles, ultimately providing the species-characteristic ovulatory quota of eggs (Fig. 6). Schwartz (10) has aptly termed this pattern the "trajectory of follicle growth." Extending the trajectory metaphor into our hypothesis outlined above, gonadotropins may be seen as providing the "thrust" and ovarian factors the "guidance" along the trajectory, not unlike some surface launched missile (Fig. 7). Clearly, without continued "thrust," the trajectory will be limited; with "thrust" in excess of the guidance system's design, the accuracy and precision of the course are compromised (7).

We shall use the term <u>recruitment</u> (Fig. 8) to indicate that a follicle has entered on this growth trajectory. Thus, under this definition, recruitment includes the entry of primordial follicles onto the trajectory, without excluding the reentry of more mature follicles which may have been transiently at rest. Pedersen's (11) studies in mice have generally been interpreted to mean that, once a follicle leaves the resting primordial pool, it must continue to mature or succumb to atresia, i.e., it does not again rest. Whether or not this is true for primates is

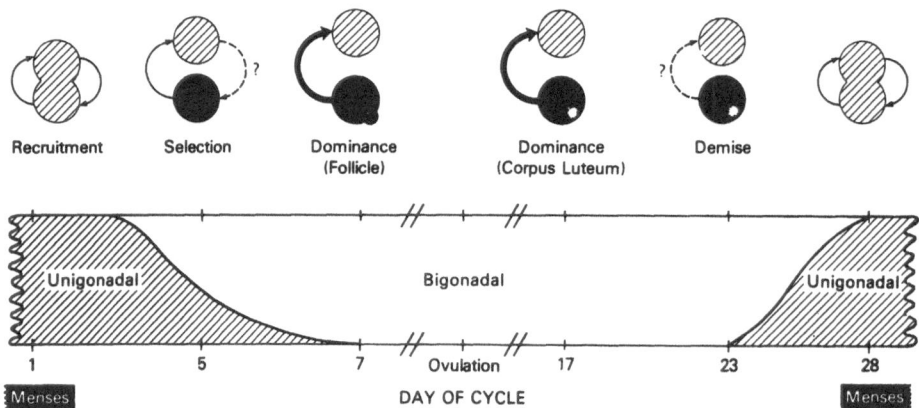

Fig. 6. In the natural menstrual cycle, either ovary may provide the dominant follicle in any given cycle. Once the dominant follicle has been selected, the two ovaries are partitioned into gametogenically active versus inactive. Ovarian function is then asymmetric.

144

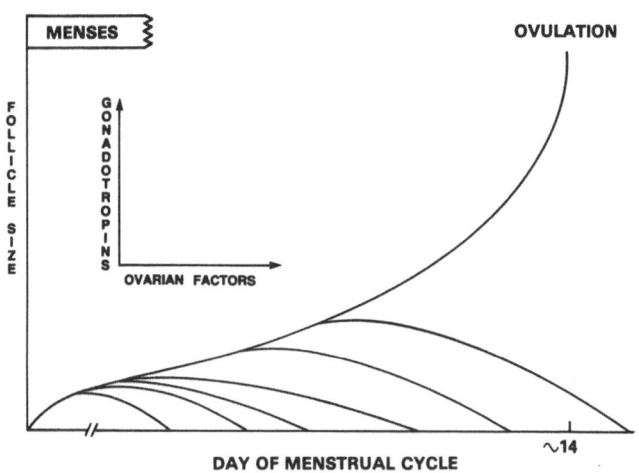

Fig. 7. Proposed relationship between gonadotropins and ovarian factors in regulating maturation or atresia along the so-called trajectory of follicle growth (from Goodman and Hodgen).

unknown, hence the broader definition used here. Since follicles at various preantral stages of development were observed in ovaries of hypophysectomized rats and rabbits (12), recruitment of primordial follicles is not wholly dependent on gonadotropins, but may be only enhanced by these hormones (13). Growing follicles are vulnerable to atresia and may depart the trajectory at any point. Thus, while an obligatory step, recruitment does not guarantee ovulation. That recruitment is a necessary, but not a sufficient, condition for ovulation is particularly important when interpreting results of experiments employing exogenous gonadotropins to stimulate follicle development, as discussed below. The term selection will be used here to indicate the final winnowing of the cohort (via atresia of "excess" follicles) down to a size equal to the species-characteristic ovulatory quota. That is, when the number of healthy follicles (i.e., with ovulatory potential) in the cohort equals the size of the ovulatory quota, then selection is complete. Implicit in this definition is the notion that the cohort may be the regulated variable rather than the fate of an individual follicle. That is, which follicles, in particular, are culled from the cohort may be due to a random process that continues until cohort size matches the ovulatory quota, in contrast to a deterministic process in which specific follicles are individually chosen according to some unknown criteria. The character (stochastic vs. deterministic) of the selection mechanism remains uncertain. What is certain, however, is that the process operates in primates with great precision; a spontaneous multiple ovulation is extremely atypical. Like recruitment, selection does not guarantee ovulation, but, given its greater temporal proximity to ovulation, selection may, with high probability, be expected to be followed by ovulation in a typical cycle. Evidence will be presented that selection is begun and is completed only during the cycle in which ovulation occurs. In contrast, the time of recruitment and, thus, the total length (duration) of the trajectory are unknown. Based on findings discussed below, the duration of the trajectory in macaques and women appears to be not less than about 2 weeks.

Clearly, the ovulatory quota in higher primates is generally unity; hence, although actual cohort size as a function of day-of-cycle is

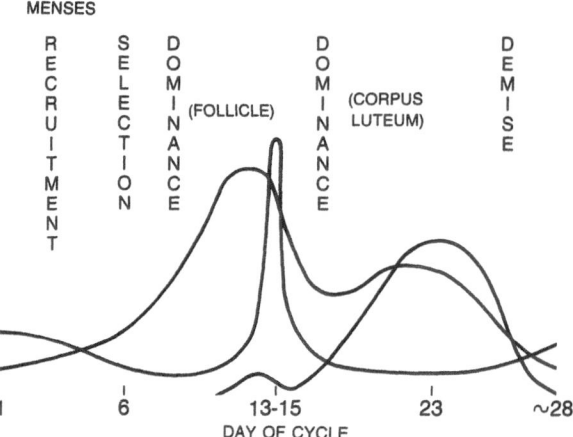

MENSES

R E C R U I T M E N T   S E L E C T I O N   D O M I N A N C E (FOLLICLE)   D O M I N A N C E (CORPUS LUTEUM)   D E M I S E

1   6   13-15   23   ~28

DAY OF CYCLE

Fig. 8. The terms used to describe the sequence of principal ovarian events during follicular maturation and corpus luteum function are temporally defined in the menstrual cycle. The curves depict idealized (stereotypical) patterns of E_2, pituitary gonadotropins, and P in peripheral circulation (from Hodgen).

unknown, the possibility of a "cohort of one" even as early as recruitment is not excluded. Even if this were true, cohort remains a meaningful construct, and it is still useful to consider recruitment and selection as distinct processes.

Although anticipating facts not yet in evidence, the term dominance is introduced here to limit our lexicography to this section. As we shall demonstrate below, the follicle destined to ovulate plays a key role in regulating the size of the ovulatory quota, at least in monkeys. That is, the follicle selected for ovulation is functionally (not merely morphologically) dominant; it inhibits the development of other competing follicles on both ovaries. As a necessary corollary, the dominant follicle (i.e., the sole follicle destined to ovulate) somehow continues to thrive in a milieu it, itself, has made inhospitable for others. Whether this capacity to thrive under these circumstances results from a unique ability of the dominant follicle which is newly acquired or from a preexisting ability originally shared by the entire cohort, but which is retained only by the dominant follicle, is unclear. That is, does the survival of the dominant follicle depend on a process of acquisition or retention of metabolic properties to resist atresia? Underpinning this issue is how the dominant follicle actually exerts its eminence. How is it spared from the very inhibition it imposes on others? As one mechanism, we hypothesize that the dominant follicle secretes a substance we call "selectron," which acts directly on the ovaries to inhibit the development of potentially competing follicles. The motivation for this hypothesis is developed in more detail below. As we have shown, the selected follicle becomes dominant about a week before ovulation. Consequently, it must maintain its dominance during the week before ovulation. Unresolved is whether the mechanism(s) by which the follicle attains dominance is the same as the mechanism(s) by which the follicle maintains dominance. The precise temporal relationship between selection and dominance is also unresolved (7).

146

GONADOTROPIC STIMULATION OF THE OVARIAN CYCLE

Blockage of the Preovulatory LH Surge

Administration of hMG preparations to adult female monkeys, either an FSH/LH combination (Fig. 9) (14) or "pure" FSH (Metrodin®, Serono) (Fig. 10) (15), produced bilateral ovarian hyperstimulation with attendant supraphysiological rises in circulating estradiol. Despite these raised estrogen levels, usually women and monkeys fail to manifest timely gonadotropin responses to estrogen-positive feedback; that is, usually these normal, intact, cycling primates do not have the expected midcycle-like LH surges, despite escalating concentrations of serum estradiol that often exceed 400 pg/ml during 12 days of FSH therapy (16). Also, we have noted that there are often no spontaneous LH surges when hMG-induced ovarian hyperstimulation occurs in postpartum monkeys. These observations fit in with the clinical finding (17) that when endocrinologically normal patients are given hMG to increase the number of follicles/ova available for IVF/ET treatment, hCG is usually required for the final maturation of these follicles. These women seldom have spontaneous LH/FSH surges, even though circulating estradiol levels exceed 300 pg/ml for several days (18).

Why is the surge mode of LH secretion not operational? Perhaps excessive secretion of one or more inhibitors of ovarian origin is driven uncontrollably by unrelenting (exogenous) FSH stimulation, thereby blocking the expected LH surges otherwise induced by estrogen-positive feedback on the hypothalamic-pituitary unit. Indeed, we have reported (19) that pretreating monkeys with charcoal-extracted porcine follicular fluid prevents both the FSH and LH surges after a conventional estrogen challenge in the follicular phase (Fig. 11). Similarly, it was shown that acute GnRH-induced release of FSH and LH was blunted when castrated monkeys were pretreated with a porcine follicular fluid extract (20).

Next, we asked whether the ovaries, undergoing exogenous stimulation with purified FSH, were obligatory for this blockade of the spontaneous LH surge, or was this inhibition due to a "short loop" feedback of FSH. FSH administration (12 days) to long-term ovariectomized monkeys did not inhibit responses to an estradiol benzoate challenge; that is, typical midcycle-like gonadotropin surges were observed. Accordingly, the occurrence of estrogen-induced FSH/LH surges in FSH-treated castrated monkeys shows that among intact monkeys the ovaries (hyperstimulated) surely participate in the blockade of estrogen-positive feedback during exogenous gonadotropin therapy. Furthermore, with hMG administration, blockade of the LH surge probably develops as a result of the actions of its FSH component (15). In contrast, when clomiphene citrate (Serophene®, Serono) is employed, a spontaneous LH usually develops, although it is frequently delayed until about cycle day 16 (Fig. 12).

With regard to hCG injection to replace the blocked LH surge, we have shown disparate effects of hCG during the late follicular phase of the primate ovarian cycle (21). More specifically, if the estrogen-induced surges of FSH and LH had been initiated, ovarian function was unaffected by hCG. In contrast, hCG given before incipient gonadotropin surges led to anovulation lasting 4-6 weeks and sometimes disruption of the tonic FSH secretion. Indeed, these findings may indicate some potential risks of premature administration of hCG to women during induced follicular maturation. Inappropriately timed (precocious) administration of hCG may actually preclude the objective; namely, to provide fertilizable oocytes and a milieu in which to nurture the embryo(s) through a normal luteal phase while achieving a fertile menstrual cycle.

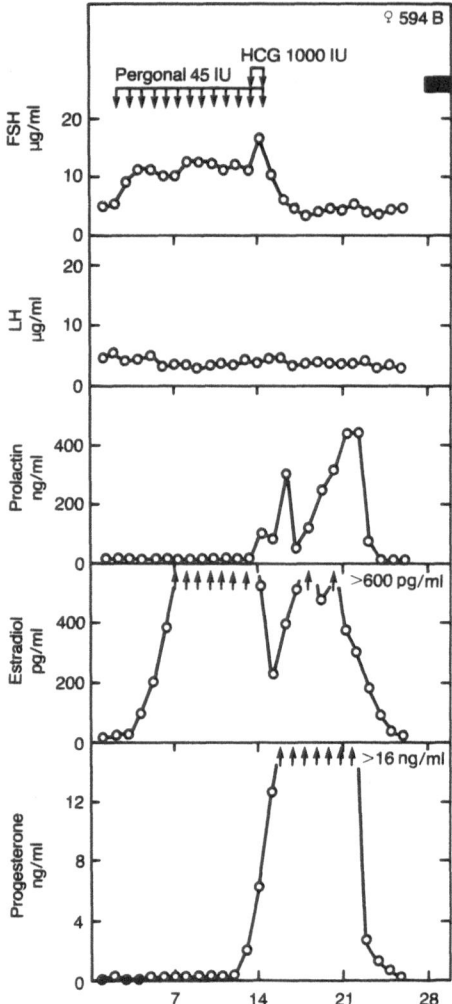

Fig. 9. HMG-induced ovarian hyperstimulation in the postpartum, non-
nursing monkeys. Note absence of an
endogenous LH surge and the induction of hyperprolactinemia (from
Goodman and Hodgen).

As illustrated in Figure 5, hMG treatment will sustain the concurrent
development of many follicles for a limited interval. Even so, only a few
quasi-synchronous follicles, such as those that begin to be responsive to
gonadotropins in the early follicular phase, can be "harvested" together
by follicular aspiration some 36-40 h after hCG injection.

If hCG is given too late, one or more of the most advanced follicles
may yield postmature (fragmented) eggs (Fig. 13) of low potential viability; conversely, if hCG is injected too soon, the follicles/eggs may be
immature (16).

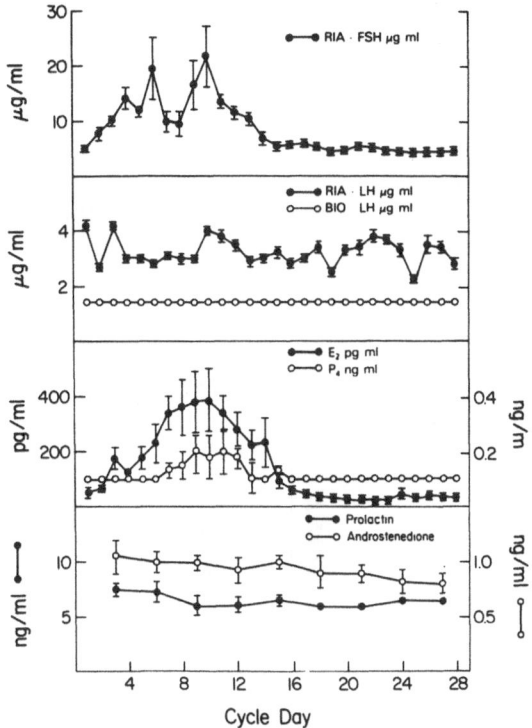

Fig. 10. Composite patterns (mean ± SE) of
serum FSH, LH, estradiol, progesterone,
androstenedione, and PRL in 5 intact monkeys
treated with FSH (25 or 50 IU daily, IM
cycle days 1-12). Note the failure of
estrogen-positive feedback for the LH surge.
Typically, FSH doses of 12.5 IU or less
daily did not produce ovarian hyperstimulation. RIA, radioimmunoassayable; BIO, bioassayable.

The Two-Cell Theory

In 1959, Falck (40) autotransplanted pure ovarian cell systems and
combinations of those cells into spayed rats. He found that estrogen
secretion was only obtained when theca cells were combined with granulosa
cells, but not in either system alone. This was further developed by
Short (22) who proposed different enzymatic capabilities of theca and
granulosa cells to explain the differences in equine follicular fluid and
luteal tissue.

Using isolated and combined human cells in vitro, Ryan et al. (23)
demonstrated that each cell type has the capacity for de novo steroid
formation from acetate. However, there was an absence of estradiol with
isolated granulosa cells. Armstrong et al., also using human cells in
vitro, developed this concept to its final form by showing granulosa cells
to be the prime site of follicular estrogen secretion and FSH to be the
regulator of that process. LH stimulated androgen production by theca
cells, and FSH stimulated aromatization of androgen to estrogen by

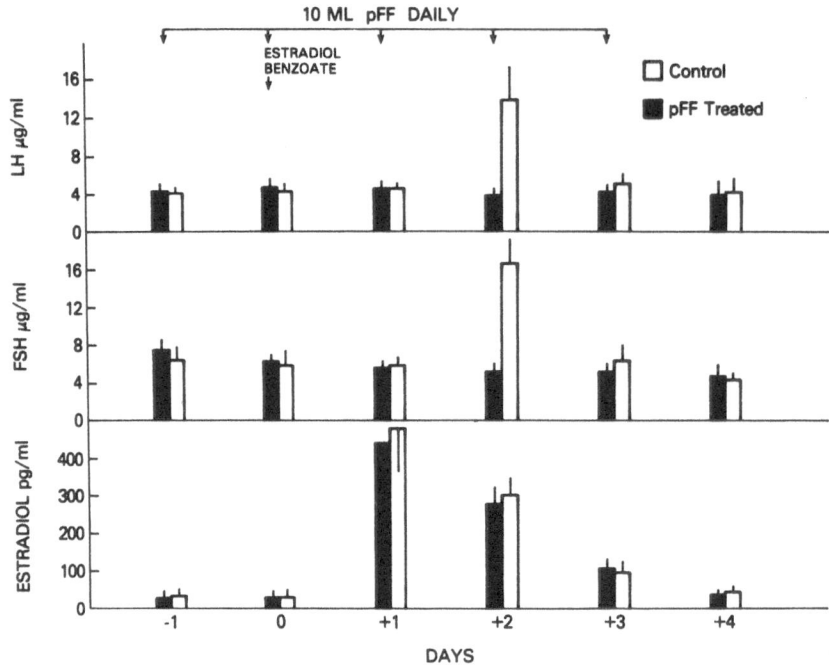

Fig. 11. Serum concentrations of LH, FSH, and E$_2$ during early-follicular-phase rhesus monkeys receiving estradiol and E$_2$ benzoate challenge (50 µg/kg) with or without pFF (extract of porcine follicular fluid/inhibin) treatment. Values shown are mean ± SE (n=5 each) (from Hodgen et al.).

granulosa cells. Therefore, a two-cell, two-gonadotropin theory of control and performance of estrogen biosynthesis was complete.

The above principles were influential on those working to develop ovulation induction agents. The two-cell theory proposed a co-equal importance to FSH and LH. When tested at an empiric 50:50 ratio of FSH to LH, it was found that urinary gonadotropins had improved efficacy over the FSH derivatives of human pituitary used prior to 1960 (24–26). Success rates in achieving ovulation in the entire spectrum of anovulatory disorders of a supraovarian origin were excellent. Furthermore, variability of response and higher than natural pregnancy loss rates were attributed to the underlying pathophysiological disorders in these patients.

With the advent of IVF/ET therapy came the first large experience with administering ovulation induction agents to women who were otherwise endocrinologically normal. In attempting to achieve multiple follicular stimulation to enhance oocyte recovery and the probability of fertilization, it became apparent that these otherwise normally cycling women showed striking differences in ovarian response to gonadotropin therapy (17). In 390 cycles stimulated by hMG in Norfolk, 107 distinct patterns of estradiol rise were distinguished (27). Furthermore, these response types tend toward a consistent pattern from cycle to cycle, thus suggesting a constancy at physiological status as opposed to a random response. With this background, we began seeking ways of reducing individual variability of responses to gonadotropin therapy based on understanding the physiological origin(s) of that variability.

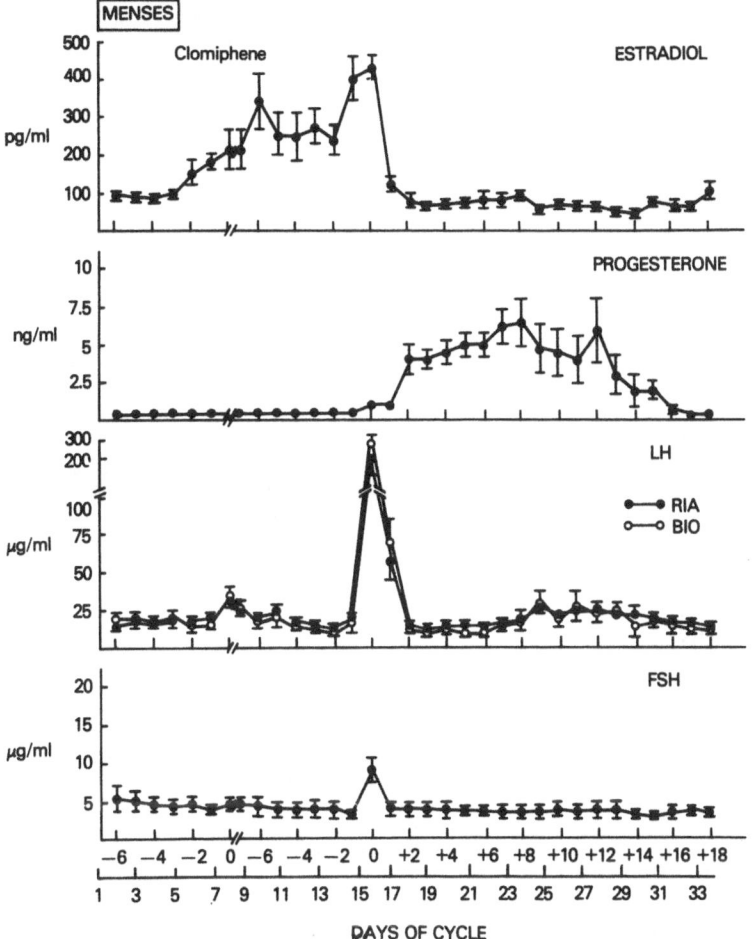

Fig. 12. Administration of clomiphene citrate (Sero-phene®, Serono) on cycle days 5 and 9 usually prompts a delayed spontaneous LH surge about cycle day 16.

Clinical experience over the last 25 years has shown that it is often easier to manage gonadotropin therapy in severely hypogonadotropic patients than those presenting anovulation of other etiologies (28). This realization has prompted other attempts at inducing a transient hypogonadotropic state in individuals undergoing ovulation induction, with the goal of achieving more uniform responses and fewer therapeutic complications for greater ultimate efficacy. Jones et al. (29) attempted pretreatment with synthetic steroids to suppress the pituitary over a 2-month interval prior to gonadotropin therapy. Fleming et al. (30) pretreated patients with a GnRH agonist before administering exogenous gonadotropin. Why have such strategies not been adopted more widely?

The above approaches have notable disadvantages: (1) Progestins are thought to inhibit folliculogenesis in the primate ovary directly (1); also, exogenous progestins modify the milieu of the uterine endometrium, cervix and fallopian tubes prematurely during the proliferative phase; and, (2) GnRH agonists actually enhance gonadotropin and estradiol secre-tion for the initial 10 to 14 days of treatment before a state of pitu-

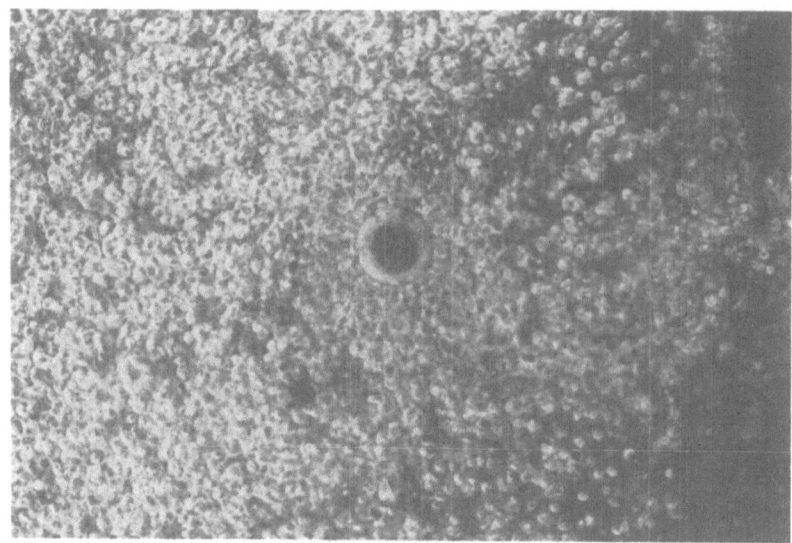

Fig. 13. A fragmented egg aspirated from a postmature follicle. Note the darkened ooplasm. Delay of the LH surge or late hCG injection can reduce ovum quality (from Hodgen).

itary suppression is attained (31,32). In contrast, the GnRH antagonist used in the present study only diminishes FSH and LH levels, without concurrent elevations of ovarian steroid secretion. Although GnRH or its analogs may influence the ovaries directly in rodents (33), persuasive evidence obtained in women and monkeys argues against a direct action of these synthetic decapeptides in the primate ovary (34,35).

Accordingly, we set out to determine whether a GnRH antagonist would reduce individual variation in response to gonadotropin therapy, through diminished functions of the hypothalamus and pituitary (Fig. 14) (36). Utilizing a strategy that employed a 17-day pretreatment with a potent GnRH antagonist (Fig. 15), followed by concurrent treatment with the GnRH antagonist plus exogenous gonadotropin therapy, either FSH and LH in equal amounts or FSH alone, the following was demonstrated in monkeys (Fig. 16).

Pretreatment with the GnRH antagonist increased the homogeneity of ovarian E_2 secretion during exogenous gonadotropin therapy, among responsive females, as compared to non-GnRH antagonist, gonadotropin-responsive subjects (Fig. 17). This constraint on individuality of responders by the GnRH antagonist suggests that an important part of the source of individual variation in response to gonadotropin therapy is supraovarian; that is, our findings indicate that hypothalamic-pituitary functions contribute substantially to the variability of ovarian response during gonadotropin treatment.

Further, there was a near even distribution of nonresponder monkeys irrespective of whether the GnRH antagonist was given. Thus, the source of relative resistance among nonresponders may derive from the ovaries themselves, as opposed to factors contributed by supraovarian components that might be influenced by the GnRH antagonist. Whether this relative refractoriness to exogenous stimulation in some females is at the receptor or humoral level remains to be determined.

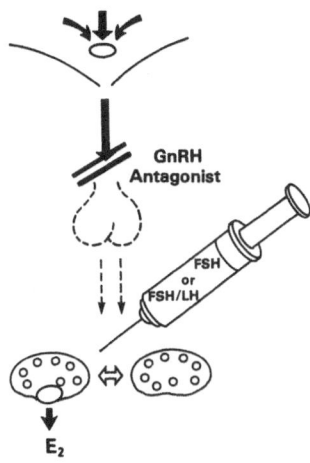

Fig. 14. Medical hypophysectomy. Reasoning
that individual variability of response may
be imparted from the hypothalamus, pituitary
and ovaries, the GnRH antagonist negates
both inhibitory and stimulatory central
factors, leaving only the variation intrin-
sic to the ovaries.

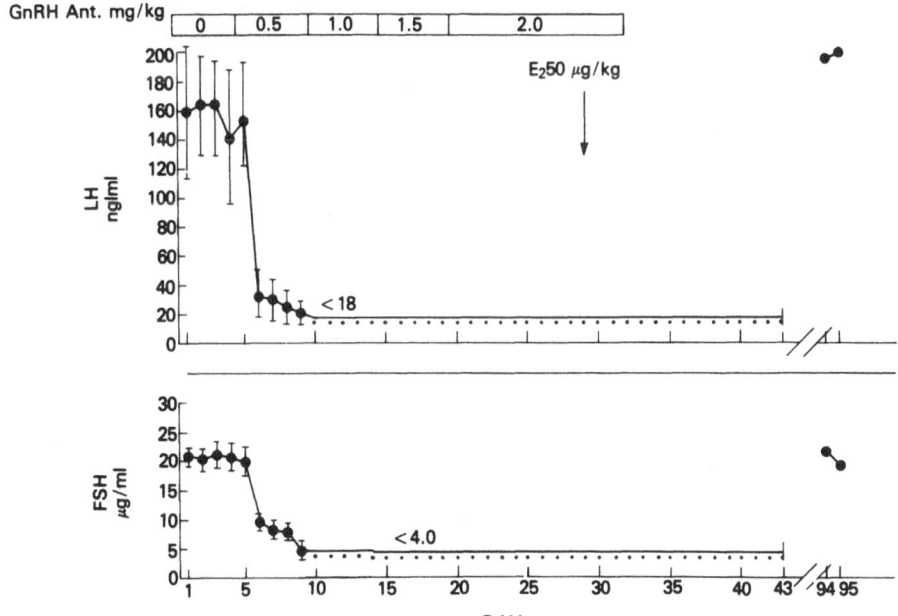

Fig. 15. Plasma LH and FSH values (mean ± SE) in 3 long-term
castrate female monkeys treated with GnRH antagonist
[(Ac-pClPhe[1],pClDPhe[2],DTrp[3],DArg[6],Dala[10])-GnRH-HCl] in increasing doses producing suppression of FSH and LH levels in serum to
or below limits of assay detection. Subjects did not respond to
an estrogen challenge test. Note full recovery of gonadotropin
secretion by 2 months after cessation of treatment (36).

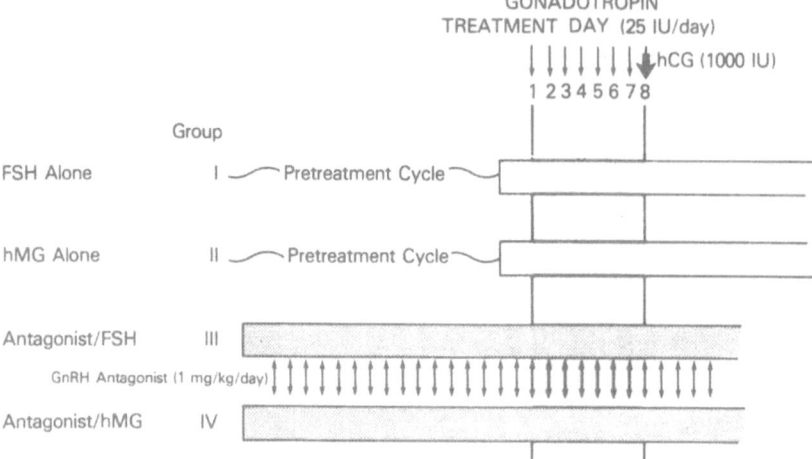

Fig. 16. Protocol for previously normal ovulatory monkeys, Groups I-IV. All subjects entered study on cycle day 3. Groups I and II received no pretreatment with GnRH antagonist; therefore, gonadotropin treatment day 1 corresponds to cycle day 3. Groups III and IV received pretreatment and concurrent treatment with the GnRH antagonist beginning on cycle day 3. For an interval of 17 days (cycle day 3-18), pretreatment with GnRH antagonist was given alone. While continuing GnRH antagonist therapy, gonadotropin treatment day 1 corresponds to cycle day 19. In all groups, FSH or hMG (25 IU/day) was given for 7 consecutive days followed by hCG 1000 IU on the 8th day. Thus, days are normalized and referred to as "Gonadotropin Treatment Days 1-8" in all groups. See Figure 17 (36).

It should be appreciated that unlike the clinical situation, the fixed protocols employed here allowed for the nonresponders not to receive more exogenous gonadotropin or, the high responders to receive less exogenous gonadotropin than others in the study, thus permitting comparison of like-treated individuals in all groups. In all likelihood, even greater conformity of subject response could be obtained with daily gonadotropin dose adjustments.

Another important finding in these experiments concerns the comparison of the different exogenous gonadotropin preparations. Here, "pure" urinary FSH was compared to a mixture of urinary FSH and LH (hMG) of even proportions. Regardless of whether GnRH antagonist was added, there was equal responsiveness of FSH alone versus hMG-treated monkeys. This is in contrast to studies in women with pituitary FSH preparations for ovulation induction which indicated lower E_2 responses when FSH was administered alone, compared to urinary preparations containing both FSH with LH (24-26). These older studies could be interpreted as supporting evidence of the two-cell theory, i.e., LH was deficient. Alternatively, the results may have been influenced by the shorter circulatory half-life of pituitary FSH compared to the longer-acting FSH entities extracted from postmenopausal urine (37).

In these primate experiments, we have also shown that "pure" FSH of urinary origin is capable of stimulating ovarian E_2 secretion at a level not dissimilar from that obtained by the same dose of a urinary hMG preparation, containing an equal ratio of FSH to LH. Furthermore, we have demonstrated undiminished ovarian estradiol production when "pure" FSH was

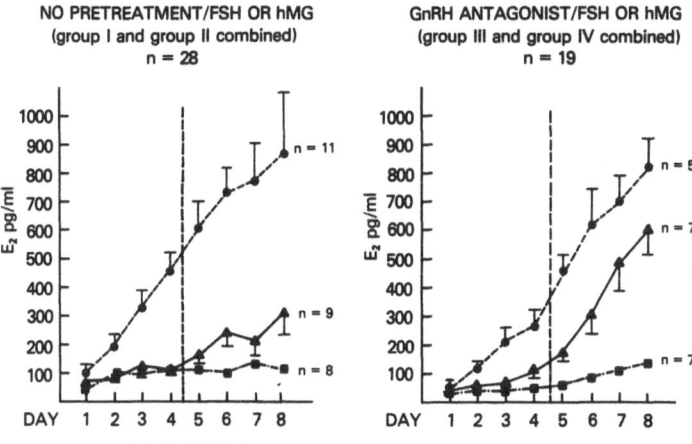

NO PRETREATMENT/FSH OR hMG
(group I and group II combined)
n = 28

GnRH ANTAGONIST/FSH OR hMG
(group III and group IV combined)
n = 19

Fig. 17. Panels represent the composite of Groups I and II versus Groups III and IV; i.e., those that did not receive and those that did receive pretreatment and concurrent treatment with the GnRH antagonist. Among responders, area under the curve (AUC) computations for days 1-4 and days 5-8 (comparing fast and slow responders analysis of variance and Kramer's modification of Duncan's multiple range test) showed a significant difference (P<0.05) between those not treated with GnRH antagonist; however, there was no significant difference (P<0.05) between responses during treatment with the GnRH antagonist. Note n equals the number of subjects for AUC analysis, whereas the number of subjects comprising daily mean E_2 values may be greater. Coefficients of variation among responders for total AUC, in Groups I-IV, were 63.1, 70.5, 43.1, and 28.3, respectively. Without GnRH antagonist (Groups I and II) or gonadotropin treatment with GnRH antagonist (Groups III and IV), the AUC coefficients of variation were 69.0 and 47.9, respectively. Thus, the GnRH antagonist significantly reduced variation of the estrogen response pattern among responding females (36).

administered in the presence of a GnRH antagonist that maintained a relative hypogonadotropic state, as regards endogenous gonadotropin secretion (Fig. 18). This does not necessarily negate the two-cell theory of ovarian steroidogenesis; however, it does open to question the previous assumptions about the relative importance of FSH and LH. In the primate ovarian cycle, it would seem that FSH is of far greater significance.

Early progesterone rise. Recent studies (38) have described a rise of plasma progesterone up to 12 h prior to initiation of the LH surge in the normal human menstrual cycle. That this progesterone elevation occurs in the absence of perceptible changes in the endogenous LH pulse amplitude or frequency may implicate an independent intraovarian mechanism that begins to shift ovarian steroidogenesis and/or secretion toward progesterone, even before initiation of the LH surge.

Collins et al. (39) used monkeys in an attempt to mimic the hyperstimulation seen among some patients who show a marked sensitivity to hMG (FSH and LH) preparation. These patients have a very early and sustained rise in serum estradiol levels. Of 16 monkeys achieving an estradiol level of 1000 pg/ml, 5 had serum progesterone values of 2 to 8

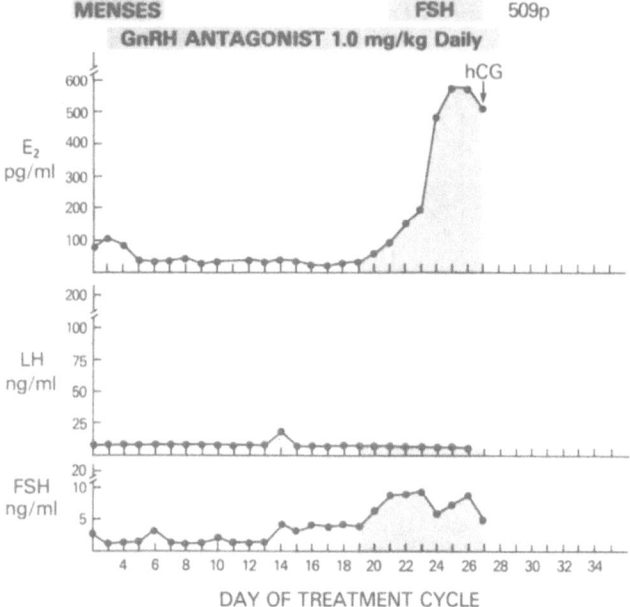

MENSES   FSH   509p

GnRH ANTAGONIST 1.0 mg/kg Daily

DAY OF TREATMENT CYCLE

Fig. 18. GnRH antagonist [(Ac-pClPhe^1,pClDhe^2,DTryp^3,DArg^6,DAla^{10})-GnRH HCl] followed by FSH therapy in intact cycling monkeys. Note suppression of endogenous gonadotropin secretion and ovarian responsiveness to FSH treatments, as indicated by elevations of estradiol (E$_2$) in serum (36).

ng/ml as much as one week prior to an LH surge. This has yet to be explored in humans, but it is suggestive that the LH component of the hMG might cause premature luteinization.

Two monkeys treated with "pure" FSH in the presence of the GnRH antagonist (36) with barely detectable LH in plasma, also had serum progesterone elevations as much as 4 days prior to hMG treatment and without an endogenous LH surge. This observation may fit with a growing body of evidence that steroidogenic shifts to progesterone can be initiated by intraovarian events, therein usurping onset of the LH surge as the initiator of these events.

Future Considerations

The new experiences gained from the familiarities of IVF/ET procedures have led to a reexamination of the physiology of the ovary and preimplantation embryo. The previously described experiments with ovulation induction suggest that newer gonadotropin preparations, with a greater emphasis on FSH, could improve the quality of ovarian stimulation. Adjunctive treatments, such as with a GnRH antagonist, offer hope that greater control and efficiency can be gained in ovulation induction by reducing the confounding problem of individual variation in response to treatment with gonadotropins.

Among the most important developments would be the technical know-how to mature the oocyte in vitro. That is, to harvest from the ovary dictyate stage oocytes for storage and subsequent maturation in an "in vitro

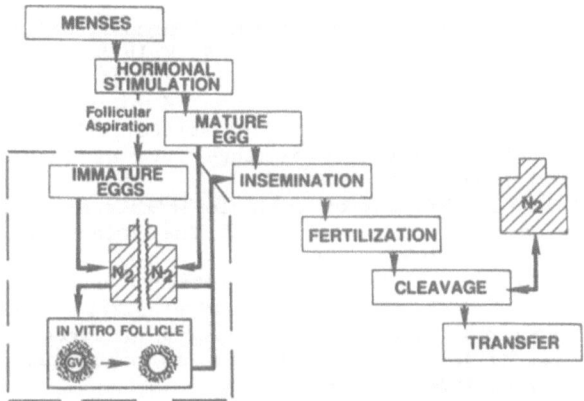

Fig. 19. Illustration of the ongoing effort to develop techniques which would permit maturation of oocytes in an "in vitro follicle."

follicle" (Fig. 19). This achievement would avert numerous ethical and legal dilemmas presented by the storage of human embryos.

A renewal of interest in intraovarian factors that affect the growth of follicles locally and feedback on the hypothalamic-pituitary axis distally has developed. In the setting of treating infertility, a greater understanding of the mechanisms involved in follicular:oocyte well-being will enhance the efficiency of IVF/ET therapies. Of equal importance is the potential for inhibition of follicular maturation and/or LH surges for contraceptive therapy by way of previously uncharacterized ovarian factors.

Now that follicular fluid, oocytes, and embryos are being observed with great frequency, this increased scrutiny can provide a better understanding of the impact of oocyte quality on early embryonic normality/abnormality. This has far-reaching implications in cytogenetics for both prenatal embryonic diagnosis and DNA therapy in the future.

REFERENCES

1. diZerega GS, Hodgen GD. Folliculogenesis in the primate ovarian cycle. Endocr Rev 1981; 2:27.
2. diZerega GS, Hodgen GD. Initiation of asymmetrical ovarian estradiol secretion in the primate ovarian cycle after luteectomy. Endocrinology 1981; 108:1233.
3. diZerega GS, Hodgen GD. Luteal phase dysfunction infertility a sequel to aberrant folliculogenesis. Fertil Steril 1981; 35:489.
4. Hodgen GD. In vitro fertilization and alternatives. JAMA 1981; 246:590.
5. Williams RF, Hodgen GD. Initiation of the primate ovarian cycle with emphasis on perimenarchial and postpartum events. In: Greep RO, ed. Reproductive physiology IV. Baltimore: University Park Press, 1983:1-55.
6. Hodgen GD. The dominant ovarian follicle. Fertil Steril 1982; 38:281.
7. Goodman AL, Hodgen GD. The ovarian triad of the primate menstrual cycle. Recent Prog Horm Res 1983; 39:1.
8. Brambell FWR. In: Parkes AS, ed. Marshall's physiology of

reproduction; vol 1, part 1. New York: Longmans, Green, 1956:397.

9. Harrison RJ, Weir BJ. In: Zuckerman S, Weir BJ, eds. The ovary; vol 1, 2nd ed. New York: Academic Press, 1977:113.

10. Schwartz NB. The role of FSH and LH and of their antibodies on follicle growth and on ovulation. Biol Reprod 1974; 10:236.

11. Pedersen T. Follicle kinetics in the ovary of the cyclic mouse. Acta Endocrinol (Copenh) 1970; 64:304.

12. Hertz R, Hisaw FL. Effects of follicle-stimulating and luteinizing pituitary extracts on the ovaries of the infantile and juvenile rabbit. Am J Physiol 1934; 108:1.

13. Lunenfeld B, Kraiem Z, Eshkol A. Structure and function of the growing follicle. Clin Obstet Gynecol 1976; 3:27.

14. Goodman AL, Hodgen GD. Postpartum patterns of circulating FSH, LH, prolactin, estradiol and progesterone in nonsuckling cynomolgus monkeys. Steroids 1978; 31:731.

15. Schenken RS, Hodgen GD. FSH induced ovarian hyperstimulation in monkeys: blockade of the LH surge. J Clin Endocrinol Metab 1983; 57:50-5.

16. Hodgen GD. Oocyte transfer and fertilization in vivo. In: Crosignini PG, Rubin BL, eds. In vitro fertilization and embryo transfer. Serono Symposia, 1983; 47:126.

17. Garcia JE, Jones GS, Acosta AA, Wright A. Human menopausal gonadotropin/human chorionic gonadotropin follicular maturation for oocyte aspiration: phase II, 1981. Fertil Steril 1983; 39:157.

18. Laufer N, DeCherney AH, Hazeltine FP, et al. The use of high-dose human menopausal gonadotropin in an in vitro fertilization program. Fertil Steril 1983; 40:734.

19. Hodgen GD, Channing CP, Anderson LD, Gagliano P, Turner CK, Stouffer RL. On the regulation of FSH secretion in the primate hypothalamic-pituitary-ovarian axis. In: Cumming IA, Funder JW, Mendelson FAO, eds. Proceedings of the sixth international congress of endocrinology. Amsterdam: Elseiver/North Holland Biomedical Press, 1980:263.

20. Rettori V, Siler-Khodr TM, Pauerstein CJ, Smith CG, Asch RH. Effects of porcine follicular fluid on gonadotropin concentrations in rhesus monkeys. J Clin Endocrinol Metab 1982; 54:500.

21. Williams RF, Hodgen GD. Disparate effects of human chorionic gonadotropin during the late follicular phase in monkeys: normal ovulation, follicular atresia, ovarian acyclicity, and hypersecretion of follicle stimulating hormone. Fertil Steril 1980; 33:64.

22. Short RV. Steroids in the follicular fluid and the corpus luteum of the mare. A "two-cell type" theory of ovarian steroid synthesis. J Endocrinol 1962; 24:59.

23. Ryan KJ, Petro Z, Kaiser J. Steroid formation by isolated and recombined ovarian granulosa and theca cells. J Clin Endocrinol Metab 1968; 28:355.

24. Jacobson A, Marshall JR. Ovulatory response rate with human menopausal gonadotropins of varying FSH-LH ratios. Fertil Steril 1969; 20:171.

25. Jewelewicz R, Warren M, Dyrenfurth I, Vende Wiele RL. Physiological studies with purified human pituitary FSH LH-FSH. J Clin Endocrinol Metab 1971; 32:688.

26. Berger MJ, Taymor ML, Karam K, Nudemberg F. The relative roles of exogenous and endogenous FSH and LH in human follicular maturation and ovulation induction. Fertil Steril 1972; 23:783.

27. Jones HW, Jones GS (Personal Communication), 1983.

28. Wentz AC. Obstet and Gynecol Survey 1983; 38:49.

29. Jones GS, Ruehsen MDM, Johanson AJ, Raiti S, Blizzard RM. Elucidation of normal ovarian physiology by exogenous gonadotropin stimulation following steroid pituitary suppression. Fertil Steril 1969; 20:14.

30. Fleming R, Adam AH, Barlow DH, Black WP, MacNaughton MC, Coutts JRT.

A new systematic treatment for infertile women with abnormal hormone profiles. Br J Obstet Gynaecol 1982; 89:80.

31. Schmidt-Gollwitzer M, Hardt W, Schmidt-Gollwitzer K, von der Ohe M, Nevinney-Stickel J. Influence on the LH–RH analog buserelin on cyclic ovarian function and on the endometrium. A new approach to fertility control? Contraception 1981; 23:187–95.

32. Werlin LB, Hodgen GD. Gonadotropin-releasing hormone agonist suppresses ovulation, menses, and endometriosis in monkeys: an individualized, intermittent regimen. J Clin Endocrinol Metab 1983; 56:844.

33. Richards JS. Maturation of ovarian follicles: actions and interactions of pituitary and ovarian hormones on follicular cell differentiation. Physiol Rev 1980; 60:51.

34. Asch RH, Sickle MV, Rettori V, et al. Absence of LH–RH binding sites in corpora luteal from rhesus monkeys (Macaca mulatta). J Clin Endocrinol Metab 1981; 53:215.

35. Clayton RN, Huhtaniemi IT. Absence of gonadotropin-releasing hormone receptors in human gonadal tissue. Nature 1982; 299:56.

36. Kenigsberg D, Littman BA, Williams RF, Hodgen GD. Medical hypophysectomy. II: Variability of ovarian response to exogenous gonadotropins. Fertil Steril 1984; 42:116.

37. Mancuso S, Dell'Acqua S, Donini P, Menini E, Bompiani A. Disappearance rate, urinary excretion and effect on ovarian steroidogenesis of highly purified urinary FSH, administered to a hypophysectomized woman. In: Bettendorf G, Insler V, eds. Clinical application of human gonadotropins. Stuttgart: G. Thieme Verlag, 1970:151–9.

38. Hoff JD, Quigley ME, Yen SSC. Hormonal dynamics at midcycle: a reevaluation. J Clin Endocrinol Metab 1983; 57:792.

39. Collins RL, Williams RF, Hodgen GD. Endocrine consequences of prolonged ovarian hyperstimulation: hyperprolactinemia, follicular atresia and premature luteinization. Fertil Steril 1984; 42:436.

40. Falck B. Site of production of oestrogen in rat ovary as studied in micro-transplants. Acta Physiol Scand 1959; 47(suppl 163).

III. CORPUS LUTEUM FUNCTION

LUTEOTROPIC ACTIONS OF LH ON THE MACAQUE CORPUS LUTEUM

Anthony J. Zeleznik and James Hutchison

Department of Physiology and OB/GYN
University of Pittsburgh School of Medicine
Pittsburgh, PA 15213

INTRODUCTION

The primate corpus luteum of the menstrual cycle secretes progesterone for 14-16 days after ovulation in the absence of an implanted
conceptus (1). In fertile cycles, the luteal life span is prolonged by
the secretion of chorionic gonadotropin by the trophoblast (2). In view
of its absolute requirement for implantation and early gestation, specific
knowledge of the regulation of the corpus luteum is important for effective control of fertility as well as correcting the pathophysiological
conditions of short and inadequate luteal phases.

In vitro studies using dispersed luteal cells and homogenates of
luteal tissue have clearly demonstrated that the corpus luteum produces
progesterone in response to LH and hCG and that this effector system is
regulated through a cell surface receptor/adenylate cyclase system (3,4).
Despite this well-established in vitro role of LH in stimulating progesterone secretion by the corpus luteum, there are conflicting views with
regard to the actual role LH plays in the regulation of progesterone
secretion and the life span of the corpus luteum in vivo (5-7). We
initiated the current work to define the role of LH during the primate
luteal phase with respect to progesterone secretion as well as its
involvement in the life span of the corpus luteum.

EXPERIMENTAL MODEL

For these studies we adopted the experimental model developed by
Knobil and colleagues (8) for the investigation of the regulation of
pituitary gonadotropin secretion and extended its application to study the
control of ovarian function. We used adult female rhesus monkeys whose
endogenous control of gonadotropin secretion was blocked by either the
placement of radiofrequency lesions in the arcuate region of the medial
basal hypothalamus (MBH) or transection of the hypothalamic-pituitary
stalk (9,10). In these animals endogenous gonadotropin secretion is
re-established and menstrual cyclicity is restored by intravenous replacement of exogenous, synthetic GnRH. With this model system, the absolute
pattern of pituitary gonadotropin secretion may be controlled directly by
the pattern by which GnRH is administered. In all studies, follicular
growth and ovulation were stimulated using a standard infusion regimen of

GnRH which is one 6-minute pulse every h which delivers GnRH at a rate of 1.25 µg/min (6 µg per pulse) as described previously (11). Details regarding modifications of this infusion regimen during the luteal phases of experimental cycles are presented in the figure legends.

ROLE OF LH IN PRODUCTION OF PROGESTERONE BY THE CORPUS LUTEUM

We investigated the role of LH in luteal progesterone production by terminating the GnRH infusion, hence pituitary LH secretion, during either the early or midluteal phase of the menstrual cycle and examined the consequences on serum progesterone concentrations (11). Results in Figure 1 (top panel) demonstrate, as described previously by Knobil and colleagues (8), that maintenance of rhesus monkeys on a fixed regimen of GnRH of 1 pulse per h results in luteal phases of 14-16 days duration which are indistinguishable from spontaneous luteal phases. When LH secretion was stopped by terminating the GnRH infusion on day 3 of the luteal phase (Figure 1, bottom panel), the rise in serum progesterone concentrations was terminated abruptly and all animals menstruated prematurely. In the absence of LH, progesterone concentrations remained undetectable throughout the entire expected duration of the luteal phase.

As shown in Figure 2, terminating the GnRH infusion (hence, pituitary LH secretion) during the midluteal phase also resulted in a prompt fall in serum progesterone and premature menstruation in all animals.

These findings provide conclusive evidence that progesterone secretion by the corpus luteum is absolutely dependent upon pituitary gonadotropins during both the early and midluteal phases of the menstrual cycle.

ROLE OF LH IN THE LIFE SPAN OF THE CORPUS LUTEUM

The results of the foregoing studies clearly show that the production of progesterone by the corpus luteum requires LH. In addition, the observation of premature menses in every animal upon curtailment of LH secretion would appear to indicate that the functional 14-17 day life span of the corpus luteum is also under the direct control of LH. However, it is not known if the cessation of progesterone secretion by the corpus luteum is equivalent to an irreversible loss of luteal function. To investigate whether the 14-16 day life span of the corpus luteum is dependent upon LH, we imposed a 3-day interruption of gonadotropic support to the corpus luteum by stopping and then reinitiating the GnRH infusion during the early, mid, and late luteal phase of the menstrual cycle (12).

Figure 3 illustrates the results of studies in which the GnRH infusion was interrupted during days 2-5 of the luteal phase. Similar to that shown in Figure 1, upon termination of the GnRH infusion there was an abrupt fall in serum LH and progesterone concentrations. The concentrations of LH and progesterone fell to below the limits of detectability of our RIAs (less than 0.2 ng/ml) during the period of GnRH withdrawal. Upon reinitiation of the GnRH infusion on day 5, there was an abrupt rise in serum LH concentrations, and progesterone concentrations increased significantly within 12 h. Thereafter the daily pattern of serum progesterone concentrations as well as the occurrence of menses was similar among both control and experimental animals.

Figure 4 shows the results of interrupting LH secretion for 3 days during the midluteal phase (days 8-11) of the menstrual cycle. Within 12 h after stopping the GnRH infusion, LH and progesterone concentrations

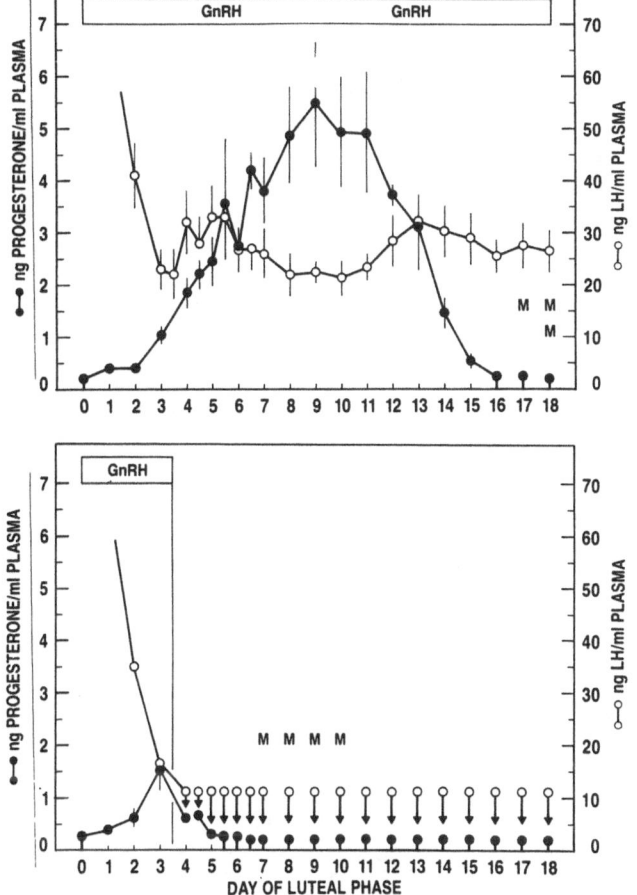

Fig. 1. Effects of terminating the GnRH infusion during the early luteal phase. The upper panel shows daily plasma progesterone and LH concentrations during control luteal phases in 4 MBH-lesioned monkeys receiving exogenous GnRH at a frequency of 1 pulse per h throughout the menstrual cycle. The lower panel shows plasma progesterone and LH concentrations in 4 MBH-lesioned monkeys when the GnRH infusion was terminated on day 3 of the luteal phase. Downward arrows from LH points and heavy vertical lines below progesterone points designate values below the sensitivities of the RIAs. The letter M indicates the first day of menses for each monkey (11).

were reduced significantly and remained below the limits of detectability throughout the 3-day period during which GnRH was withheld. However, restoring LH secretion by resuming the GnRH infusion in day 11 was followed by a resumption in progesterone secretion. Progesterone concentrations during the initial 36 h following the restoration of GnRH were approximately 40% of that seen at comparable times of control cycles. Thereafter the daily pattern of progesterone concentrations was indistinguishable from those of control cycles. Although premature menses was

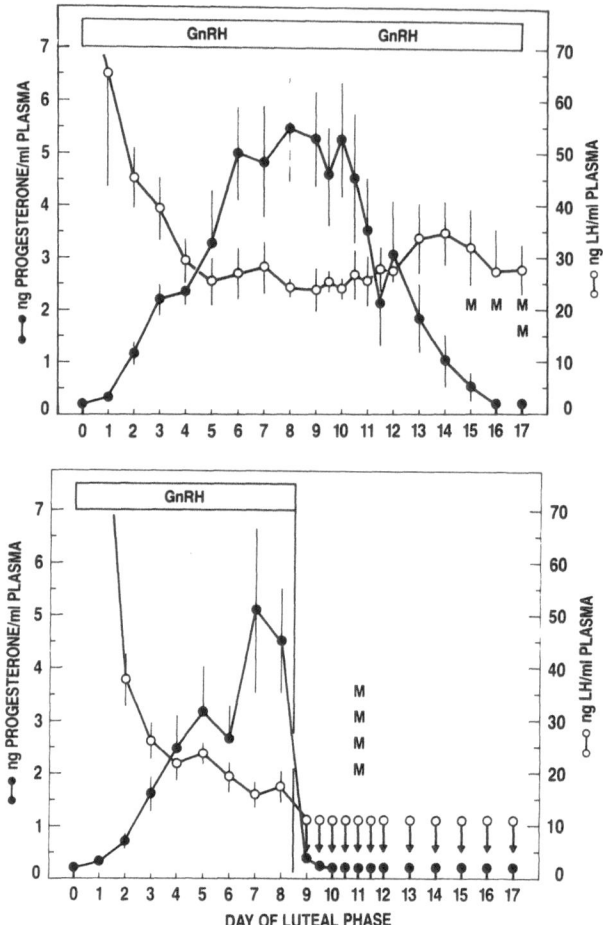

Fig. 2. Effects of terminating the GnRH
infusion during the midluteal phase. The
upper panel illustrates serum progesterone and
LH concentrations in control cycles. The
bottom panel illustrates serum progesterone
and LH concentrations in monkeys when the GnRH
infusion was terminated on day 8. See legend
to Figure 1 for details. Reproduced from
reference 11 with permission.

evident in 3 of 4 animals, renewed progesterone production was evident in
all animals and the duration of progesterone secretion, measured from the
time of ovulation, was similar in control and experimental animals. Thus,
the 14- to 16-day "luteal clock" continued to run despite a 3-day
withdrawal of LH.

It is obvious from data shown in Figures 3 and 4 that the restoration
of GnRH resulted in acute increases in plasma LH concentrations which were
3-5 times greater than those seen during control cycles. To determine
whether the restoration of luteal function was due solely to the height-
ened LH response following reinitiation of the GnRH infusion, we performed
a third study in which GnRH was withdrawn on day 13 and reinitiated on day
16, the expected time of luteal regression. Results in Figure 5 show that

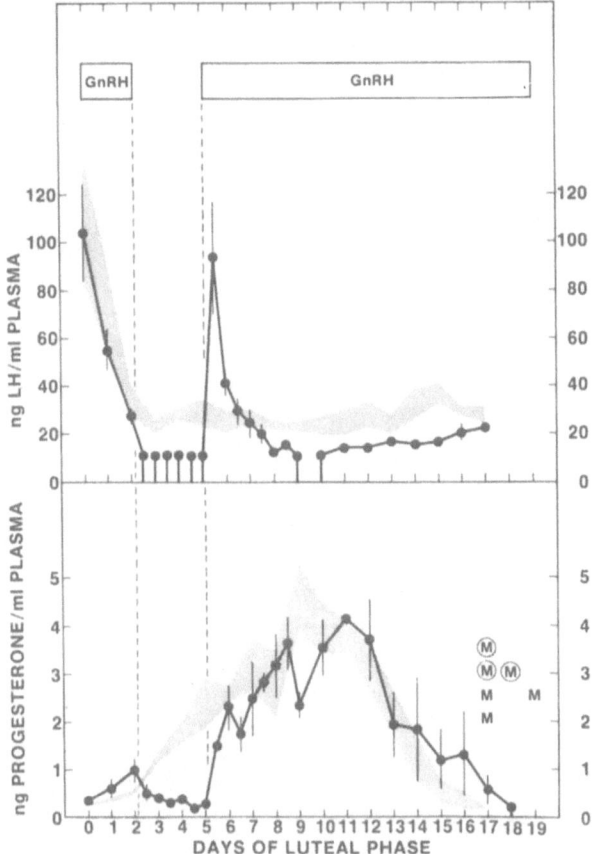

Fig. 3. Effects of a transient withdrawal of gonadotropic support during the early luteal phase. The upper panel shows LH concentrations and the lower panel shows progesterone concentrations in control and experimental animals. The shaded areas encompass 1 standard error about the mean of hormone concentrations during control cycles in which the GnRH infusion was maintained at 1 pulse per h throughout the menstrual cycle. The solid lines illustrate daily and bidaily hormone concentrations in experimental cycles in which the GnRH infusion was stopped and then reinitiated on day 5. M stands for the first day of menses in experimental cycles. Reproduced from reference 12 with permission.

although there was a large rise in LH concentrations following the reinitiation of GnRH treatment on day 16, the corpus luteum failed to respond with an increase in progesterone secretion.

These results demonstrate that although progesterone secretion is absolutely dependent upon the presence of LH, the maintenance of the functional capacity of the corpus luteum to produce progesterone is less dependent upon LH. Thus, it appears that there may be separate and perhaps independent regulatory mechanisms involved in the acute control of

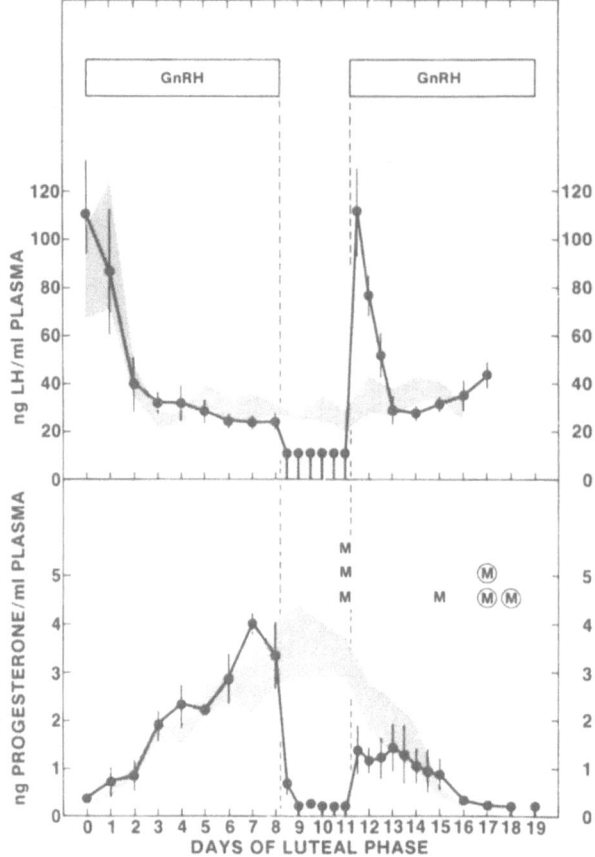

Fig. 4. Effects of a transient withdrawal of gonadotropic support during the midluteal phase. Details are the same as in Figure 3. In experimental cycles, the GnRH infusion was stopped on day 8 and reinitiated on day 11. Reproduced from reference 12 with permission.

steroid production by the corpus luteum and the maintenance of the 14- to 16-day life span of the corpus luteum.

ARE CHANGES IN LH SECRETION CAUSAL TO THE ONSET OF SPONTANEOUS LUTEOLYSIS?

Results shown in the previous sections indicate that luteal steroidogenesis is absolutely dependent upon LH. In view of these findings, it is of interest to determine whether the fall in luteal steroidogenesis which accompanies luteal regression could be due to alterations in pituitary LH secretion. Recent studies in both humans and macaques have shown that a dramatic decrease in the frequency of LH pulses occurs during the mid to late luteal phase which coincides with the declining progesterone concentrations associated with luteal regression (13,14).

To answer this question we conducted a study in which a GnRH pulse frequency like that seen during the late luteal phase (1 pulse every 8 h)

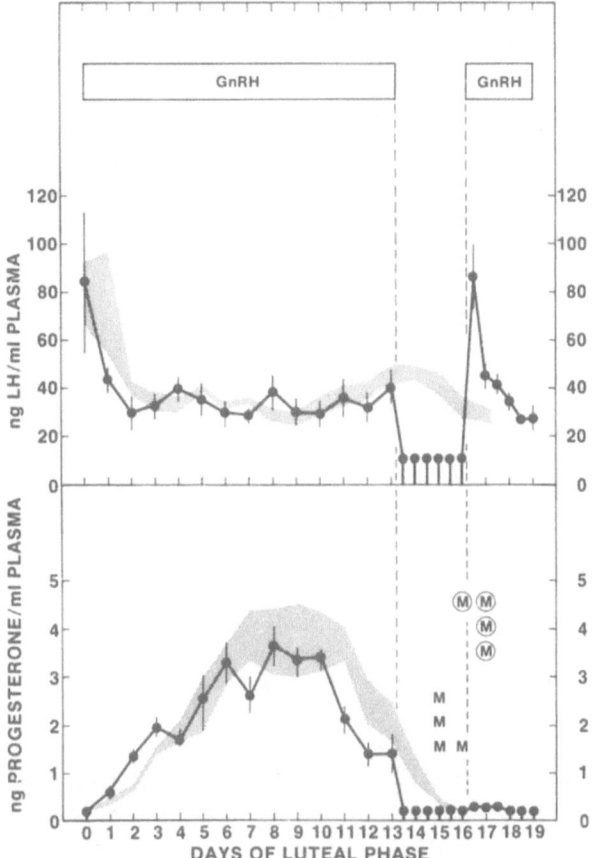

Fig. 5. Effect of a transient withdrawal of gonadotropic support during the late luteal phase. Details are the same as in Figure 3. In experimental cycles, the GnRH infusion was stopped on day 13 and reinitiated on day 16.

was initiated shortly after ovulation (15). We examined the pattern of progesterone and the onset of luteal regression in the presence of this slow pulse frequency. If a change in LH pulse frequency could be causal to luteal regression, we would expect to observe premature luteal regression in the presence of a slow LH pulse frequency. Figure 6 illustrates daily serum progesterone concentrations in 4 rhesus monkeys in which the GnRH, hence LH, pulse frequency was changed from 1 pulse per h to 1 pulse per 8 h on day 3 of the luteal phase. Despite the imposition of this slow LH pulse frequency very early in the luteal phase, serum progesterone concentrations progressively rose to typical midluteal phase concentrations and 3 of 4 animals had luteal phases of normal duration.

Thus, it appears that the major alteration in LH secretion that occurs during the mid to late luteal phase in itself is not causal to the onset of luteolysis. Further, our observations and those of others (8) that luteal phases of normal duration also occur in the presence of a rapid (1 per h) pulse frequency strongly suggest that spontaneous luteal regression is not due to an alteration in pulsatile LH secretion.

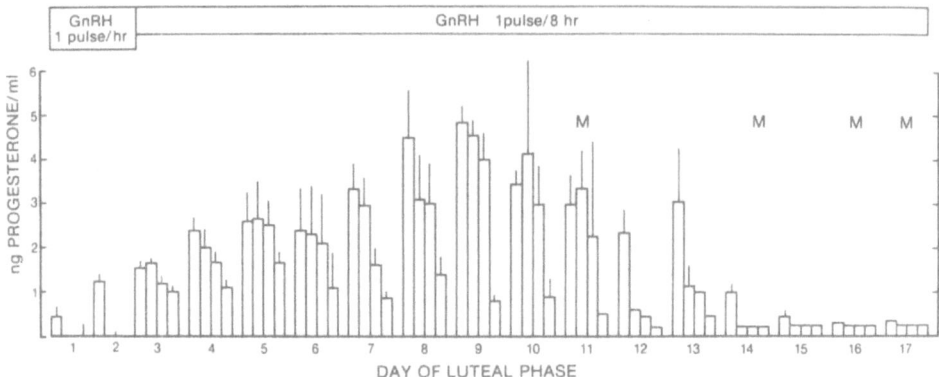

Fig. 6. Daily plasma progesterone concentrations during the luteal phase of the menstrual cycle in animals whose GnRH pulse frequency was changed to 1 pulse per 8 h on day 3 of the luteal phase. The individual bars over each day reflect plasma progesterone concentrations obtained 30, 60, 120, and 240 min after the morning GnRH pulse. The letter M denotes the day of menses in each of 4 animals. Reproduced from reference 15 with permission.

SITE OF ACTION AND POSSIBLE ROLE OF ESTROGEN IN INITIATING LUTEAL REGRESSION

Administration of estrogen or its synthetic agonist diethylstilbestrol during the luteal phase of humans and nonhuman primates causes premature luteal regression (16,17). The possibility that estrogen is an endogenous luteolysin is attractive in view of the temporal association between rising concentrations of estrogen in luteal tissue and blood and the onset of spontaneous luteal regression in nonfertile cycles (18,19). However, this hypothesis has been questioned because neither the administration of aromatase inhibitor (20) nor estrogen antagonists (21,22) prolong the functional life span of the corpus luteum. In addition to uncertainties regarding the physiological role of estrogen-induced luteolysis, the site of action of estradiol (hypothalamic-pituitary axis or directly at the ovary) is uncertain (23,24).

We investigated the phenomenon of estrogen-induced luteolysis in GnRH treated rhesus monkeys in an attempt to determine the site of action of estrogen in causing luteal regression as well as to provide information regarding estrogen's role as a physiological luteolysin.

Figure 7 shows the effects of estrogen administration to rhesus monkeys whose gonadotropin secretion was maintained by pulsatile infusion of exogenous GnRH at a frequency of 1 pulse per h (25). Placement of estrogen-containing Silastic capsules on day 6 of the luteal phase produced plasma estradiol concentrations of approximately 150 pg/ml, within the range of other studies which demonstrated estrogen-induced luteolysis (23). Immediately following the insertion of estrogen capsules, there was a transient fall in serum LH and progesterone concentrations. However, progesterone concentrations rose to normal values within 4 days after insertion of capsules and thereafter were similar to control (nonestrogen-treated) animals.

In additional studies, the effects of estrogen were studied in animals where GnRH pulse frequency was set at 1 pulse per 8 h to determine if estrogen would cause luteal regression in the presence of a slow LH

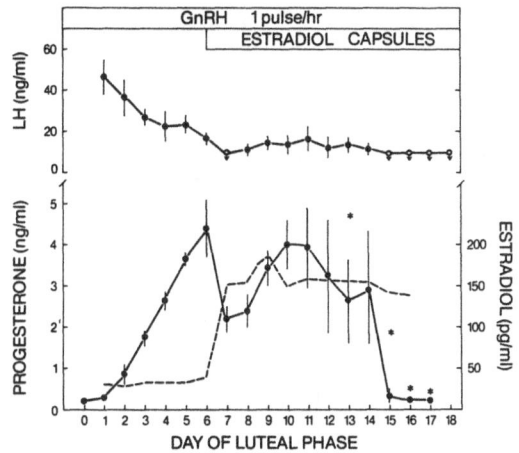

Fig. 7. Effect of exogenous estradiol on corpus luteum function in menstrual cycles driven by exogenous GnRH at a pulse frequency of 1 pulse per h. Estradiol capsules were inserted subcutaneously on day 6 of the luteal phase. The upper panel shows plasma LH concentrations. The lower panel shows plasma progesterone concentrations (solid line) and estradiol concentrations (interrupted line) [n = 4].

pulse frequency like that seen during the mid to late luteal phase. Again, as shown in Figure 8, estrogen did not cause premature luteolysis, even in the presence of a reduced LH pulse frequency.

These findings indicate that estrogen does not cause luteolysis by acting directly at the level of the ovary. If the ovary was the site of action of estrogen, we would have expected to observe premature luteolysis in these studies. The findings also appear to rule out a pituitary site of action of estrogen because estrogen failed to cause luteolysis when exogenous GnRH was provided. By exclusion, we therefore conclude that the primary means by which estrogen promotes luteal regression is through its effects on GnRH secretion by the hypothalamus.

SUMMARY

The two goals of this research were to elucidate the roles of LH in the control of progesterone secretion by the corpus luteum and on the regulation of its 14- to 16-day life span. With respect to the first issue, our results clearly demonstrate that the acute regulation of progesterone production is absolutely dependent upon LH. These findings are consistent with studies in which the dynamics of LH secretion were correlated with those of progesterone secretion during the luteal phase (14). In these studies, it was shown that during the mid to late luteal phase when the LH pulse frequency is reduced to 1 pulse per 4 to 8 h, there is nearly a 1:1 concordance between LH pulses and secretory episodes of progesterone secretion.

The second issue, whether LH is involved in the regulation of the life span of the corpus luteum and spontaneous luteal regression, is likely not to have a simple solution. Our results show that total

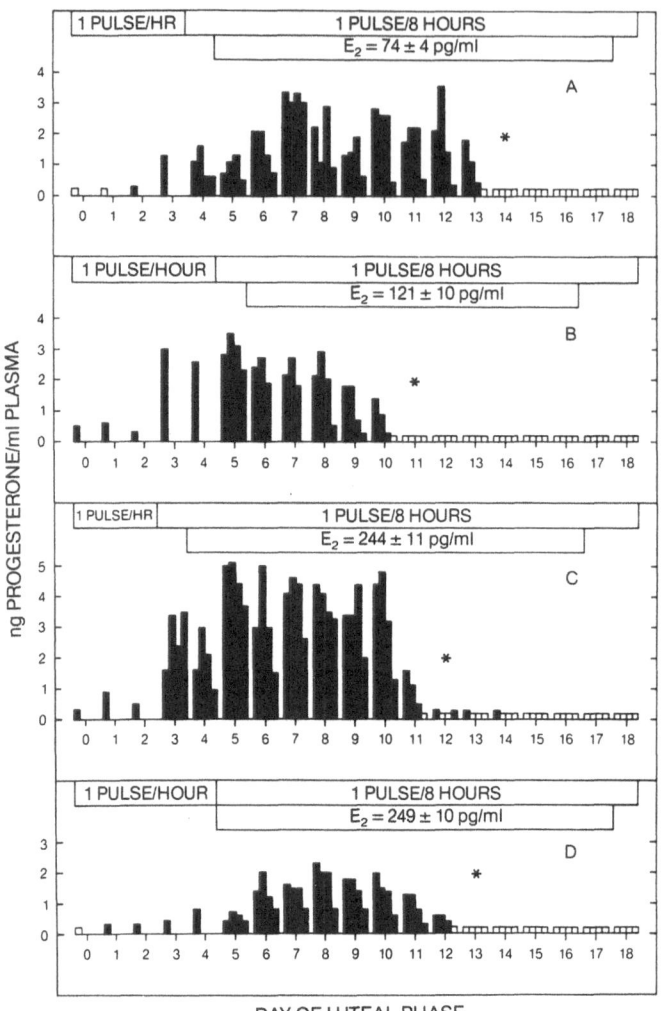

Fig. 8. Effect of exogenous estradiol on corpus luteum function in menstrual cycles driven by exogenous GnRH at a pulse frequency of 1 pulse per 8 h. Each panel (A-D) shows data from individual animals. Following insertion of estradiol implants, blood samples were removed 30, 60, 120, and 240 min after the morning GnRH pulse. Daily progesterone concentrations are presented as a group of 4 bars representing values obtained at the respective times. The asterisks represent the day plasma progesterone concentrations fell to values below the limit of detectability (<0.2 ng/ml). Reproduced from reference 25 with permission.

deprivation of LH results in premature menstruation which is consistent with the notion that LH plays an important role in maintenance of the life span of the corpus luteum. Further, it is well known that the LH-like placental hormone, chorionic gonadotropin, is capable of extending the life span of the corpus luteum well beyond 14-16 days (26).

On the basis of the aforementioned findings, it would not be unreasonable to conclude that LH plays an important role in the maintenance of the life span of the corpus luteum. On the other hand, our data also indicate that changes in LH secretion like those seen during the spontaneous luteal phase do not cause luteal regression. These observations indicate that although LH is important for luteal steroidogenesis, luteal regression may occur independent of changes in LH secretion. In this regard, the notion of a 14-day "luteal clock" which runs to some extent independently of luteal steroid production, could account for our data, especially the studies in which a 3-day withdrawal of gonadotropin secretion neither shortened nor lengthened the life span of the corpus luteum. Thus, in this situation, the "clock" continued to run despite the fact that steroid production was curtailed.

The obvious key to understanding the cause of luteal regression will be to determine whether the demise of the corpus luteum is a process akin to aging in which the activity of biologically important metabolic pathways decline with finite half-lives or whether luteolysis is an active process mediated by local secretion or internal production of luteolytic agents. Our finding that estrogen fails to cause luteal regression in the presence of exogenous GnRH appears to rule out a local luteolytic role of estrogen. Whether other agents such as prostaglandins or ovarian peptides (27,28) play a physiological role on the onset of luteal regression remains to be determined.

REFERENCES

1. Knobil E. On the regulation of the primate corpus luteum. Biol Reprod 1973; 8:246-58.
2. Atkinson LE, Hotchkiss J, Fritz GR, Surve AH, Neill JD, Knobil E. Circulating levels of steroids and chorionic gonadotropin during pregnancy in the rhesus monkey with special attention to the rescue of the corpus luteum in early pregnancy. Biol Reprod 1975; 12:335-45.
3. Cameron JL, Stouffer RL. Gonadotropin receptors of the primate corpus luteum. I. Characterization of ^{125}I-labeled human luteinizing hormone and human chorionic gonadotropin binding to luteal membranes from the rhesus monkey. Endocrinology 1982; 110:2059-67.
4. Eyster KM, Stouffer RL. Adenylate cyclase in the corpus luteum of rhesus monkeys. I. General properties and optimal assay conditions. Endocrinology 1985; 116:1543-51.
5. Van de Wiele RL, Bogumil J, Dryenfurth I, et al. Mechanisms regulating the menstrual cycle in women. Recent Prog Horm Res 1970; 26:63-87.
6. Mougdal NR, MacDonald GJ, Greep RO. Role of endogenous LH in maintaining corpus luteum function of the monkey. J Clin Endocrinol Metab 1972; 35:113-6.
7. Asch RH, Moustapha AS, Braunstein GD, Pauerstein CJ. Luteal function in hypophysectomized rhesus monkeys. J Clin Endocrinol Metab 1982; 55:154-61.
8. Knobil E, Plant TM, Wildt L, Belchetz PE, Marshall G. Control of the rhesus monkey menstrual cycle: permissive role of gonadotropin releasing hormone. Science 1980; 207:1371-3.
9. Plant TM, Krey LC, Moosey J, McCormack JT, Hess DL, Knobil E. The arcuate nucleus and the control of gonadotropin and prolactin secretion in the female rhesus monkey. Endocrinology 1978; 102:52-62.
10. Carmel PW, Araki S, Ferin M. Pituitary stalk portal blood collection in rhesus monkeys: evidence for pulsatile release of gonadotropin releasing hormone. Endocrinology; 99:243-8.

11. Hutchison JS, Zeleznik AJ. The rhesus monkey corpus luteum is dependent in pituitary gonadotropin secretion throughout the luteal phase of the menstrual cycle. Endocrinology 1984; 115:1780-6.
12. Hutchison JS, Zeleznik AJ. The corpus luteum of the primate menstrual cycle is capable of recovering from a transient withdrawal of pituitary gonadotropin support. Endocrinology 1985; 117:1043-9.
13. Filicori M, Butler JP, Crowley WF Jr. Neuroendocrine regulation of the corpus luteum in the human. J Clin Invest 1984; 73:1638-47.
14. Ellinwood WE, Normal RL, Spies HG. Changing frequency of pulsatile luteinizing hormone and progesterone secretion during the luteal phase of the menstrual cycle of rhesus monkeys. Biol Reprod 1984; 31:714-22.
15. Hutchison JS, Zeleznik AJ. Effects of different gonadotropin pulse frequencies on corpus luteum function during the menstrual cycle of rhesus monkeys. Endocrinology 1986; 119:1964-71.
16. Karsch FJ, Krey LC, Weick RF, Dierschke DJ, Knobil E. Functional luteolysis in the rhesus monkey: the role of estrogen. Endocrinology 1973; 92:1148-52.
17. Gore BZ, Caldwell BU, Speroff L. Estrogen induced human luteolysis. J Clin Endocrinol Metab 1973; 36:615-7.
18. Hotchkiss J, Atkinson LE, Knobil E. Time course of serum estrogen and luteinizing hormone concentration during the menstrual cycle of the rhesus monkey. Endocrinology 1971; 89:177-83.
19. Butler WR, Hotchkiss J, Knobil E. Functional luteolysis in the rhesus monkey: ovarian estrogen and progesterone during the luteal phase of the menstrual cycle. Endocrinology 1975; 96:1509-12.
20. Ellinwood WE, Resko JA. Effect of inhibition of estrogen synthesis during the luteal phase on function of the corpus luteum in rhesus monkeys. Biol Reprod 1983; 28:636-44.
21. Albrecht ED, Haskins AL, Hodgen GD, Pepe GJ. Luteal function in baboons with administration of the antiestrogen ethamoxytiphetol (MER-25) throughout the luteal phase of the menstrual cycle. Biol Reprod 1981; 25:451-7.
22. Westfahl PK, Resko JA. The affects of clomiphene in luteal function in the nonpregnant cynomolgus macaque. Biol Reprod 1983; 29:963-9.
23. Karsch FJ, Sutton GP. An intra-ovarian site for the luteolytic action of estrogen in the rhesus monkey. Endocrinology 1976; 98:553-61.
24. Schoonmaker JN, Bergman KS, Steiner RA, Karsch FJ. Estradiol-induced luteal regression in the rhesus monkey: evidence for an extraovarian site of action. Endocrinology 1982; 110:1708-15.
25. Hutchison JS, Kubik CJ, Nelson PB, Zeleznik AJ. Estrogen induces premature luteal regression in rhesus monkeys during spontaneous menstrual cycles, but not in cycles driven by exogenous gonadotropin releasing hormone. Endocrinology 1987; 120 (in press).
26. Ottobre JS, Stouffer RC. Persistent versus transient stimulation of the macaque corpus luteum during prolonged exposure to human chorionic gonadotropin: a function of age of the corpus luteum. Endocrinology 1984; 114:2175-82.
27. Auletta FJ, Kamps DL, Pories S, Bisset J, Gibson M. An intracorpus luteum site for the luteolytic action of prostaglandin $F_{2\alpha}$ in the rhesus monkey. Prostaglandins 1984; 27:285-98.
28. Auletta FJ, Paradis DK, Wesley M, Duby RT. Oxytocin is luteolytic in the rhesus monkey (<u>Macaca mulatta</u>). J Reprod Fertil 1984; 72:406.

LUTEOLYSINS AND MECHANISMS OF LUTEOLYSIS

H. R. Behrman, R. F. Aten, J. J. Ireland, L. K. Soodak,
J. R. Pepperell, and B. Musicki

Reproductive Biology Section, Departments of
Obstetrics/Gynecology and Pharmacology, Yale University
School of Medicine, New Haven, CT 06510

INTRODUCTION

A fundamentally important event in reproduction is luteolysis because without a decrease in progesterone secretion, there can be no gonadotropin-dependent ovarian differentiation and cyclic function. Until the last two decades, virtually nothing was known of the mechanisms of luteolysis. or of the agents that regulate such processes. It was the pioneering work of researchers at the Upjohn Company which led to the finding that prostaglandin (PG) $F_{2\alpha}$ was luteolytic in the laboratory rat (1). This eicosanoid produces luteal regression in a host of domestic and laboratory animals. $PGF_{2\alpha}$ is generally regarded to be the major physiological uterine luteolysin in domestic species (2), but $PGF_{2\alpha}$ is not an effective luteolysin in women. Thus, in the human, progress in understanding the mechanisms of luteolysis has not been as rapid. Nevertheless, from studies using ovarian cells from diverse species, an understanding of the nature of luteolysins and the mechanisms of luteolysis in the human may ultimately be realized.

In this chapter, we describe a working hypothesis of the nature of luteolysins and the mechanisms of luteal regression. We apologize beforehand to those whose publications have not been included in this chapter. However, many reviews have been referenced in order to provide the reader access to specific articles. Much of the discussion in this review focuses on functional luteolysis, which begins within a minute or less in response to luteolysins such as $PGF_{2\alpha}$. Also discussed are the endocrine processes that appear to regulate $PGF_{2\alpha}$ secretion and delivery to the corpus luteum, as well as the cellular mechanism of $PGF_{2\alpha}$ action in the luteal cell. Recent evidence is summarized for a novel antigonadotropic peptide in the corpus luteum of diverse species including the human being. Finally, evidence is described for a gonadotropin-dependent process of initiation of structural luteolysis which is based on LH-induced depletion of ATP.

DEFINITIONS

Luteolysis is defined as a sustained decrease in the ability of the corpus luteum to secrete progesterone. Historically, however, luteolysis is a process that is comprised of two events. The first process, functional luteolysis, involves a sustained loss in progesterone synthesis and secretion. The second process, structural luteolysis, is the involution and degeneration of the corpus luteum. In some species such as the hamster and cow, a rapid structural involution of the corpus luteum occurs almost in parallel with functional luteolysis. In other species such as the rat, the structure persists after progesterone secretion has abated, and 20α-dihydroprogesterone, an inactive metabolite, is secreted instead.

LUTEOLYSIS IN NONPRIMATES

A distinctive feature of the many domestic and laboratory animals is that the removal of the uterus prolongs the estrous cycle by extending the function of the corpus luteum (3). These early observations sparked the search for a uterine luteolysin which culminated in the discovery of $PGF_{2\alpha}$. In the primate, however, there appears to be no effect of hysterectomy on the functional life span of the corpus luteum (4). $PGF_{2\alpha}$ is luteolytic in virtually all domestic animals (2), and it is selectively delivered from the uterine vein to the ovarian artery by a unique vascular arrangement that permits diffusion of small molecular species across the vessel walls (3).

Estrogen and Oxytocin Regulate Uterine $PGF_{2\alpha}$ Secretion

Control of uterine luteolysin secretion in the ruminant is regulated by at least two ovarian factors. Estrogen (5) of follicular origin (6) and oxytocin (7) of luteal origin (8) are known to be luteolytic. However, only recently has the significance of these early findings been woven into a framework for understanding the regulation of synthesis and secretion of uterine $PGF_{2\alpha}$. A description of this hypothesis is shown in Figure 1, which is a summary of recent reports (8,9).

Estrogen induces differentiation of the uterus, increases the capacity of the uterus for prostaglandin secretion, and induces the appearance of uterine oxytocin receptors (9). If a sufficient number of oxytocin receptors are induced, occupancy of these receptors by oxytocin acutely stimulates the arachidonic cascade which results in $PGF_{2\alpha}$ synthesis and secretion (10). $PGF_{2\alpha}$, released into the uterine vein, is transported selectively to the corpus luteum, where it initiates the luteolytic proc-

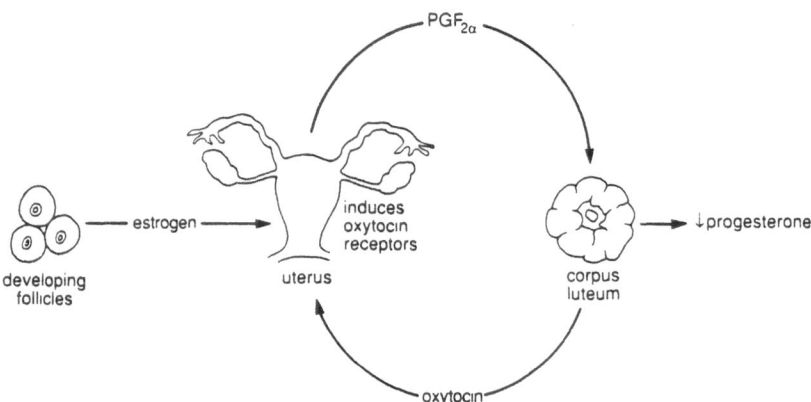

Fig. 1. Summary of the interactions between estrogen, oxytocin and $PGF_{2\alpha}$ in the regulation of luteolysis in the ewe.

ess (8) and stimulates oxytocin secretion from the corpus luteum (11). The major sources of oxytocin in the corpus luteum are the large luteal cells (12); oxytocin release is pulsatile (8) due to the episodic release of $PGF_{2\alpha}$ from the uterus (13). It appears, however, that $PGF_{2\alpha}$ does not directly stimulate release of oxytocin from luteal cells in isolated tissue slices of ovine corpora lutea (14). Thus, secondary mediators may control oxytocin secretion by $PGF_{2\alpha}$ in vivo.

A direct inhibitory effect of oxytocin on gonadotropin-dependent progesterone secretion has been reported in luteal tissue (15,16). However, several laboratories have been unable to confirm these reports with isolated luteal tissue or cells (summarized in 8). We also found no direct inhibitory effect of oxytocin on gonadotropin-sensitive secretion of progesterone in luteinized granulosal cells of women (Polan ML, DeCherney A, and Behrman HR, unpublished observations). Since oxytocin is not directly luteolytic, the primary mechanism of action of oxytocin in luteolysis appears to be stimulation of $PGF_{2\alpha}$ secretion from the uterus (8).

$PGF_{2\alpha}$ Is an Antigonadotropic Hormone

The corpus luteum is completely dependent on gonadotropic hormones for maintenance of function, but luteal regression is not due to a decrease in circulating levels of gonadotropin. Therefore, it seems likely that luteal regression may be due to an inability of gonadotropin to maintain luteal function, and that a luteolysin may function as an antigonadotropic agent. Evidence for this conclusion is based on studies in the rat in which $PGF_{2\alpha}$ antagonizes the steroidogenic response of an acute injection of LH (17). Subsequent studies showed that $PGF_{2\alpha}$ acts directly at the ovarian level (17,18), that it does not compromise ovarian or luteal blood flow (17,19) and that it blocks the action of gonadotropin (20,21). A summary of the antigonadotropic actions of $PGF_{2\alpha}$ in the rat is shown in Figure 2.

One process by which $PGF_{2\alpha}$ blocks the action of LH is by inducing a loss of LH receptors in the corpus luteum (18,22,23). However, progesterone secretion is reduced hours before a decrease in LH receptor content occurs (23). Therefore, downregulation of LH receptors induced by $PGF_{2\alpha}$ in vivo must be an effect, but not the initial cause, of luteolysis. This induced loss of LH receptors probably ensures that regression is irreversible once it occurs.

A second process by which $PGF_{2\alpha}$ blocks the action of LH is by impaired delivery of the hormone to the luteal cell, an effect that is rapid and only seen in vivo (24). The time course for inhibition of gonadotropin uptake by $PGF_{2\alpha}$ in the corpus luteum directly parallels the decrease in progesterone secretion (24). This effect is not seen in isolated luteal cells (21,25) or in LH receptor-enriched rat luteal plasma membranes (18,21,26). Since $PGF_{2\alpha}$ also inhibits prolactin uptake by rat

1. Impaired uptake of gonadotropin within the corpus luteum.
   (rapid in vivo response)

2. Desensitization of luteal LH receptors by:
   a) Mediator-dependent inhibition of adenylate cyclase
      activation by LH. (rapid and occurs in isolated cells)

   b) Mediator-dependent inhibition of LH receptor
      microaggregation. (rapid and occurs in isolated cells)

3. Down-regulation of luteal LH receptors by inhibition of
   prolactin action. (slow in vivo response)

Fig. 2. Antigonadotropic actions of $PGF_{2\alpha}$ in the rat.

luteal tissue (18), and because $PGF_{2\alpha}$ does not affect blood flow to the corpus luteum (17,19), it appears that inhibition of hormone uptake by $PGF_{2\alpha}$ may be due to impaired capillary transfer of gonadotropin, possibly due to closure of capillary clefts. Further studies are necessary to resolve the in vivo mechanism of this action of $PGF_{2\alpha}$.

A third mechanism by which $PGF_{2\alpha}$ abrogates LH action is by interruption of the intracellular signal (cyclic AMP) that mediates the action of LH. Physiological concentrations of $PGF_{2\alpha}$ acutely inhibit the cyclic AMP and steroidogenic response of isolated luteal cells to LH, independent of an effect on LH receptor binding activity or cyclic AMP degradation (21,26). $PGF_{2\alpha}$ does not directly inhibit LH-sensitive adenylate cyclase activity in rat luteal membranes (21). Therefore, it seems likely that some agent must mediate the intracellular action of $PGF_{2\alpha}$ following its binding to specific membrane receptors (27).

Another mechanism of the antigonadotropic action of $PGF_{2\alpha}$ is associated with acute changes in LH receptor dynamics on luteal cells. LH receptor movement and changes in the membrane arrangement of LH receptors appear to be necessary for the expression of LH action in luteal cells. For example, by high resolution ultrastructural analysis we found that LH receptors are rapidly organized into small aggregates that increase in size as ferritin-LH binding and progesterone production increase (28,29). Acute exposure of rat luteal cells to $PGF_{2\alpha}$ prevents this aggregation, but does not abolish the characteristic pattern (29). In addition, $PGF_{2\alpha}$ prevents LH-induced upregulation of LH receptors by a process that involves unmasking of cryptic membrane receptors (30). In contrast, treatment of cells with microfilament-directed drugs disperses microaggregates and abolishes LH-stimulated cyclic AMP and progesterone production (31). Thus, LH receptors are organized into discrete structural and functional domains such that following binding to LH, receptor movement and activation of adenylate cyclase occurs. The initial action of $PGF_{2\alpha}$ appears to result in a decrease in membrane fluidity, which reduces the ability of LH receptors to aggregate and to activate adenylate cyclase. Reduced membrane fluidity at luteal regression and in response to $PGF_{2\alpha}$ has been confirmed by fluorescent probe analysis (32).

Taken together, these results indicate that $PGF_{2\alpha}$ blocks the action of LH by an indirect mechanism that is rapid in onset and occurs only in the intact cell. An intracellular mediator of $PGF_{2\alpha}$ must, therefore, be invoked which somehow prevents the activation of adenylate cyclase by the occupied LH receptor. The acute antigonadotropic response to $PGF_{2\alpha}$ appears to be linked to inhibition of the lateral movement of occupied LH receptors into microaggregates that are necessary for the action of LH to be expressed. However, these findings do not preclude additional actions of $PGF_{2\alpha}$ which block coupling reactions between the LH receptor and the catalytic subunit of adenylate cyclase, and which are necessary for activation of enzyme activity.

Calcium--A Cellular Mediator of $PGF_{2\alpha}$ Action

The evidence that calcium mediates the action of $PGF_{2\alpha}$ has yet to be substantiated, but results from several indirect studies point to this conclusion. Early studies from this laboratory (33) showed that acute shifts in the major monovalent cations, Na^+ and K^+, in rat luteal cells are probably not involved in the acute luteolytic response to $PGF_{2\alpha}$. The basis for this conclusion is that changes in, or inhibition of, cell depolarization produced by reducing extracellular Na^+, increasing extracellular K^+, or incubating the cells with tetrodotoxin have no $PGF_{2\alpha}$-like, luteolytic effect (33). In contrast, incubation of luteal cells with ouabain, an inhibitor of Na^+, K^+-ATPase, or monensin, a monovalent cationophore with high selectivity for Na^+, produces a marked and dose-related inhibition of LH-dependent cyclic AMP and progesterone production (33). Like that seen with $PGF_{2\alpha}$, both drugs elicit these effects only in the intact cell, with no effect on LH receptor binding activity or cyclic AMP degradation (33). These effects of ouabain and monensin are dependent on the presence of extracellular sodium, as expected, but their antigonadotropic effects are also dependent on the presence of extracellular calcium (33). From these and other results, we concluded that intracellular sodium exchanges for extracellular calcium, and that an increase in intracellular calcium inhibits the action of LH in the luteal cell (33).

We examined, therefore, the effects of calcium on luteal cell function by treatment with A23187, a calcium ionophore (25). Calcium ionophore produces a marked and dose-related decrease in LH-stimulated cyclic AMP accumulation like that seen with $PGF_{2\alpha}$. Identical responses are also seen with a more specific calcium ionophore, ionomycin (Cross, Soodak and Behrman, unpublished observations). This effect of A23187 is dependent on the presence of extracellular calcium, consistent with the action of this drug as a calcium ionophore. Like $PGF_{2\alpha}$, A23187 has no effect on LH receptor binding activity, LH-sensitive adenylate cyclase activity or cyclic AMP degradation. In other studies on rat luteal cells (33), we examined the effect of removing extracellular calcium as well as blocking influx of calcium through voltage-dependent calcium channels with Verapamil. Removal of extracellular calcium or treatment with Verapamil has no effect on the response to $PGF_{2\alpha}$. Therefore, an influx of extracellular calcium does not appear to be involved in the acute antigonadotropic response to this luteolysin.

For calcium to mediate the action of luteolysins, an increase in intracellular calcium must, therefore, arise from within the cell. One possibility is that a high affinity calcium pump may sequester calcium into intracellular organelles and act in concert with the plasma membrane pump (34) to maintain low levels of calcium inside the cell. Thus, a decrease in calcium sequestration or a decrease in calcium extrusion from the cell could increase intracellular calcium. To examine this possibility, we measured high affinity calcium-ATPase activity in purified plasma membranes and in microsome-enriched membranes (35). Treatment of animals or luteal cells with $PGF_{2\alpha}$ inhibited high affinity calcium-ATPase activity microsomes, but not in the plasma membrane fraction of luteal tissue (35). It is not known whether this effect mediates the response to $PGF_{2\alpha}$.

Recent studies indicate that products of phosphoinositol (PI) turnover such as inositol 1,4,5-trisphosphate (IP_3) may serve a role in mediating hormone-induced release of sequestered calcium from microsomes of liver cells (36). $PGF_{2\alpha}$ stimulates PI turnover in rat luteal cells (37,38), and this response is associated with an increase in IP_3 formation, presumably due to the action of phospholipase C activity (38). Similar findings have been reported with bovine luteal cells in which $PGF_{2\alpha}$ stimulates release of IP_3 within 10 sec, and this response is followed by a sustained increase in intracellular calcium levels that lasts for several minutes (39).

Thus, it appears that $PGF_{2\alpha}$ binds to specific receptors in the plasma membrane of luteal cells and rapidly stimulates the intracellular release of IP_3 from phosphoinositides. IP_3, in turn, produces a rapid release of calcium within the cell, probably from microsomes, by a mechanism that may be linked to inhibition of a high affinity and ATP-dependent calcium pump. As a consequence, intracellular calcium levels are elevated and antigonadotropic responses are initiated. This proposed mechanism is summarized in Figure 3.

Calcium Inhibits Luteal Adenylate Cyclase Activity

To evaluate if calcium has direct antigonadotropic effects in luteal cells, studies were carried out with purified plasma membranes. Calcium directly inhibits activation of adenylate cyclase by LH at concentrations in the low micromolar range, but it has no effect on LH receptor binding activity or cyclic AMP degradation (25). Levels of free calcium of 500 nM, which are within the physiological range, were also inhibitory and this inhibition is reversible (40). We concluded, therefore, that calcium blocks interaction of the occupied receptor with adenylate cyclase and thereby prevents enzyme activation. The major difference between the action of calcium and $PGF_{2\alpha}$, however, is that calcium produces this effect directly in membranes, whereas an intact cell is necessary to elicit this effect with $PGF_{2\alpha}$.

Protein Kinase C Activation Mimics the Action of $PGF_{2\alpha}$

In the past few years, a novel protein kinase has been described, protein kinase C, which is activated by phosphatidyl serine, calcium and diglyceride. Diglyceride markedly increases the affinity of the enzyme for calcium and phosphatidylserine (41). Since IP_3 is released by hydrolysis of phosphatidylinositol 4,5-bisphosphate (PIP_2) by phospholipase C, it is evident that another product of this same reaction is diglyceride. Therefore, the necessary components are present in luteal cells for activation of protein kinase C.

Indeed, the enzyme is present in the bovine corpus luteum (42), and it has an inhibitory action in swine granulosa cells (43). Moreover, phorbol esters, which mimic the action of diglyceride in activation of protein kinase C (44), produces a $PGF_{2\alpha}$-like effect in rat luteal cells

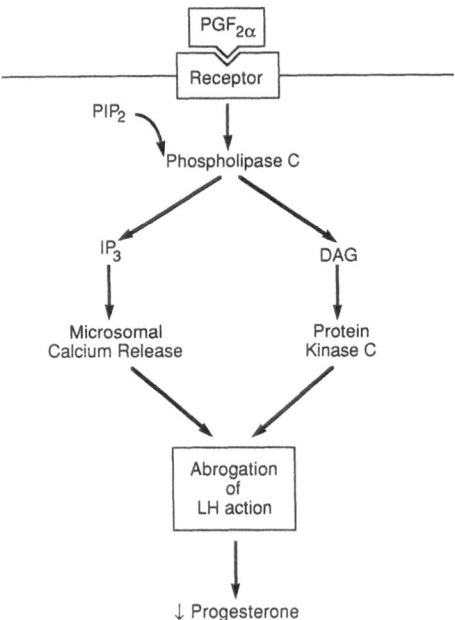

Fig. 3. Cellular mechanism of $PGF_{2\alpha}$-induced luteolysis. PIP_2 = phosphatidylinositol 4,5-bisphosphate; IP_3 = inositol 1,4,5,-trisphosphate; DAG = diacylglycerol.

(45). Therefore, it is possible that the antigonadotropic actions of $PGF_{2\alpha}$ may be mediated not only by calcium, but also by diglyceride-dependent protein phosphorylation. However, it is not known if these two potential mediators of $PGF_{2\alpha}$ are dependently linked or whether only one pathway plays the major role in the luteolytic process. We also have no idea of the nature of the acceptor protein that is phosphorylated by the action of protein kinase C. A summary of these proposed mechanisms of $PGF_{2\alpha}$ action is shown in Figure 3.

LUTEOLYSIS IN PRIMATES

The nature of luteolysins, the regulation of luteolysin secretion and the mechanisms of luteolysis in the primate, in particular the human primate, are virtually unknown. It is still commonplace to read in modern gynecologic textbooks that luteolysis in women is due to preprogrammed cell death. However, emerging evidence indicates that the primate shares many of the similarities of other animals in the endocrine parameters that regulate corpus luteum function and luteal regression.

First, the function of the human corpus luteum is dependent upon LH and in its absence, such as after hypophysectomy, corpus luteum function ceases unless LH is frequently administered (46). LH is known to be released in a pulsatile manner (47), and the pulse-frequency of LH secretion is reduced during the luteal phase, particularly in the periluteolytic period (48). But, recent evidence shows that the duration of luteal function in the nonhuman primate is unaffected by large reductions in the pulse-frequency of LH secretion (49). Thus, luteal regression in the primate, as in other animals, is not due to a lack of availability of LH.

Second, LH sensitivity of adenylate cyclase is decreased in the regressing primate corpus luteum (50), as in other animals (21,26). The primate thus seems to share an antigonadotropic mechanism of luteolysis similar to that seen in lower animals. Luteolysis in the primate, as in other animals, appears to be due to an induced refractoriness of the luteal cell to gonadotropic hormone action rather than to a decrease in gonadotropin secretion.

Third, the primate ovary contains oxytocin like lower animals (51), and oxytocin has been reported to be luteolytic in the primate (52). But in contrast to other animals (5-14), the significance of luteal oxytocin with regard to luteolysis in the primate is not apparent because the presence, or absence, of the uterus has no effect on the duration of the luteal phase (4). Thus, a utero-ovarian, positive-feedback interaction between luteal oxytocin and uterine $PGF_{2\alpha}$ secretion does not seem to be a relevant mechanism for regulation of luteolysis in the primate. Although a direct antigonadotropic effect of high levels of oxytocin has been reported in isolated cells (15,16), others have not seen a similar effect (8). These findings, however, do not preclude the possibility of intraovarian actions of oxytocin that may induce local release of antigonadotropic agents.

A luteolytic role of $PGF_{2\alpha}$ in women remains equivocal despite the presence of $PGF_{2\alpha}$ (53) and its receptors (54) in the human corpus luteum. Also, there are reports which show antigonadotropic effects of this prostanoid in isolated human luteal tissue (55). However, there is little luteolytic effect of $PGF_{2\alpha}$ following systemic injection in women, and direct intraluteal administration of $PGF_{2\alpha}$ produces only a transient suppression of progesterone secretion (56). In the nonhuman primate, a luteolytic effect of $PGF_{2\alpha}$ occurs following administration into the ovarian artery (57), and inhibition of prostaglandin biosynthesis with indomethacin extends the luteal phase of the monkey (58). However, treatment of women with inhibitors of prostaglandin biosynthesis has little effect on the duration of the luteal phase (59). Thus, substantial evidence indicates that $PGF_{2\alpha}$ may not be a relevant luteolysin in the human, although it may serve such a role in lower primates.

Estrogen produces a luteolytic effect in most species, including the human. For example, in the rhesus monkey, estradiol reduces luteal function when injected directly into the corpus luteum, but has no effect when administered systemically or when injected into the ovarian stroma (60). Estrone of luteal origin is suggested to play a luteolytic role in the rhesus monkey, based on the finding that it is elevated in ovarian venous blood prior to the onset of menses (61). However, it is difficult to reconcile a luteolytic action of estrogen with the fact that estrogen is produced by the primate corpus luteum throughout the luteal phase. In contrast, the corpus luteum of other species does not produce estrogen. We do not know if estrogen is a physiological luteolysin in the primate but if it is, we know little with regard to its mechanism of induction of functional luteolysis. It is possible that estrogen may intereact in some manner with release and modulation of intraovarian oxytocin, or perhaps induce the synthesis and/or release of unknown luteolysins in the primate ovary.

NEW DEVELOPMENTS

A Novel Antigonadotropic Ovarian Protein

We recently identified a novel ovarian protein (62) that displays marked antigonadotropic activity against LH in rat luteal cells (63) and against FSH in rat granulosal cells (64). This protein has been partially purified (62), and it is present in the ovaries of diverse species such as the rat (62), ewe and cow (64), and human (65). This protein is selectively enriched in bovine luteal and granulosal tissue, but little activity is seen in the theca and stroma (66), and no activity is seen in follicular fluid, ovarian venous serum or jugular plasma (64,66). Therefore, we suggest that this protein may play a paracrine or autocrine antigonadotropic role in the ovary and, by such a process, it may play a role in follicular atresia and luteolysis.

The rationale for our search for such a protein arose from the finding that the rat ovary contains high affinity receptors for GnRH (67). We (68), and others (67), found that GnRH, like $PGF_{2\alpha}$, elicits antigonadotropic activity in rat luteal cells. We, therefore, used a GnRH receptor preparation from rat ovaries, and a specific RIA for GnRH, to assay and to isolate GnRH and GnRH-like proteins from ovarian extracts. Although we expected to find GnRH in the rat ovary, none was found. To our surprise, we discovered a protein that avidly binds to the so-called GnRH receptors of the rat ovary. This protein is physically, chemically and immunologically different from authentic GnRH, and a wide variety of other known peptides, and evokes marked antigonadotropic activity (62-66). The HPLC characteristics of this protein in human and rat ovarian extracts and the antigonadotropic activity of bovine ovarian extracts in isolated rat luteal cells are shown in Figure 4.

The evidence for antigonadotropic proteins is not limited to mammalian species. Evidence for antigonadotropic agents that inhibit egg development in insects, such as the cockroach, was first published in 1935 (69). Since then, reports for antigonadotropic agents that inhibit egg development in the eye gnat, decapod crustaceans, the housefly and mosquitoes have appeared (reviewed in 70). Recently, a protein was purified from ovaries of the mosquito, referred to as oostatic hormone (2200

daltons), which blocks egg development by a direct action on the ovary
(70). We suggest that the recently identified ovarian antigonadotropic
peptide of mammals may be a member of this class of regulatory proteins.
However, complete characterization will be necessary to determine if these
proteins share similarities in their structure and mechanism of action.
Thus, autocrine and paracrine antigonadotropic hormones produced by the
ovary appear to represent ancient regulatory processes for control of
ovarian function.

LH Depletes Luteal ATP: A Mechanism of Structural Luteolysis?

The maintenance of ATP levels is critical for optimum function of all
cells because this essential substrate drives most, if not all, vital
reactions in cells. Under conditions that deplete cell ATP, such as
hypoxia, a cascade of reactions begins which lead to cell damage and,
ultimately, death due to pathologic elevations of intracellular calcium
(71). The origin of calcium includes release from microsomes and
mitochondria, as well as influx from the extracellular fluid (71). An
increase in intracellular calcium activates phospholipases A_1, A_2 and C
that further elevate intracellular levels of calcium, which leads,
ultimately, to cell death (71). A summary of these responses is shown in
Figure 5.

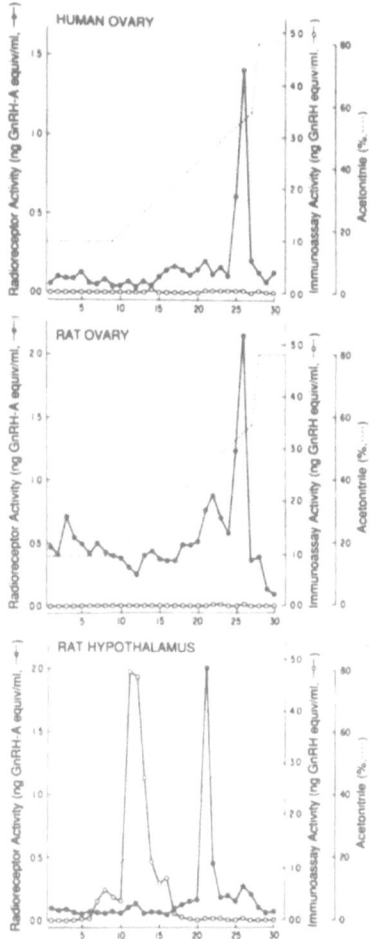

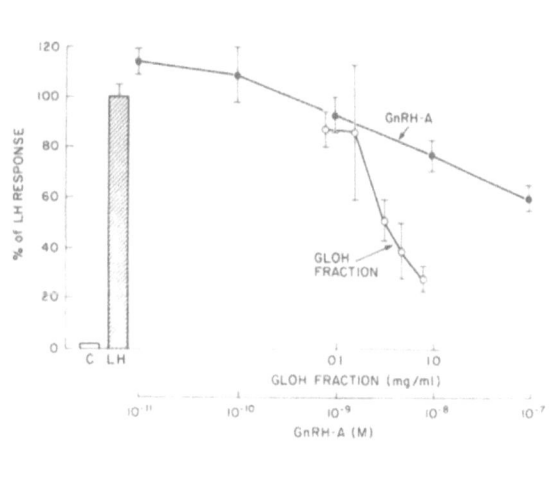

Fig. 4. Presence of GnRH-like ovarian
hormone (GLOH) in extracts of human and
rat ovary and antigonadotropic activity
of bovine GLOH in rat luteal cells.
Note difference between GnRH and hypothalamic GnRH-like protein from human
and rat GLOH and the absence of GnRH
immunoactivity of human and rat GLOH.
Antigonadotropic activity represents
inhibition of LH-sensitive cyclic AMP
accumulation with GLOH and a GnRH
agonist. From 63 and 65.

It seems reasonable, therefore, that the initiation of structural luteolysis may arise due to processes that interfere with maintenance of optimum levels of ATP in the luteal cell. In fact, following the initiation of luteal regression in the rat, a significant depletion of luteal ATP occurs in vivo, coincident with a rise in serum levels of LH, but not FSH (Soodak and Behrman, unpublished observations). However, a similar depletion of ATP does not occur within 2 h of a luteolytic dose of $PGF_{2\alpha}$, or 24 h after hypophysectomy (73). Depletion of luteal ATP in the rat occurs in a dose-dependent manner within 2 h of injection of LH (73); this effect occurs within 5 min of LH injection, it is maximal within 30 min and is sustained for up to 24 h (73).

In many tissues, such as muscle, large changes in the levels of ATP are buffered by a reservoir of high energy phosphate sequestered in cells as phosphocreatine. However, rat luteal cells have virtually no such reserves because the corpus luteum has little creatine phosphate or creatine phosphokinase to buffer decreases in ATP levels (74). For this reason, ATP levels in the corpus luteum in the rat are subject to marked changes. Based on these results, we suggest that the levels of ATP in the mid- and late-stage corpus luteum of the rat are under sensitive endocrine control and that an increase in LH secretion places the corpus luteum at risk because it depletes this essential substrate.

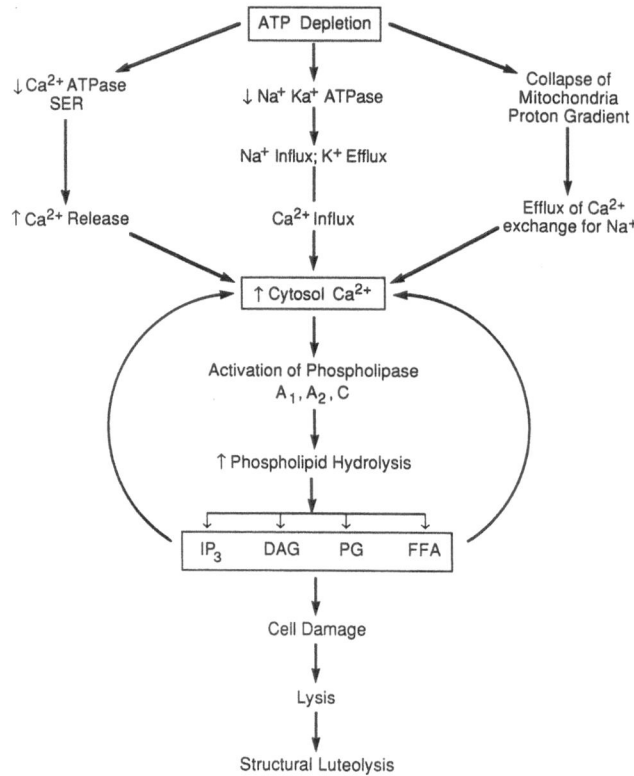

Fig. 5. Proposed metabolic consequences of ATP depletion in luteal cells. Ca^{2+} ATPase = high affinity calcium pump; SER = smooth endoplasmic reticulum; IP_3 = inositol 1,4,5-trisphosphate; DAG = diacyclclycerol; PG = prostaglandin; FFA = free fatty acid.

An increase in LH levels occurs after initiation of functional luteolysis, due to the loss in negative feedback-control by progesterone. This increase in LH secretion depletes luteal ATP and compromises the ability of the luteal cells to maintain low intracellular levels of calcium. An excessive decrease in cell levels of ATP initiates a cascade of events that further elevate calcium to pathological levels in the cells. As a consequence, cell death and structural luteolysis ensue. These events, we suggest, probably continue until LH levels are reduced, LH receptors are depleted, or responses to LH are totally abated. It should be noted, however, that evidence for LH depletion of ATP is only documented in the rat. To our knowledge, this effect of LH has not been examined in any other species. A summary of a working hypothesis of luteolysis is shown in Figure 6.

SUMMARY

We propose that the process of functional luteolysis is due to an induced loss in the ability of luteal cells to response to gonadotropic hormones, primarily LH. $PGF_{2\alpha}$ serves a luteolytic role in nonprimates by this process. This effect of $PGF_{2\alpha}$ appears to be mediated by calcium, which is released within the luteal cell by phosphatidyl inositol-derived products following binding of $PGF_{2\alpha}$ to specific membrane receptors. Elevation of calcium levels alone directly inhibits activation of LH-sensitive adenylate cyclase in luteal membranes. However, recent evidence

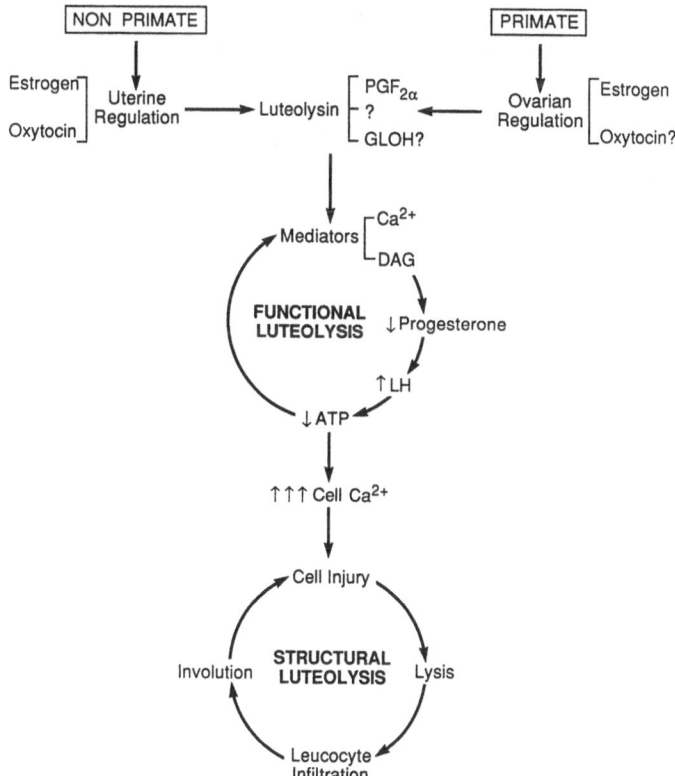

Fig. 6. An integrated working model of functional and structural luteolysis.

shows that diglyceride-mediated protein phosphorylation may also play a role in luteolysis, since activation of protein kinase C with phorbol ester mimics the effect of $PGF_{2\alpha}$. Luteal peptides may also play a role in luteolysis. Oxytocin, of luteal origin, appears to promote luteolysis in the ewe by stimulation of uterine $PGF_{2\alpha}$ secretion. A novel ovarian protein was recently identified in luteal and ovarian extracts of the rat, cow, ewe and human which elicits marked antigonadotropic activity in rat luteal cells. This protein is not detected in follicular fluid or peripheral serum, but it avidly binds to GnRH receptors of the rat ovary. However, this protein is different from GnRH and other known proteins and, based on its distribution and biological activity, it may serve a role in luteolysis. Finally, an endocrine-dependent process for initiation of structural luteolysis in the rat via LH-induced depletion of ATP is proposed. By this mechanism, the rising levels of LH that follow functional luteal regression result in ATP depletion in the corpus luteum and, as a consequence, precipitate events that lead to cell lysis and involution of the corpus luteum.

ACKNOWLEDGMENTS

This work was supported by NIH-HD-15403 and NIH-HD-10718. The authors express their appreciation to Ms. Cindy Davis for preparation of the manuscript and to TradeScript for editorial assistance.

REFERENCES

1. Pharriss BB, Wyngarden LJ. The effect of prostaglandin $F_{2\alpha}$ on the progestagen content of ovaries from pseudopregnant rats. Proc Soc Exp Biol Med 1969; 130:92-4.
2. Thatcher WW, Bazer FW, Sharp DC, Roberts RM. Interrelationships between uterus and conceptus to maintain corpus luteum function in early pregnancy: sheep, cattle, pigs, and horses. J Anim Sci 1986; 62(suppl 2):25-46.
3. Horton EW, Poyser NI. Uterine luteolytic hormone: a physiological role for prostaglandin $F_{2\alpha}$. Physiol Rev 1976; 56:595-651.
4. Neill JD, Johansson ED, Knobil E. Failure of hysterectomy to influence the normal pattern of cyclic progesterone secretion in the rhesus monkey. Endocrinology 1969; 84:464-7.
5. Wiltbank JN, Ingalls JE, Rowden WW. Effects of various forms and levels of estrogens alone and in combinations with gonadotrophins on the estrous cycle of beef heifers. J Anim Sci 1961; 20:341-6.
6. Fogwell RL, Cowley JA, Wortman JA, Ames NK, Ireland JJ. Luteal function in cows following destruction of ovarian follicles at midcycle. Theriogenology 1985; 23:389-98.
7. Armstrong DT, Hansel W. Alteration of the bovine estrous cycle with oxytocin. J Dairy Sci 1959; 42:533-42.
8. Flint APF, Sheldrick EL, Theodosis DT, Wooding FBP. Ovarian peptides: role of luteal oxytocin in the control of estrous cyclicity in ruminants. J Anim Sci 1986; 62(suppl 2):62-71.
9. Soloff MS. Regulation of oxytocin action at the receptor level. In: Bottari S, Thomas JP, Vokaer A, Vokaer R, eds. Uterine contractility. New York: Mason Publishing, 1982:261-4.
10. Roberts JS, McCracken JA, Gavagan JE, Soloff MS. Oxytocin-stimulated release of prostaglandin $F_{2\alpha}$ from ovine endometrium in vitro: correlation with estrous cycle and oxytocin-receptor binding. Endocrinology 1976; 99:1107-14.
11. Flint APF, Sheldrick EL. Ovarian secretion of oxytocin is stimulated by prostaglandin. Nature 1982; 297:587-8.
12. Rogers RJ, O'Shea JD, Findlay JK, Flint APF, Sheldrick EL. Large

luteal cells the source of oxytocin in the sheep. Endocrinology 1983; 113:2302-4.

13. Thorburn GD, Cox RI, Currie WB, Restall BJ, Schneider W. $PGF_{2\alpha}$ and progesterone concentration in utero-ovarian venous plasma of the ewe during the estrous cycle and pregnancy. J Reprod Fertil 1973; (suppl 18):151-8.

14. Hirst JJ, Rice GE, Jenkin G, Thorburn GD. Secretion of oxytocin and progesterone by ovine corpora lutea in vitro. Biol Reprod 1986; 35:1106-14.

15. Tan GJS, Tweedale R, Biggs JSG. Effects of oxytocin on the bovine corpus luteum of early pregnancy. J Reprod Fertil 1982; 66:75-8.

16. Tan GJS, Tweedale R, Biggs JSG. Oxytocin may play a role in the control of the human corpus luteum. J Endocrinol 1982; 95:65-70.

17. Behrman HR, Macdonald GJ, Greep RO. Regulation of ovarian choles-terol esters: evidence for the enzymatic sites of prostaglandin-induced loss of corpus luteum function. Lipids 1971; 6:791-6.

18. Behrman HR, Grinwich DL, Hichens M, Macdonald GJ. Effect of hypophysectomy, prolactin and $PGF_{2\alpha}$ on LH and prolactin binding in vivo and in vitro in the corpus luteum. Endocrinology 1978; 103:349-57.

19. Pang CY, Behrman HR. Acute effects of $PGF_{2\alpha}$ on ovarian and luteal blood flow, luteal gonadotropin uptake in vivo and gonadotropin binding in vitro. Endocrinology 1981; 108:2239-44.

20. Behrman HR, Ng TS, Orczyk GP. Interactions between prostaglandins and gonadotropins in corpus luteum function. In: Moudgal NR, ed. Gonadotropins and gonadal function. New York: Academic Press, 1974:332-44.

21. Thomas JP, Dorflinger LJ, Behrman HR. Mechanism of the rapid antigonadotropic action of prostaglandins in cultured luteal cells. Proc Natl Acad Sci USA 1978; 75:1344-8.

22. Hichens M, Grinwich DL, Behrman HR. $PGF_{2\alpha}$-induced loss of corpus luteum receptors. Prostaglandins 1984; 7:449.

23. Grinwich DL, Hichens M, Behrman HR. Control of the LH receptor by prolactin and $PGF_{2\alpha}$ in rat corpora lutea. Biol Reprod 1976; 14:212-8.

24. Behrman HR, Hichens M. Rapid block of gonadotropin uptake by corpora lutea in vivo induced by $PGF_{2\alpha}$. Prostaglandins 1976; 12:83-95.

25. Dorflinger LJ, Albert PJ, Williams AT, Behrman HR. Calcium is an inhibitor of LH-sensitive adenylate cyclase in the luteal cell. Endocrinology 1984; 114:1208-15.

26. Dorflinger LJ, Luborsky JL, Gore SD, Behrman HR. Inhibitory characteristics of $PGF_{2\alpha}$ in the rat luteal cell. Mol Cell Endocrinol 1983; 33:225-41.

27. Wright K, Pang CY, Behrman HR. Luteal membrane binding of $PGF_{2\alpha}$ and sensitivity of corpora lutea to $PGF_{2\alpha}$-induced luteolysis in pseudopregnant rats. Endocrinology 1980; 106:1333-7.

28. Luborsky JL, Behrman HR. LH receptor antiserum interacts with LH receptors but does not change hormone binding. Biochem Biophys Res Commun 1979; 90:1407-13.

29. Luborsky JL, Dorflinger LJ, Wright K, Behrman HR. $PGF_{2\alpha}$ inhibits LH-induced increase in LH receptor binding to isolated rat luteal cells. Endocrinology 1984; 115:2210-6.

30. Luborsky JL, Slater WT, Behrman HR. LH receptor aggregation: modification of ferritin-LH binding and aggregation by $PGF_{2\alpha}$ and ferritin LH. Endocrinology 1984; 115:2217-26.

31. Luborsky JL. Molecular interactions and cell surface receptor rearrangement in response to LH binding [Abstract]. 67th Meeting Endocrine Society, 1985:226.

32. Carlson JC, Buhr MM, Gruber MY, Thompson JE. Compositional and physical properties of microsomal membrane lipids from regressing rat corpora lutea. Endocrinology 1981; 108:2124-8.

33. Gore SD, Behrman HR. Alteration of transmembrane sodium and potassium gradients inhibits the action of LH in the luteal cell. Endocrinology 1984; 114:2020-31.

34. Verma AK, Penniston JT. A high affinity calcium-stimulated and magnesium-dependent ATPase in rat corpus luteum plasma membrane fractions. J Biol Chem 1981; 256:1269-75.

35. Albert PJ, Preston SL, Behrman HR. Prostaglandin-induced luteolysis linked to inhibition of calcium pump activity [Abstract]. 7th International Congress of Endocrinology 1984:340.

36. Burgess GM, Godfrey PP, McKinney JS, Berridge MJ, Irvine RF, Putney JW. The second messenger linking receptor activation to internal calcium release in liver. Nature 1984; 309:63-6.

37. Raymond V, Leung PCK, Labrie F. Stimulation by $PGF_{2\alpha}$ of phosphatidic acid-phosphatidyl inositol turnover in rat luteal cells. Biochem Biophys Res Commun 1983; 116:39-46.

38. Leung PCK, Minegishi T, Ma F, Zhou F, Ho-Yuen B. Induction of polyphosphoinositide breakdown in rat corpus luteum by prostaglandin $F_{2\alpha}$. Endocrinology 1986; 119:12-8.

39. Davis JS, Weakland LL, Weiland DA, Farese RV, West LA. Prostaglandin $F_{2\alpha}$ stimulates phosphatidylinositol 4,5-bisphosphate hydrolysis and mobilizes intracellular Ca^{2+} in bovine luteal cells. Proc Natl Acad Sci USA 1987; 84:3728-32.

40. Behrman HR, Albert PJ, Preston SL. Calcium-inhibition of luteal adenylate cyclase is blocked by GTP. Biol Reprod 1984; 30(suppl 1):58.

41. Takai Y, Kishimoto A, Kikkawa U, Mori T, Nishizuka Y. Unsaturated diacylglycerol as a possible messenger for the activation of calcium-activated, phospholipid-dependent protein kinase system. Biochem Biophys Res Commun 1979; 91:1218-24.

42. Davis JS, Clark MR. Activation of protein kinase in the bovine corpus luteum by phospholipid and Ca^{2+}. Biochem J 1983; 214:569-74.

43. Veldhuis JD, Demers LM. An inhibitory role for the protein kinase C pathway in ovarian steroidogenesis. Biochem J 1986; 239:505-11.

44. Van Duuren BL, Sivak A. Tumor-promoting agents from croton tiglium L and their mode of action. Cancer Res 1968; 28:2349-56.

45. Sender Baum M, Rosberg S. A phorbol ester, phorbol 12-myristate 13-acetate, and a calcium ionophore, A23187, can mimic the luteolytic effect of prostaglandin $F_{2\alpha}$ in isolated luteal cells. Endocrinology 1987; 120:1019-26.

46. Vande Wiele RL, Bogumil J, Dyrenfurth I, et al. Mechanisms regulating the menstrual cycle in women. Recent Prog Horm Res 1970; 26:63.

47. Yen SSC, Tsai CC, Naftolin F, Vandenberg G, Ajabor L. Pulsatile patterns of gonadotropin release in subjects with and ovarian function. J Clin Endocrinol Metab 1972; 34:671-5.

48. Reame N, Sauder SE, Kelch RP, Marshall JC. Pulsatile gonadotropin secretion during the human menstrual cycle: evidence for altered frequency of gonadotropin-releasing hormone secretion. J Clin Endocrinol Metab 1984; 59:328-37.

49. Hutchison JS, Nelson PB, Zeleznik AJ. Effects of different pulse frequencies on corpus luteum function during the menstrual cycle of rhesus monkeys. Endocrinology 1986; 119:1964-71.

50. Eyster KM, Ottobre JS, Stouffer RL. Adenylate cyclase in the corpus luteum of the rhesus monkey. III. Changes in basal and gonadotropin-sensitive activities during the luteal phase of the menstrual cycle. Endocrinology 1985; 117:1571-7.

51. Schaeffer JM, Liu J, Hsueh AJW. Presence of oxytocin and arginine-vasopressin in human ovary, oviduct and follicular fluid. J Clin Endocrinol Metab 1984; 59:970-3.

52. Auletta FJ, Paradis DK, Wesley M, Duby RT. Oxytocin is luteolytic in the rhesus money (Macaca mulatta). J Reprod Fertil 1984; 72:401-6.

53. Challis JRG, Calder AA, Dilley S, et al. Production of prostaglan-

dins E and F by corpora lutea, corpora albicantes and stroma of the human ovary. J Endocrinol 1976; 68:401-8.

54. Powell WS, Hammerstrom S, Samuelsson B, Sjoberg B. Prostaglandin $F_{2\alpha}$ receptor in human corpora lutea. Lancet 1974; 1:1120.

55. Dennefors B, Sjoren A, Hamberger L. Progesterone and 3',5'-monophosphate formation by isolated human corpora lutea of different ages. Influence of human chorionic gonadotropin and prostaglandins. J Clin Endocrinol Metab 1982; 55:102-7.

56. Korda AR, Shutt DA, Smith ID, Shearman RP, Lyneham RC. Assessment of possible luteolytic effect of intraovarian injection of prostaglandin $F_{2\alpha}$ in the human. Prostaglandins 1975; 9:443-9.

57. Auletta FJ, Speroff L, Caldwell BV. Prostaglandin $F_{2\alpha}$ induced steroidogenesis and luteolysis in the primate corpus luteum. J Clin Endocrinol Metab 1973; 36:405-7.

58. Auletta FJ, Caldwell BV, Speroff L. Estrogen-induced luteolysis in the rhesus monkey: reversal with Indomethacin. Prostaglandins 1976; 11:745-52.

59. Gibson M, Auletta FJ. Effect of prostaglandin synthesis inhibition on human corpus luteum function. Prostaglandins 1986; 31:1023-8.

60. Karsch FJ, Sutton GP. An intraovarian site for the luteolytic action of estrogen in the rhesus monkey. Endocrinology 1976; 98:553-61.

61. Butler WR, Hochkiss J, Knobil E. Functional luteolysis in the rhesus monkey: ovarian estrogen and progesterone during the luteal phase of the menstrual cycle. Endocrinology 1975; 96:1509-12.

62. Aten RF, Williams AT, Behrman HR. Ovarian gonadotropin-releasing hormone-like protein(s): demonstration and characterization. Endocrinology 1986; 118:961-7.

63. Aten RF, Ireland JJ, Weems CW, Behrman HR. Presence of gonadotropin-releasing hormone-like proteins in bovine and ovine ovaries. Endocrinology 1987; 120:1727-33.

64. Aten RF, Ireland JJ, Behrman HR. The ovarian GnRH-like protein is antigonadotropic in both .rat luteal and granulosa cells [Abstract]. 69th Annual Meeting of the Endocrine Society, Indianapolis, IN, 1987.

65. Aten RF, Polan ML, Bayless R, Behrman HR. A gonadotropin-releasing hormone (GnRH)-like protein in human ovaries: similarity to the GnRH-like protein of the rat. J Clin Endocrinol Metab 1987; 64:1288-93.

66. Ireland JJ, Aten RF, Behrman HR. Selective localization of the antigonadotropic GnRH-like protein in corpora lutea of the bovine ovary [Abstract]. Biol Reprod 1987; 36(suppl 1).

67. Clayton RN, Harwood JP, Catt KJ. Gonadotropin-releasing hormone analog binds to luteal cells and inhibits progesterone production. Nature 1979; 282:90-2.

68. Behrman HR, Preston SL, Hall AH. Cellular mechanism of the antigonadotropic action of luteinizing hormone-releasing hormone in the corpus luteum. Endocrinology 1980; 107:656-64.

69. Iwanov PP, Mescherskaya KA. Die physiologischen besonderheiten der geschlechtlich unreifen insecktenovarien und die zyklischen veranderungen ihrer eigenschaften. Zool Jb (Physiol) 1935; 55:281-8.

70. Borovsky D. Isolation and characterization of highly purified mosquito oostatic hormone. Arch Insect Biochem Physiol 1985; 2:333-49.

71. Hochachka PW. Defense strategies against hypoxia and hypothermia. Science 1986; 231:234-41.

72. Behrman HR, Aten RF, Luborsky JL, Polan ML, Miller JGO, Soodak LK. Purines, prostaglandins and peptides: nature and mechanisms of local assist and assassin agents in the ovary. J Anim Sci 1986; 62(suppl 2):14-24.

73. Soodak LK, Macdonald GJ, Behrman HR. LH—a regulator of adenosine release in the rat corpus luteum. Biol Reprod 1986; 34(suppl 1).

74. Cross JC, Soodak LK, Musicki B, Behrman HR. Absence of detectable phosphocreatine in rat luteal cells. Am J Physiol 1987 (in press).

THE ROLE OF PROSTAGLANDINS AND CATECHOLAMINES

FOR HUMAN CORPUS LUTEUM FUNCTION

Lars Hamberger, Mats Hahlin, and Bo Lindblom

Department of Obstetrics and Gynecology, University of
Goteborg, S-413 45 Goteborg, Sweden

INTRODUCTION

In many animal species as well as in women, the function of the
corpus luteum appears to be regulated by both luteotropic and luteolytic
factors.   The limited accessibility to well-defined human tissue has
impaired studies on the human corpus luteum, and most knowledge, therefore, is based on extrapolations from measurements of steroids in the
ovarian vein blood, or in the systemic circulation. Since a countercurrent system carrying steroids and prostaglandins (PGs) from the utero-
ovarian vein to the ovarian artery has been demonstrated both in animals
(1) and in women (2), an intraovarian hormonal environment is created
different from that of the periphery. This local milieu appears to be
important for follicular development, ovulation and corpus luteum formation and function, which can be regarded as a dynamic sector within the
ovary. However, there exists also a more static compartment, represented
by primordial follicles and stromal cells. In the following, we will
focus the discussion upon factors regulating the corpus luteum function
during its life span. Crudely, these influences can be divided into
distant factors, e.g., gonadotropins, and local factors, represented by
PGs and catecholamines. Since we recently reviewed the gonadotropic
regulation of human corpus luteum function (3), the current presentation
will be restricted to the above-mentioned local factors. The intimate
interrelation between these two regulatory systems, however, must be kept
in mind.

PROSTAGLANDIN E_2

PGE_2 is one of the major luteotropic factors in women, both in the
sterile cycle and in early pregnancy. PGE_2 is synthesized by the human
corpus luteum (4,5) and the content is of the same magnitude as that of
$PGF_{2\alpha}$ (6), at least in certain phases of the corpus luteum life span.
Receptors for PGE_2 have been demonstrated in the corpus luteum of the menstrual cycle (7). PGE_2 may also reach the corpus luteum through the
circulation, but no data support the theory that PGE_2 exerts its effect
through changes in the corpus luteum blood flow. Following the endogenous
gonadotropic peak preceding ovulation, a relative refractoriness to LH and
hCG can be registered in the early corpus luteum (8). At this phase (1 to
2 days postovulation), PGE_2 seems to be a more potent stimulator of cAMP
formation than hCG, when the hormones are administered at maximal

concentrations (Fig. 1). If these two hormones are administered in low concentrations which do not, per se, stimulate cAMP formation, the combination of hormones causes a highly stimulatory effect (Fig. 2). PGE_2 thus shows a clear potentiation of the hCG effect or vice versa.

In the midluteal phase of a natural cycle, the effect of hCG at a maximal concentration is generally more pronounced than that of PGE_2 and a combined administration causes an additive, but not a potentiated effect (Fig. 3) (9). This is the case for both cAMP and progesterone formation, as was first pointed out by Marsh and LeMaire (10).

In early pregnancy, the human corpus luteum responds to PGE_2 in vitro with increased cAMP and progesterone formation of the same magnitude as in the natural cycle, while the tissue's reactivity to hCG is relatively weak (Table 1) (11). Against this background it is tempting to speculate that PGE_2 produced by the conceptus or endometrium may at least partly be responsible for the sustained elevated levels of progesterone around implantation and during the first two or three weeks of pregnancy.

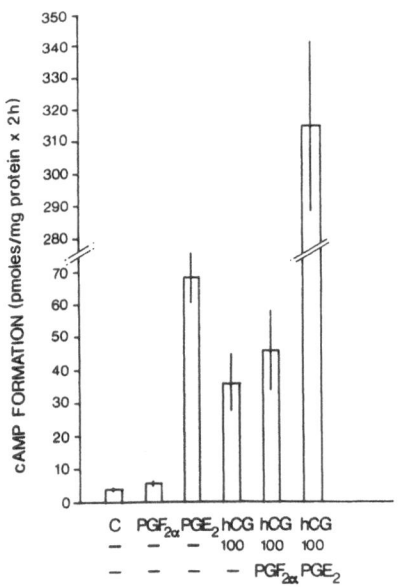

Fig. 1. Effects of $PGF_{2\alpha}$ (1 µg/ml), PGE_2 (1 µg/ml) and hCG (100 IU/ml), alone and in combination, on tissue cAMP production in isolated human corpus lutea of the early luteal phase after a 1-h incubation period. Each bar represents the mean of 12-30 observations. Vertical lines indicate the SEM. The effects of PGE_2, hCG, hCG plus $PGF_{2\alpha}$, and hCG plus PGE_2 vs. the controls (C) are statistically significant (P<0.05, P<0.01, P<0.01 and P<0.01, respectively). Data from reference 31.

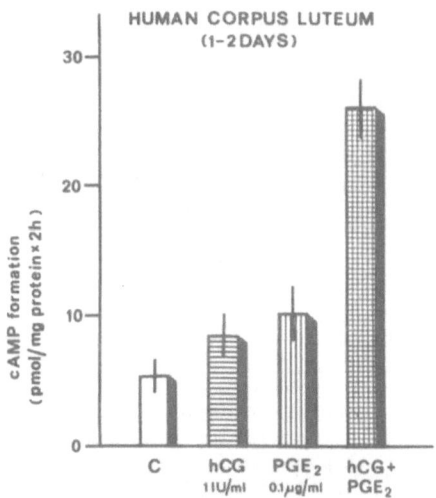

Fig. 2. Influence of hCG and PGE_2, alone or
in combination, on cAMP formation by a very
early corpus luteum. The effect of the
combined influence vs. the control is significant ($P<0.01$). Vertical lines indicate
± SEM.

PROSTAGLANDIN I_2

PGI_2 has been postulated to be of physiological importance, especially in the early luteal phase and around the time for implantation.
Both the myometrium and the endometrium have been shown to contain high
concentrations of PGI_2, and it cannot be excluded that the countercurrent
system between the utero-ovarian vein and ovarian artery can transport
this labile PG to the corpus luteum. PGI_2 can also be formed by the human
corpus luteum as reported by Liedkite and Seifer (12). In experiments on
corpus lutea from the goat, it was recently reported that PGI_2 could
stimulate progesterone formation (13). A stimulatory effect on cAMP

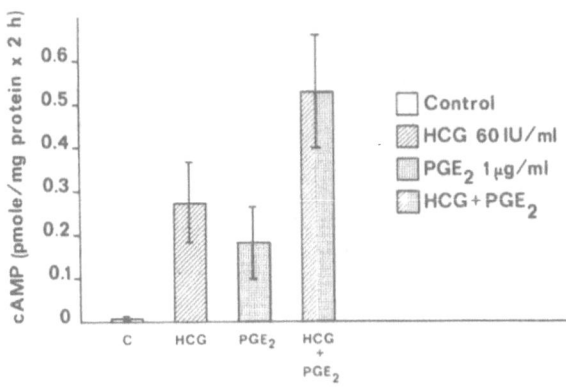

Fig. 3. Effect of hCG and PGE_2, alone and
in combination, on the cAMP release into the
incubation medium from an 8-day old corpus
luteum. Data from reference 9.

Table 1. Influence of PGE_2 and hCG on progesterone release into the incubation media after a 2-h incubation period by the human corpus luteum of mid- and late-luteal phase of the menstrual cycle and of early pregnancy.

	PGE_2 1 µg/ml (% of control)[a]	hCG 10 IU/ml (% of control)[a]
Midluteal phase[b] (18)[c]	137 ± 11.3*	176 ± 8.6**
Late luteal phase[b] (7)[c]	159 ± 34.2	205 ± 35.9*
Early pregnancy[b] (9)[c]	146 ± 12.8*	127 ± 11.1

[a] Values given are percentage of control and represent the mean ± SEM. The stimulatory effect of PGE_2 vs. control is significant ($P < 0.05$) in midluteal phase and early pregnancy. The stimulatory effect of hCG vs. control is significant ($P < 0.01$, $P < 0.05$, respectively) in midluteal phase and late luteal phase. No other comparisons are statistically significant.
[b] The control value 100% corresponds to 709, 245, 682 ng progesterone/mg protein, respectively.
[c] The number of corpus lutea is given in parentheses.

formation was reported some years ago from our laboratory (14) (Fig. 4) in dispersed human luteal cells, although its potential physiological importance at that time was unclear. Like PGE_2, PGI_2 may be of physiological importance in the early luteal phase and partly responsible for the more rapid rise in serum progesterone registered in IVF pregnancies compared to IVF cycles where no pregnancy occurs (15).

PROSTAGLANDIN $F_{2\alpha}$

The mechanism(s) underlying functional luteolysis in the human is still unknown. In several animal species, there is strong evidence that $PGF_{2\alpha}$ is the essential luteolytic agent. Thus, Behrman et al. (16) already in 1971 reported in experiments on the rat corpus luteum that $PGF_{2\alpha}$ could block the acute stimulation of progesterone secretion induced by LH. Later, Lahav et al. (17) found a similar interaction between $PGF_{2\alpha}$ and LH on cAMP formation in corpus lutea from early pregnant rats. Our group was the first to demonstrate that LH- or hCG-stimulated cAMP and progesterone formation in slices of human corpus luteum from the midluteal phase could be counteracted by $PGF_{2\alpha}$ (Fig. 5, 6). In specimens from young corpus lutea, $PGF_{2\alpha}$ does not seem to interfere with LH and hCG, either on cAMP or on progesterone formation. Human corpus lutea of early and midluteal phases contain and produce similar amounts of $PGF_{2\alpha}$ (4), and receptors for $PGF_{2\alpha}$ have been located in the human corpus luteum in all phases of the natural cycle (17).

CATECHOLAMINES

Both in the rat and in the human, catecholamines can exert luteotropic effects on the corpus luteum in terms of increased cAMP and progesterone formation (18,19). It has also been reported that PMSG-induced rat corpus lutea rapidly acquire β-adrenergic receptors during the first days after their formation and that the β-adrenergic receptors decline thereafter (20). Concomitant with this decline, a decrease is

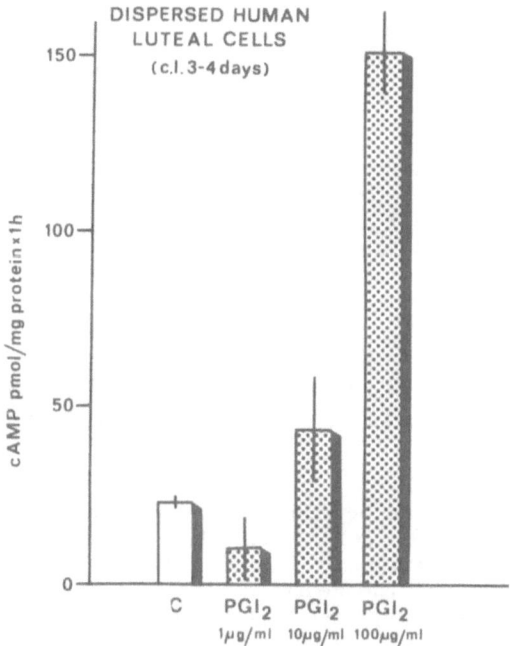

Fig. 4. Cyclic AMP formation by dispersed human luteal cells from an early human corpus luteum. The cells were incubated for 1 h in the absence or presence of PGI_2 methyl esther in various concentrations. Vertical lines indicate ± SEM. Data from reference 14.

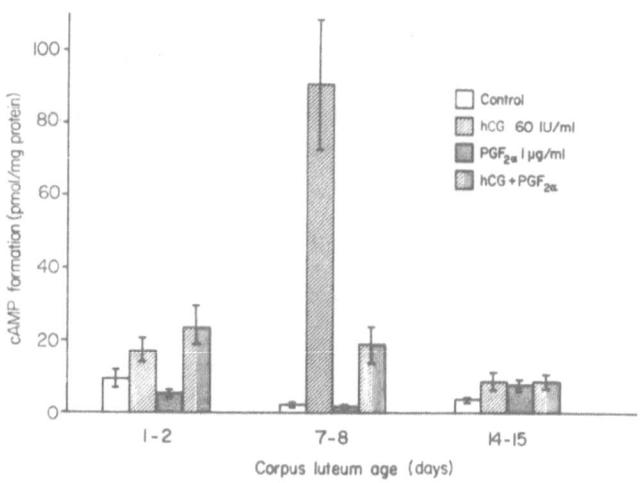

Fig. 5. Effects of hCG and $PGF_{2\alpha}$, alone and in combination, on the cAMP production of isolated human corpus lutea of different ages. Each group of columns represents values from 3-4 patients. Vertical lines represent ± SEM. Data from reference 9.

195

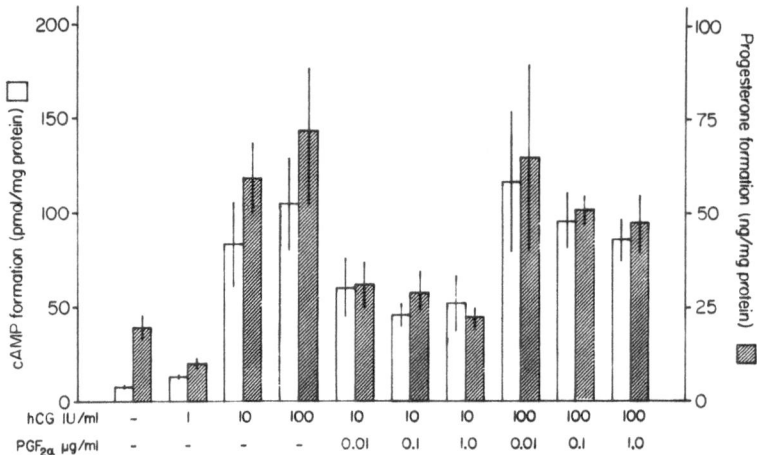

Fig. 6. Interaction between various concentrations of hCG (10-100 IU/ml) and PGF$_{2\alpha}$ (0.01-1.0 µg/ml) on cAMP and progesterone formation in a human corpus luteum from the midluteal phase of the menstrual cycle. Incubation time 2 h. Vertical lines represent ± SEM. Data from reference 31.

seen in the response to β-adrenergic agonists in the rat corpus luteum (21). In spite of numerous reports on β-adrenergic effects on corpus luteum metabolism in animals, only few reports concerning the occurrence of catecholamines in this tissue have been published (22,23). In these studies the determinations were performed on corpus lutea at one specific age. In a recent study from our laboratory (21), it was demonstrated that the endogenous levels of both adrenaline and noradrenaline (NA), measured by HPLC according to Keller et al. (24) and modified by Jonsson et al. (25), were low in the early luteal phase. Around day 7 following ovulation, the tissue content of NA increased two- to threefold. These determinations were performed both in corpus lutea from PMSG-treated rats, but also in the human corpus luteum (Fig. 7). The tissue content of adrenaline seems low and unaltered during the entire luteal phase.

Prior to ovulation, the membrana granulosa of a preovulatory follicle is avascular and not innervated. Following rupture, however, the blood flow in the corpus luteum increases tremendously, probably due to the lack of neuronal control of the blood vessels. In studies on PMSG-treated rats, a noradrenergic innervation of the vessels appears concomitant with a decrease in the blood flow (26). Whether the NA in the corpus luteum only emanates from vascular innervation or from avascular compartments as well cannot be evaluated from the above-mentioned experiments.

In experiments on cell suspensions of human luteal cells, Richardson and Masson (27), as well as Casper et al. (28), failed to demonstrate a stimulatory effect of catecholamines on cAMP and progesterone formation. In 1984 we reported a stimulatory effect by NA on progesterone formation in intact tissue specimens of human corpus lutea in the early luteal phase (26). The difference in preparation techniques may well be responsible for this discrepancy.

GONADOTROPINS AND CATECHOLAMINES

A synergism between catecholamines and gonadotropins on cAMP and progesterone formation seems to exist in the early and midluteal phases in

196

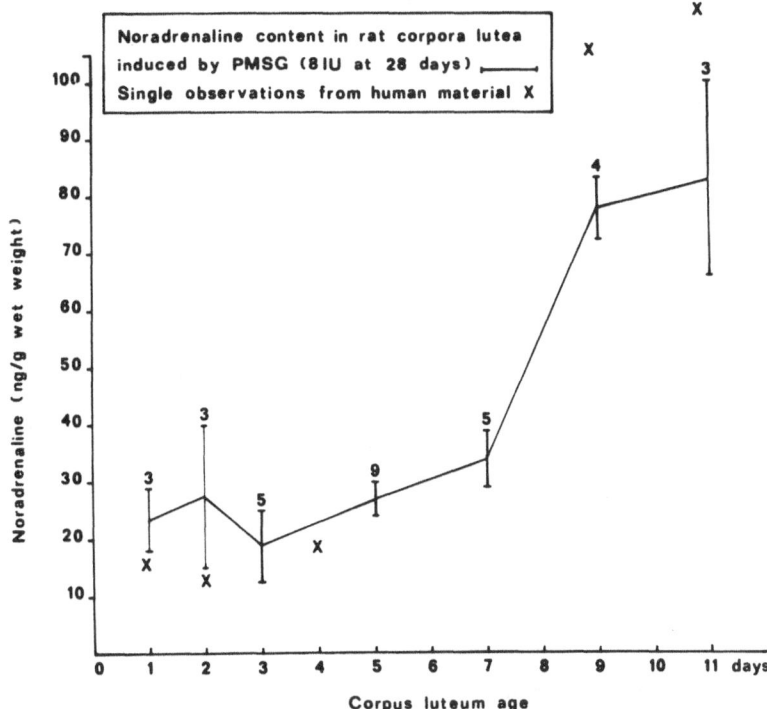

Fig. 7. Levels of NA, determined biochemically by use of
HPLC, in isolated rat corpus lutea of different ages.
Also indicated in the figure are individual observations
from isolated human corpus lutea (dots).   Data from
reference 21.

the human corpus luteum in vitro.   In 1980 we reported (14) that NA
(1 µg/ml), in combination with hCG (60 IU/ml), caused a dramatic increase
in cAMP formation compared to hCG alone in specimens of corpus lutea
isolated 1 to 3 days postovulation (Fig. 8).   Recently, we reported a
similar synergism between hCG and isoproteronol in experiments on cultured
granulosa cells between day 4 and 6 in culture (Fig. 9) (8).   In this
experimental situation, no significant effect on basal progesterone
secretion was found when isoproteronol was added alone.

GONADOTROPINS AND PROSTAGLANDINS

As mentioned earlier, a potentiation of the gonadotropin effect in
the presence of PGE_2 seems to exist in the very early luteal phase.   Later
in the natural cycle, hCG and PGE_2 have additive effects.   In a recent
study from this laboratory (11), it was shown that PGE_2 caused a more
rapid increase in progesterone formation than did hCG.   However, the
duration of the stimulatory effect was significantly shorter for PGE_2 than
for hCG.   These data were based on both incubation and superfusion experiments.   The explanation for this difference in type of effect may be due
to different cell populations in the corpus luteum specimens which has
been demonstrated both morphologically and functionally (29,30).

197

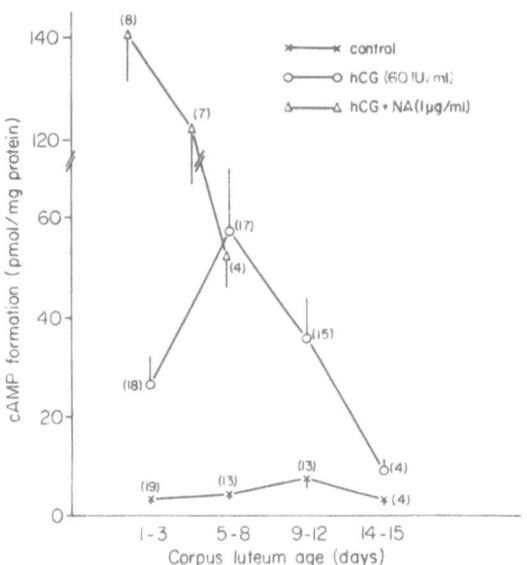

Fig. 8. Tissue cAMP in specimens (10–15 mg wet weight) of corpus lutea from various ages incubated for 2 h. Vertical lines indicate ± SEM. The effects of hCG and hCG + NA are highly significant (P<0.001). Data from reference 14.

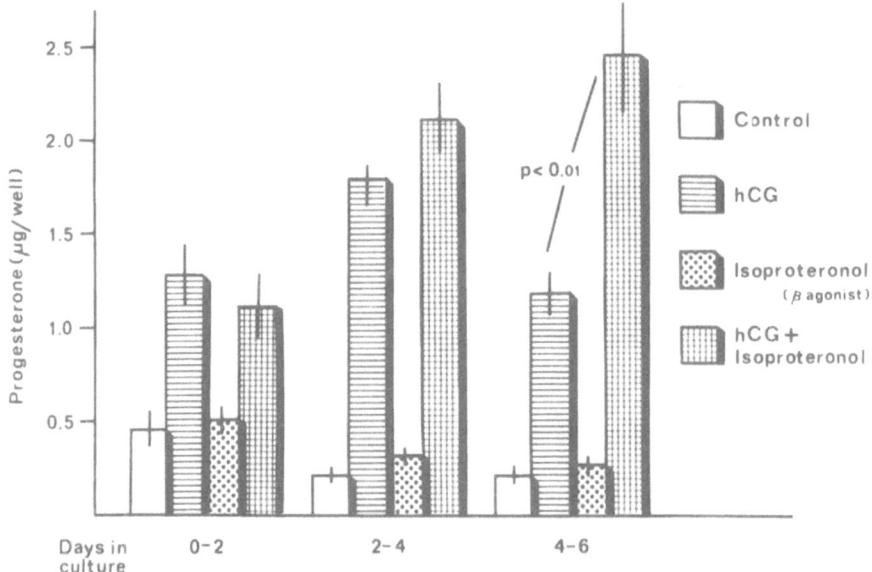

Fig. 9. Effects of hCG and isoproteronol on progesterone secretion. Granulosa cells from hMG–hCG–stimulated patients were cultured with hCG (10 IU/ml), isoproteronol (10^{-7}M) or a combination thereof. Mean ± SEM of 3 to 4 replicates per group are shown. **P<0.01 (with analysis of variance) compared to hCG alone. Data from reference 8.

The interaction(s) between catecholamines and $PGF_{2\alpha}$ is more complicated. The antigonadotropic effect of $PGF_{2\alpha}$ exists only in the corpus luteum of the mid- or late-luteal phases (31,32) while in the early corpus luteum (1 to 5 days postovulation), $PGF_{2\alpha}$ does not interfere with basal or gonadotropin-induced cAMP and progesterone formation (Fig. 5). As mentioned above, the amounts of endogenous catecholamines appeared to be low in corpus lutea of the early luteal phase of the rat and the human (21). The hypothesis that vascular innervation is a prerequisite for PG-induced luteolysis in the human corpus luteum was put forward (14). Specimens of early corpus lutea were incubated in the presence of hCG, $PGF_{2\alpha}$ or NA and in various combinations. It was found that $PGF_{2\alpha}$ could exert its antigonadotropic effects also in young corpus lutea if the medium was fortified with NA (Fig. 10). To demonstrate the importance of catecholamines further, specimens from older corpus lutea were preincubated with reserpine to deplete the tissue of catecholamines. In this situation, $PGF_{2\alpha}$ could no longer counteract the stimulatory influence by hCG on cAMP formation (Fig. 11).

In an additional series of experiments (33), we exposed corpus lutea of the midluteal phase to the β-adrenoreceptor blocker propranolol concomitant with hCG and $PGF_{2\alpha}$. The antigonadotropic effects of $PGF_{2\alpha}$ on cAMP and progesterone were then abolished (Fig. 12, 13). In conclusion, our data strongly indicate that the presence of adrenergic innervation and β-receptor stimulation is a prerequisite for the antigonadotropic effect of $PGF_{2\alpha}$. These findings can also explain why attempts to demonstrate the luteolytic effects of $PGF_{2\alpha}$ in dispersed human luteal cells have been unsuccessful (28). Tissue integrity with preserved luteal innervation is essential to demonstrate the luteolytic action of $PGF_{2\alpha}$ in human corpus lutea of the midluteal phase.

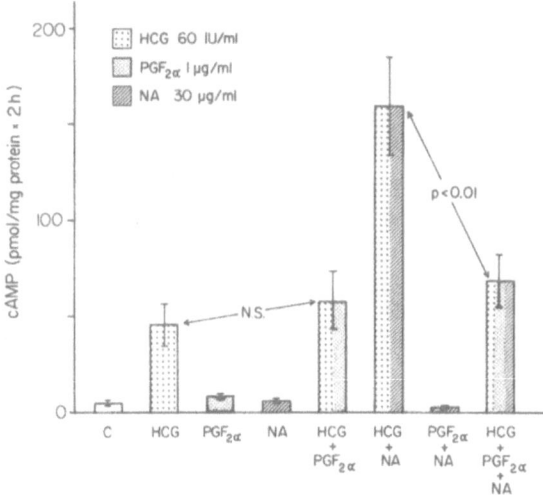

Fig. 10. CAMP formation in 1-2-day-old human corpus lutea (2 patients). Effects of hCG, $PGF_{2\alpha}$, and NA in various combinations on tissue cAMP after 2-h incubation. Vertical lines indicate ± SEM. Significances are indicated in the figure. Data from reference 14.

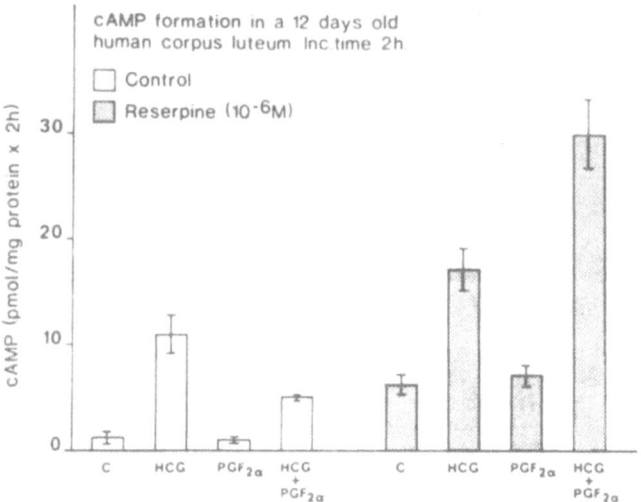

Fig. 11. Comparison between the effects of hCG, $PGF_{2\alpha}$ or their combination in a corpus luteum preincubated for 60 min in buffer containing reserpine (10^{-6}M). The significant antagonistic effect induced by $PGF_{2\alpha}$ (open bars) is turned into a stimulatory effect in the presence of reserpine (hatched bars). Vertical lines indicate ± SEM. Data from reference 14.

CLINICAL APPLICATIONS

Based on our in vitro results on corpus luteum function, a few clinical trials have been conducted. In the first series of experiments (34), a PGF analog (ICI 81.008) was administered as vaginal suppositories in the early and midluteal phases of natural cycles (Fig. 14). It was found that serum progesterone was significantly decreased compared to the control cycle. Each woman served as her own control. These data indicate an antigonadotropic, i.e., a luteolytic, effect which is in accordance with the in vitro studies on the human corpus luteum. It may be hypothesized that PGF analogues are able to regulate fertility.

In another trial, $PGF_{2\alpha}$ or 15-methyl-$PGF_{2\alpha}$ was injected into the corpus lutea of patients with an early ectopic pregnancy (35). An additional injection of PG was performed directly into the affected oviduct. The described procedure resulted in a rapid decline of hCG and a termination of the ectopic pregnancy without further intervention (Fig. 15). These preliminary results point to the possibility of utilizing $PGF_{2\alpha}$ or its analogs for termination of ectopic pregnancy. In contrast to systemic administration, the local injections did not cause any adverse effects.

An expanded knowledge of the mechanism of action for PGs and catecholamines on human corpus luteum function will certainly open new possibilities for interfering with corpus luteum function in the menstrual cycle and in early pregnancy.

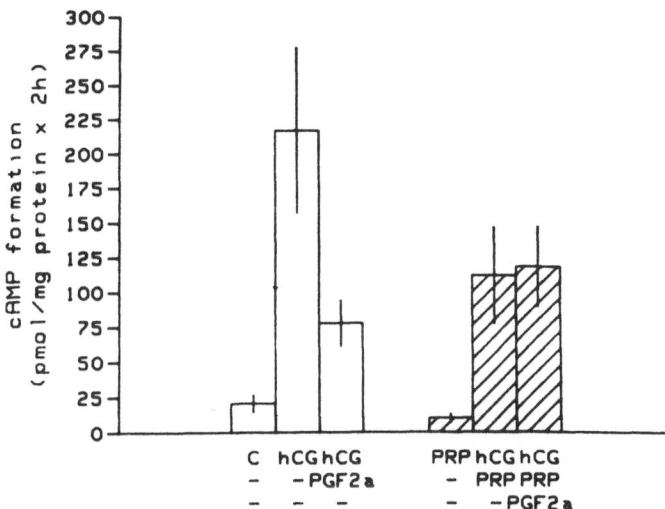

Fig. 12. Effects of hCG (100 IU/ml), PGF$_{2\alpha}$ (1 μg/ml)
and propranolol (PRP) (1 μg/ml), 4×10^{-6}M), alone or in
the combinations indicated, on cAMP formation by isolated human corpus lutea of midluteal phase after a
2-h incubation period. Each bar represents the mean
of 14-15 observations. Vertical lines indicate SEM.
In the left group (open bars, absence of PRP), the
effects of hCG vs. control and of hCG and PGF$_{2\alpha}$ vs.
hCG alone are statistically significant (P<0.01 and
P<0.05, respectively). In the right group (hatched
bars, presence of PRP), the effects of hCG and PRP vs.
PRP alone and of hCG in combination with PGF$_{2\alpha}$ and PRP
vs. PRP alone are significant (P<0.05). Data from
reference 14.

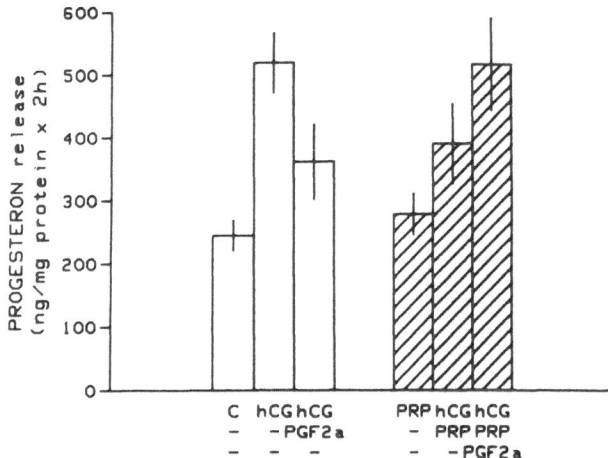

Fig. 13. Effects of hCG (100 IU/ml) and propranolol (PRP) (1 µg/ml), 4×10^{-6}), alone or in the combinations indicated, on the release of progesterone into the incubation medium after a 2-h incubation period of human corpus lutea of the midluteal phase. Each bar represents the mean of 27-37 observations. Vertical lines indicate SEM. In the left group (open bars, absence of PRP), the effects of hCG vs. control and of hCG and $PGF_{2\alpha}$ vs. hCG alone are statistically significant (P<0.01 and P<0.05, respectively). In the right group (hatched bars, presence of PRP), the stimulatory effect of hCG in combination with $PGF_{2\alpha}$ and PRP vs. PRP alone is significant (P<0.01), while no other differences in progesterone release are statistically significant. Data from reference 33.

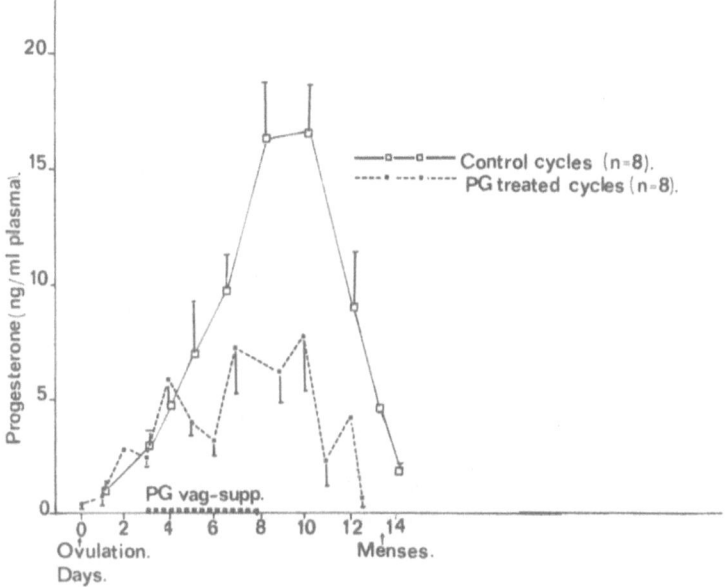

Fig. 14. Serum progesterone levels in 4 volunteers during the secretory phase in control and experimental cycles. In the experimental cycle, 2 vaginal suppositories (500–600 μg ICI 81.008) were administered to each subject with a fixed interval of 24 h at various times after ovulation. The treatment caused both a reduction of progesterone formation and shortening of the luteal phase. Data from reference 34.

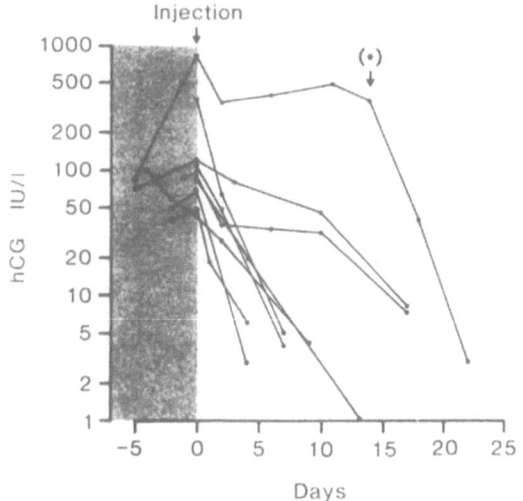

Fig. 15. Serum hCG concentration (log scale) in 9 patients with ectopic pregnancy treated with local $PGF_{2\alpha}$ injections. Data from reference 35.

ACKNOWLEDGMENTS

For typing the manuscript our thanks are due to Mrs. Ann-Louise Dahl. Certain illustrations were designed by Mrs. Marianne Wedblad. Supported by grants from The Swedish MRC (No. 2873).

REFERENCES

1. McCracken JA, Carlsson JC, Glew ME, et al. Prostaglandin identified as a luteolytic hormone in sheep. Nature New Biol 1972; 238:129-34.
2. Bendz A, Lundgren O, Hamberger L. Countercurrent exchange of progesterone and antipyrine between human utero-ovarian vessels and of antipyrine between the female vessels in the cat. Acta Physiol Scand 1982; 114:611-5.
3. Hamberger L, Hahlin M, Hillensjo T, Johanson C, Sjogren A. Luteotrophic and luteolytic factors regulating human corpus luteum function. Ann NY Acad Sci 1987 (in press).
4. Challis JRG, et al. Production of prostaglandin E and F by corpora lutea, corpora albicantes and stroma from the human ovary. J Endocrinol 1976; 68:401-8.
5. Pathvardhan VV, Linthier A. Luteal phase variations in endogenous concentrations of prostaglandins PGE and PGF and in the capacity for their in vitro formation in the human corpus luteum. Prostaglandins 1985; 30:91-8.
6. Vijayakumar R, Walters WA. Human luteal tissue prostaglandins, 17β-estradiol and progesterone in relation to the growth and genescence of the corpus luteum. Fertil Steril 1983; 29:298-303.
7. Fitz TA, Mayan MH, Sawyer HR, Niswender GD. Characterization of two steroidogenic cell types in the ovine corpus luteum. Biol Reprod 1982; 27:703-11.
8. Hillensjo T, Sjogren A, Strander B, et al. Effect of gonadotropins on progesterone secretion by cultured granulosa cells obtained from human preovulatory follicles. Acta Endocrinol (Copenh) 1985; 110:401-7.
9. Hamberger L, Nilsson L, Dennefors B, Khan I, Sjogren A. Cyclic AMP formation of isolated human corpora lutea in response to hCG-interference by $PGF_{2\alpha}$. Prostaglandins 1979; 17:615-21.
10. Marsh JM, LeMaire WJ. Cyclic AMP accumulation and steroidogenesis in the human corpus luteum: effect of gonadotropins and prostaglandins. J Clin Endocrinol Metab 1974; 38:99-106.
11. Hahlin M, Dennefors B, Johansson C, Hamberger L. Luteotrophic effects of PGE_2 on the human corpus luteum of the sterile cycle and in early pregnancy. J Clin Endocrinol Metab (submitted).
12. Liedkite M, Seifert B. Biosynthesis of prostaglandins in human ovarian tissue. Prostaglandins 1978; 16:825-33.
13. Band V, Kharbanda SM, Marugesan K, Farooq A. Prostacyclin and steroidogenesis in goat ovarian cell types in vitro. Prostaglandins 1986; 31:509-25.
14. Hamberger L, Dennefors B, Hamberger B, et al. Is vascular innervation a prerequisite for PG induced luteolysis in the human corpus luteum? In: Samuelsson B, Ramwell W, Pauletti P, eds. Advances in prostaglandin and thromboxane research. New York: Raven Press, 1980; 8:1365-8.
15. Jones HW, Seegar Jones G, Andrew MC, et al. Aspects of the programme for in vitro fertilization in Norfolk. In: Crosignani PG, Rubin BL, eds. In vitro fertilization and embryo transfer. London: Academic Press, 1983:365-71.
16. Behrman HR, Yoshinaga K, Greep RO. Extraluteal effects of prostaglandins. Ann NY Acad Sci 1971; 180:426-35.
17. Lahav M, Frend A, Lindner HR. Abrogation by prostaglandin $F_{2\alpha}$ of LH

stimulated cyclic AMP accumulation in isolated rat corpora lutea of pregnancy. Biochem Biophys Res Commun 1976; 68:1294-1300.

18. Selstam G, Rani S, Nordenstrom K, Norjavaara E, Rosberg S, Ahren K. Development of sensitivity to catecholamines in granulosa and luteal cells. In: McKerns KW, Aakwaag A, Hansson V. Regulation of target cell responsiveness. New York: Plenum Press, 1985:37-53.

19. Spicer LJ. Catecholaminergic regulation of ovarian function in mammals. Life Sci 1986; 39:1701-11.

20. Norjavaara E, Rosberg S, Gafvels M, Selstam G. β-adrenergic receptor concentration in corpora lutea of different ages obtained from pregnant mare serum gonadotropin-treated rats. Endocrinology 1984; 114:2154-9.

21. Selstam G, Norjavaara E, Rosberg S, Khan I, Hamberger L. Catecholamine content and adenylate cyclase activity in corpora lutea of different ages of the PMSG treated immature rat. Fertil Steril 1987 (in press).

22. Ben-Jonathan N, Arbogast LA, Rhoades TA, Bahr JM. Norepinephrine in the rat ovary. Outogeny and de novo synthesis. Endocrinology 1984; 115:1426-31.

23. Selstam G, Norjavaara E, Tegenfelt T, Lundberg S, Sandstrom C, Persson S-A. Partial denervation of the ovaries by transection of the suspensory ligament does not inhibit ovulation in rats treated with PMSG. Anat Rec 1985; 213:392-5.

24. Keller B, Oke A, Mefford E, Adams RN. Liquid chromatographic analysis of catecholamines. Routine assays for regional brain mapping. Life Sci 1976; 19:995-1004.

25. Jonsson G, Hallman H, Mefford E, Adams RN. In: Fuxe K, Goldstein M, Hokfelt B, Hokfelt T, eds. Central adrenaline neurons—basic aspects and cardiovascular functions. Oxford: Pergamon Press, 1980:59-71.

26. Dennefors B, Hamberger L, Hillensjo T, et al. Aspects concerning the role of prostaglandins for ovarian function. Acta Obstet Gynecol Scand Suppl 1982; 113:31-41.

27. Richardson M, Masson GM. Progesterone production by disperse cells from human corpus luteum: stimulation by gonadotropins and $PGF_{2\alpha}$; lack of response to adrenaline or isoprenaline. J Endocrinol 1980; 87:247-54.

28. Casper RF, Cofferell MA. The effects of adrenergic and cholinergic agents on progesterone production by human corpus luteum in vitro. Am J Obstet Gynecol 1984; 148:663-9.

29. Crisp TM, Dessouky A, Denys FR. The fine structure of the human corpus luteum of early pregnancy and during the progestational phase of the menstrual cycle. Am J Anat 1970; 127:37-70.

30. Fitz TA, Hoyer PB, Niswender GD. Interaction of prostaglandins with subpopulation of ovine luteal cells. I. Stimulatory effects of prostaglandins E_1, E_2, and I_2. Prostaglandins 1984; 28:119-26.

31. Dennefors BL, Sjogren A, Hamberger L. Progesterone and cAMP formation by isolated human corpora lutea of different ages: influences of human chorionic gonadotropins and prostaglandins. J Clin Endocrinol Metab 1982; 55:102-7.

32. Pathwardhan VV, Lanthier A. Effect of prostaglandin $F_{2\alpha}$ on the hCG stimulated progesterone production by human corpora lutea. Prostaglandins 1984; 27:465-73.

33. Bennegard B, Dennefors B, Hamberger L. Interaction between catecholamine and prostaglandin $F_{2\alpha}$ in human luteolysis. Acta Endocrinol (Copenh) 1984; 106:533-7.

34. Hamberger L, Kallfelt B, Forshell S, Dukes M. A luteolytic effect of prostaglandin $F_{2\alpha}$ analogue in nonpregnant women. Contraception 1980; 22:383-8.

35. Lindblom B, Hahlin M, Kallfelt B, Hamberger L. Local $PGF_{2\alpha}$ injection for termination of ectopic pregnancy. Lancet 1987; 1:4:776-7.

REGULATION OF THE PRIMATE CORPUS LUTEUM

DURING EARLY PREGNANCY

Richard L. Stouffer, Joseph S. Ottobre* and
Catherine A. VandeVoort

Division of Reproductive Biology and Behavior, Oregon
Regional Primate Research Center, Beaverton, Oregon, and
*Department of Dairy Science, Ohio State University,
Columbus, Ohio

In women and many nonhuman primates, the life span of the corpus luteum during the nonfertile menstrual cycle is limited to approximately 2 weeks. However, the interval of luteal function is extended when conception and pregnancy follow ovulation. The so-called "rescue" (1) and continued function of the corpus luteum in early pregnancy is essential until the endocrine activities, notably progesterone production, are assumed by the placenta. Ovariectomy or lutectomy prior to the development of placental steroidogenesis causes abortion unless progesterone supplements are provided (2). The luteal-placental shift occurs near the end of the third week of gestation in rhesus monkeys (3) and at 6 weeks in women (2). Hence, the corpus luteum of the fertile cycle must function for an additional 1-4 weeks to ensure continued pregnancy in these species.

It is widely accepted that the life span of the corpus luteum is prolonged in early pregnancy by chorionic gonadotropin (CG), a glycoprotein hormone secreted by the developing syncytiotrophoblast (1,2). Circulating CG is first detected in women around 9 days after ovulation, rises to peak levels at 8-12 weeks of gestation, and then declines to lower but detectable levels throughout the remainder of pregnancy. The role, if any, for CG after the first few weeks of pregnancy is unknown. Interestingly, the duration of CG production in monkeys is much shorter than in humans. Macaque CG is no longer detected in circulating blood, urine concentrates, or placental extracts after the 40th day of pregnancy (4). The precise stage at which the embryo begins secreting CG and when the corpus luteum is first exposed to this hormone is ill-defined. The earliest detection of CG in the peripheral circulation at 9-11 days after ovulation appears to coincide with the initial attachment of the blastocyst and trophoblast formation (5). However, there are scattered reports of CG in ovarian venous blood or in concanavalin-A extracts of urine up to 3 days before its detection in peripheral blood (6). Thus, a possible earlier role of CG from the pre-implantation blastocyst should be considered (5).

Several experimental approaches indicate that CG plays a vital role in the maintenance of the corpus luteum during early pregnancy. In 1975, Moudgal and co-workers (7) reported that passive immunization of monkeys with anti-LH/CG antiserum prior to the luteal-placental shift caused a rapid decline in serum progesterone levels and pregnancy termination. Likewise, active immunization with modified forms of hCG or its β subunit produced infertility in women (8) and nonhuman primates (9) despite normal ovulatory cycles. In an elegant study, Thau and Sundaram (10) showed that the antifertility effect of CG antibodies in rhesus macaques was due to the prevention of extended luteal function in early pregnancy. Administration of a synthetic progestin, medroxyprogesterone acetate (MPA), to animals with anti-CG antibodies restored fertility to control levels. The progesterone patterns in MPA-treated monkeys indicated that the typical increase due to the rescue of the corpus luteum in early pregnancy did not occur, but the later rise due to placental synthesis was normal. Thus, CG is essential for corpus luteum rescue and indirectly promotes placental/embryonic development after implantation via the stimulation of luteal progesterone production.

There are numerous reports that exogenous CG acutely increases circulating progesterone levels and extends the life span of the corpus luteum of the menstrual cycle in women (11,12) and nonhuman primates (13,14). After the development of specific radioimmunoassays for CG, investigators employed longer treatment regimens to mimic the patterns and levels of endogenous CG in early pregnancy. Wilks and Noble (15) and our laboratory (16) demonstrated that a 10-day regimen of increasing doses of hCG beginning on day 8-10 of the luteal phase elicited changes in luteal function in rhesus monkeys which were characteristic of early pregnancy (1; see Figure 1): (a) the temporal response, levels and patterns of progesterone secretion were remarkably similar; (b) the life span of the corpus luteum was extended; and, (c) nonsteroidogenic activities, such as relaxin production (discussed later, 17) were enhanced. Thus, CG in the absence of other embryonic or placental factors (18), appears capable of rescuing the corpus luteum in early pregnancy. Treatment of nonpregnant rhesus monkeys with hCG in the described manner offers a suitable model for studying the mechanisms involved in the regulation of the primate corpus luteum by CG in early gestation. This model overcomes the problems associated with breeding and monitoring conception in primates. Also, the interval from initial CG exposure to subsequent luteal responses can be timed precisely.

THE MECHANISM OF ACTION OF CG

Although gonadotropic activity was discovered in the urine of pregnant women in 1927 by Aschheim and Zondek (19), the chemical, biologic, and immunologic properties of this substance now known as hCG were not unraveled until the past two decades (20). Human CG is a member of the glycoprotein family of hormones, which includes luteinizing hormone (LH), follicle-stimulating hormone (FSH), and thyroid stimulating hormone (TSH). These hormones consist of two noncovalently-associated subunits, designated α and β. The primary structures of the α-subunits in these hormones are identical. There is also substantial homology between the β subunits of hLH and hCG; 89 of the amino acid residues in β-hLH share identical positions in the NH_2-terminal sequence of β-hCG. However, β-hCG contains an additional 30 amino acids at the COOH-terminus and additional oligosaccharide chains on serine residues. Consequently, hCG is estimated to be the largest gonadotropin (37,000 kD) with the greatest proportion (30% by weight) of carbohydrate content.

In virtually every system studied, the effects of administered hCG closely resemble those of the pituitary gonadotropin, LH (20). Due to its relative abundance, hCG is used in place of LH in clinical and research situations to promote a number of ovarian events, including meiotic

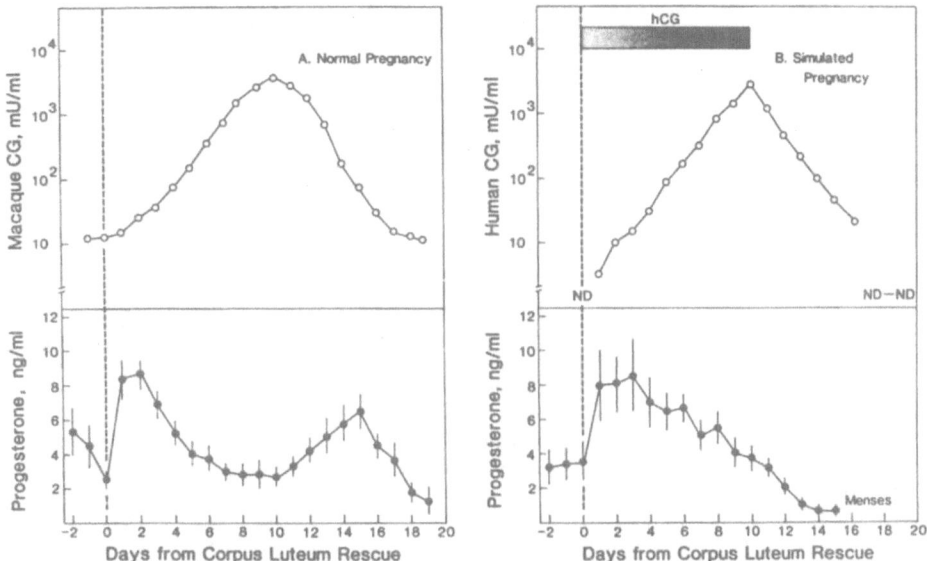

Fig. 1. Composite of progesterone and CG levels circulating in rhesus monkeys during actual early pregnancy (A) or during administration of increasing doses of hCG for 10 days (B) to simulate the pattern of macaque CG in normal pregnancy. Data (mean ± SE) are normalized to the day before rescue of the corpus luteum (day 0). Note the temporal relationship between progesterone and CG patterns. The second peak in circulating progesterone on day 16 of normal pregnancy is of placental origin. Adapted from reports of Knobil (1; Fig. 1a) and Ottobre and Stouffer (16; Fig. 1b).

maturation of oocytes, ovulation, and the development and function of the corpus luteum (21,22). Studies in our laboratory on the initial steps in gonadotropin action indicate that the macaque corpus luteum contains a single population of receptors which bind both hLH (but not nonprimate LH preparations, 23) and hCG with equally high affinity (equilibrium dissociation constant, $K_d \approx 1 \times 10^{-10}$ M) throughout the luteal phase of the menstrual cycle (24,25), and in our simulated model of early pregnancy (26). Moreover, both hLH and hCG stimulate adenylate cyclase and cyclic AMP secretion by macaque luteal membranes (27) and enhance progesterone secretion by dispersed luteal cells during short-term incubations in vitro (28). Research on human luteal tissue (29,30) generally supports the concept that LH and CG share a common receptor which regulates luteal cells at least in part via cAMP-mediated processes.

In an earlier chapter in this monograph, Zeleznik reviewed the importance of pituitary LH in the control of the corpus luteum of the menstrual cycle. Several investigators have demonstrated that LH is secreted from the pituitary in an episodic manner and that the frequency of LH pulses slows during the luteal phase of the menstrual cycle in women (31) and monkeys (32). However, recent studies indicate that varying the LH pulse frequency within the range observed during the menstrual cycle (1 pulse per 60-90 min to 1 pulse per 8 h) did not alter the functional life span of the corpus luteum. Zeleznik noted that premature reduction of the LH pulse frequency in the early luteal phase failed to elicit premature luteolysis in rhesus monkeys (33). Conversely, maintenance of high-frequency LH pulses during the luteal phase in monkeys (34) or women (35) did not prevent timely luteolysis. These observations suggest that a decrease in pituitary LH support is not the primary cause of luteal regression during the menstrual cycle. Moreover, increasing the frequency of LH pulses over a physiologic range will not extend the life span of the corpus luteum.

Within this framework, it remains to be determined how the production of another LH-like hormone, namely hCG, rescues the corpus luteum in early pregnancy. Perhaps it is related to differences in the secretion or circulating patterns of LH and CG during the late luteal phase. To date, the rapid sampling methods which led to the discovery of pulsatile LH secretion by the pituitary have not been employed to closely monitor CG patterns during pregnancy initiation. However, it is unlikely that CG patterns mimic those of LH during the late luteal phase (Fig. 2). The intermittent pulses of LH translate into intervals of gonadotropin support and deprivation for the corpus luteum which correlate positively with luteal steroidogenic activity. Since CG has a much longer half-life than LH in the bloodstream (20) and is produced in increasing amounts by the developing syncytiotrophoblast (5), CG may circulate continuously and in rising levels which ultimately obscure any remaining vestige of LH pulses (Fig. 2). Thus, the placenta may offer uninterrupted (as opposed to episodic) and increasing levels of luteotropic support for the corpus luteum. Whether such qualitative and quantitative differences in circulating gonadotropin are the primary factors in the rescue of the corpus luteum in early pregnancy await experimentation. Also, there may be important differences in the mechanisms of action of LH and CG in the primate corpus luteum. To date, most studies on gonadotropin action have focused on acute responses; little is known about later effects on cellular parameters, including hormone production, growth or differentiation. Niswender and co-workers have several lines of evidence which indicate that the movement and fate of ovine LH-receptor complexes on ovine luteal cells is markedly different from that of receptors occupied with hCG (36). These findings may explain why a short (15-min) exposure to hCG stimulated progesterone secretion by ovine luteal cells for a prolonged period of time (>6 h), whereas a similar pulse of oLH enhanced steroidogenesis only briefly (36). Whether a more persistent interaction and response to gonadotropin of placental, as opposed to pituitary, origin occurs in primate target tissues, is unknown. Further studies are clearly needed which compare the mechanisms of LH and CG action in species where these are both endogenous hormones.

Equally puzzling is the relationship of the CG signal to the luteolytic processes which normally occur within the corpus luteum at the end of the menstrual cycle. The factors and mechanisms responsible for luteolysis in primates are poorly understood. Until the physiologic events in luteal regression are documented, we can only speculate that CG either prevents a luteolytic "signal" from occurring or overcomes an existing signal by a quantum increase in luteotropic support. Evidence for the operation of both such mechanisms exists in nonprimate species during maternal recognition of pregnancy (37).

THE TRANSIENT RESPONSE OF THE CORPUS LUTEUM TO CG

With the first exposure to CG in early pregnancy, the levels of circulating progesterone in rhesus monkeys quickly rise above those seen in the normal menstrual cycle (Fig. 1a). Shortly thereafter, the progesterone concentration declines despite the continued presence—indeed, rising levels—of CG. A similar biphasic response is observed in women, although the interval of maximal progesterone levels is extended somewhat (38). This phenomenon also occurs in monkeys during an hCG treatment regimen designed to simulate the pattern and levels of CG in early preg-

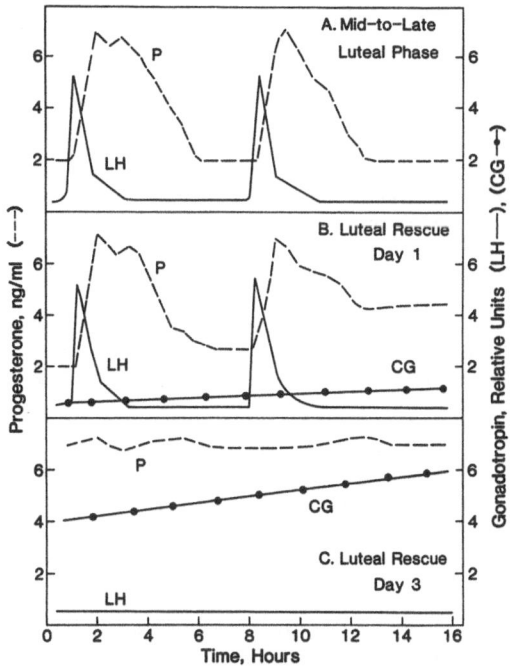

Fig. 2. Schematic representation of progesterone and gonadotropin (LH and CG) levels
circulating in rhesus monkeys during the
mid-to-late luteal phase of the nonfertile
(A) menstrual cycle and as postulated
following initial (day 1) and 3 days of CG
exposure during rescue of the corpus luteum
in the fertile cycle (B, C). Whereas LH is
secreted in intermittent pulses (1 pulse
every 8 h) by the pituitary, the developing
trophoblast may secrete increasing amounts
of CG which circulate for long intervals due
to its protracted half-life. Whether these
possible differences between LH and CG
exposure are sufficient to explain the
rescue of the corpus luteum by an LH-like
hormone is unknown. Data in top panel (A)
is adapted from Ellinwood et al. (32).

nancy (Fig. 1b). The mechanisms responsible for the transient response to
CG are unknown, although several hypotheses have been presented.

In 1972, Neill and Knobil (13) proposed that after the initial
response to CG, the corpus luteum of early pregnancy became refractory to
further stimulation by the continued high levels of gonadotropin.
Evidence from our laboratory (39) that luteal cells from the rhesus monkey
no longer respond to hCG in vitro with increased progesterone production
by day 22 of pregnancy (~13 days exposure to endogenous CG) supported this
hypothesis. Neill and Knobil originally postulated that the refractory
state was due to the depletion of precursors for progesterone secretion
following the initial steroidogenic response to CG. In the past decade,
investigators have determined that many factors control the rate of
progesterone production by the corpus luteum, including the availability

and metabolism of external sources of cholesterol. In the human corpus luteum, it appears that progesterone synthesis is dependent on low density lipoprotein (LDL) cholesterol in the circulation (40,41). Research in various systems indicates that LDL is taken up through a receptor-mediated endocytotic pathway and cholesterol is liberated for use by the cell. Golos and co-workers (42) provided important insight into the control mechanisms in luteal tissue when they reported that the expression of LDL receptors by luteinized granulosa cells from women was regulated by two pathways: (a) a stimulatory pathway involving hCG action and probably mediated via cAMP, and (b) an inhibitory pathway mediated by cholesterol. Conceivably, the availability of circulating LDL, the expression of LDL receptors, or the intracellular metabolism of lipoprotein in luteal cells could be insufficient to maintain progesterone synthesis during early pregnancy. Significant alterations in cholesterol metabolism/storage likely occur, since histologic studies (43) observed a rapid depletion of lipid droplets in many luteal cells during early pregnancy. Whether such changes are causes or effects of the gonadotropin refractory state of the corpus luteum must also be established.

Alternatively, the transient response to CG in early pregnancy may represent the delayed, but now predominant, activation of luteolytic processes normally observed at the end of the menstrual cycle. In a review published in 1973, Knobil (1) proposed a "self-destruct mechanism" whereby a secretory product of the primate corpus luteum elicits luteolysis during the cycle. The candidate nominated was estrogen. Since the concentrations of estradiol and estrone remain elevated during early pregnancy, Knobil also hypothesized a role for estrogens in the transient response of the corpus luteum to CG. Neither the described luteolytic role for estrogens (44) nor their intraluteal site of action (45) has been supported by recent investigations on rhesus monkeys during the menstrual cycle. Nevertheless similar approaches, such as administering an aromatase inhibitor (44) to evaluate estrogen's role in early pregnancy, have not been reported. Other products of the corpus luteum, including $PGF_{2\alpha}$ (46) or oxytocin (47) may regulate the functional life span of the corpus luteum during the menstrual cycle, and possibly in early pregnancy. However, definitive studies establishing their physiologic importance and comparing their actions during luteolysis in the menstrual cycle and in the transient response to CG in early pregnancy are needed.

During the course of our experiments on the LH/CG receptor-adenylate cyclase system in the corpus luteum of rhesus monkeys, other researchers reported the loss of gonadotropin receptors (36) and diminished gonadotropin-stimulated adenylate cyclase activity (48) in luteal tissue from domestic animals and rodents following in vivo administration of a large bolus of LH or CG. These events, termed "down-regulation of receptors" and "desensitization of adenylate cyclase" occur in many target tissues in response to elevated levels of peptide or protein hormones. We postulated that similar changes in the gonadotropin receptor-adenylate cyclase system could play an important role in the development of a refractory state in the primate corpus luteum to the rising levels of CG in early pregnancy. The nonpregnant rhesus monkey given increasing amounts of hCG for up to 10 days beginning near the typical time of implantation in the luteal phase of the cycle (Fig. 1b) was employed as a model for early pregnancy. The steroidogenic response during the initial exposure (≤24 h) to CG in vivo was not associated with any apparent change in the gonadotropin receptor-adenylate cyclase system (49,50). Subsequently, the number of available CG receptors declined concomitant with the fall in circulating progesterone (Fig. 3); moreover, the affinity of the remaining receptors for CG was reduced after 6-10 days of treatment. However, the decline in available receptor sites was balanced by a marked increase in sites occupied with administered CG. Thus, CG exposure did NOT result in downregulation or loss of receptors per se. Rather, there was remarkable constancy of the total (available + occupied) receptor population within the corpus luteum despite dramatic changes in circulating gonadotropin and progesterone secretory activity in simulated early pregnancy. Nevertheless, the functional capacity of the remaining available receptors and those occupied with administered CG was questionable.

Studies on the adenylate cyclase system in luteal tissue from simulated early pregnancy (Fig. 4; 50) indicated that the ability to respond to gonadotropin in vitro was impaired after 3 days of hCG treatment—even though our earlier investigations observed appreciable numbers of available receptors at this stage. By 6-10 days of hCG treatment, cAMP production in vitro was insensitive to gonadotropin. Notably, the nonhormonal activators, forskolin and guanine nucleotides, as well as prostaglandins PGE_2, D_2, and I_2, continued to stimulate adenylate cyclase activity throughout simulated early pregnancy. We concluded that the various membrane components of the adenylate cyclase system were present, functional, and capable of transducing signals from PG receptors, but NOT

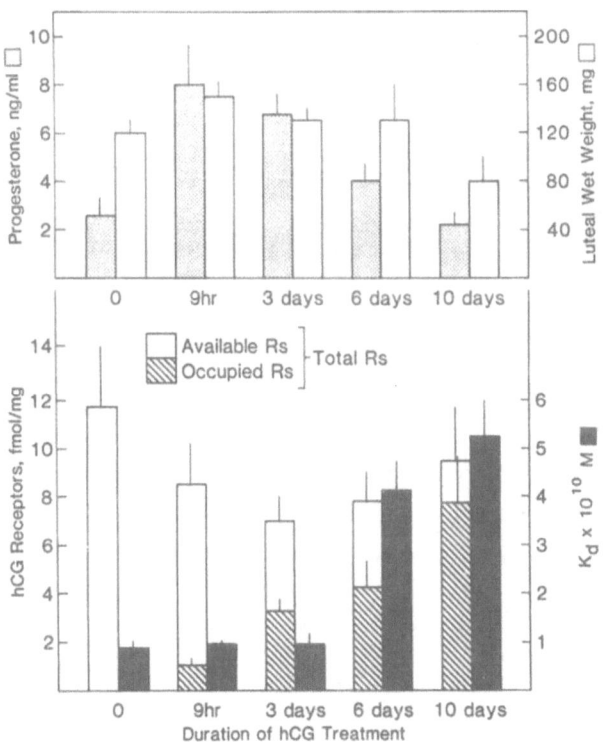

Fig. 3. Summary of the changes in the concentrations of available, occupied, and total receptors (Rs) for CG and the affinity constant of available CG receptors in the corpus luteum of rhesus monkeys during simulated early pregnancy. Corpora lutea (n = 4 or 5 per group) were removed at various intervals after onset of hCG treatment. For comparison, the levels of serum progesterone and luteal wet weight are included (top panel). See the text for discussion. Data are derived from references 26,49.

gonadotropin receptors, after the initial stages of CG exposure. We hypothesize that homologous (50) desensitization of the adenylate cyclase system occurred in the macaque corpus luteum in simulated early pregnancy. The functional, if not physical, uncoupling of gonadotropin receptors from their effector systems (e.g., adenylate cyclase) may be an important mechanism regulating the transient response of the primate corpus luteum to CG in early pregnancy.

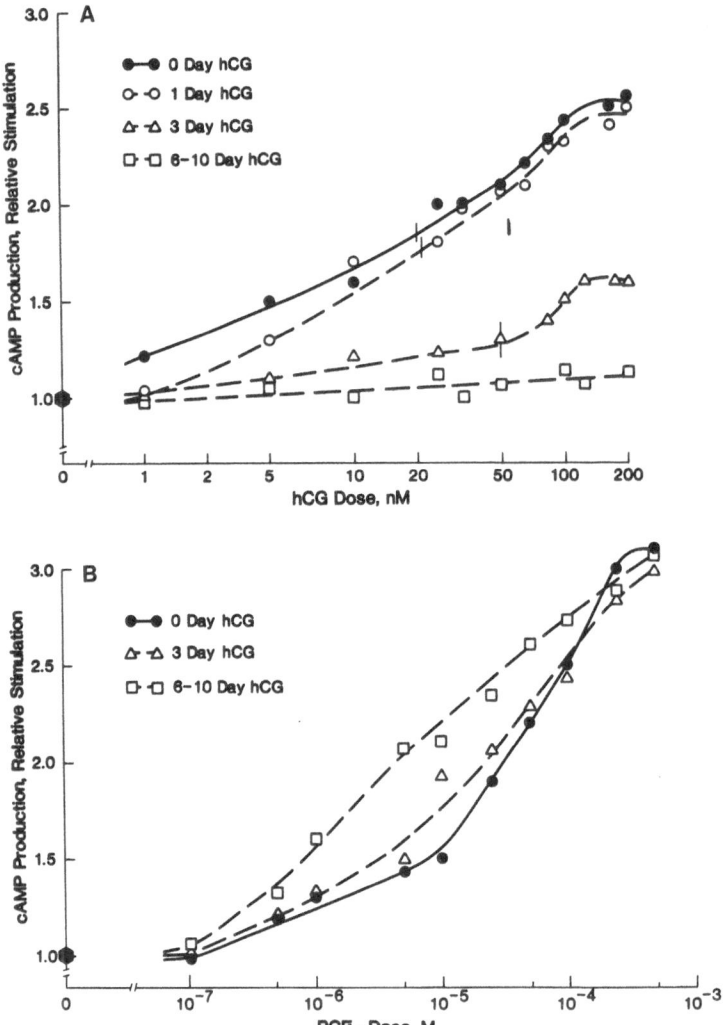

Fig. 4. Dose-response curves for hCG (A) and PGE_2 (B) stimulation of adenylate cyclase in homogenates of luteal tissue obtained from rhesus monkeys during simulated early pregnancy. Corpora lutea (n = 3 or 4 per group) were removed at various intervals after onset of hCG treatment. Data are expressed as stimulation relative to activity of 50 µl GTP alone (control value of 1). See text for discussion. Data derived from reference 50.

Further studies in our laboratory provided compelling evidence that certain responses of the corpus luteum to CG were not transitory in nature. When rhesus monkeys received the standard 10-day regimen of increasing doses of hCG beginning 3 days earlier in the luteal phase (5-6 days after the midcycle LH surge), there was a persistent rather than transient increase in circulating progesterone levels (Fig. 5). The reason(s) for the disparate response of the younger corpus luteum to CG is not known. However, it is clear that whatever mechanisms result in the transient response of the corpus luteum to CG around the typical time of implantation, these processes are inoperative or thwarted earlier in the luteal phase.

In addition, not all secretory activities of the macaque corpus luteum during actual (1) or simulated (Fig. 6) early pregnancy parallel

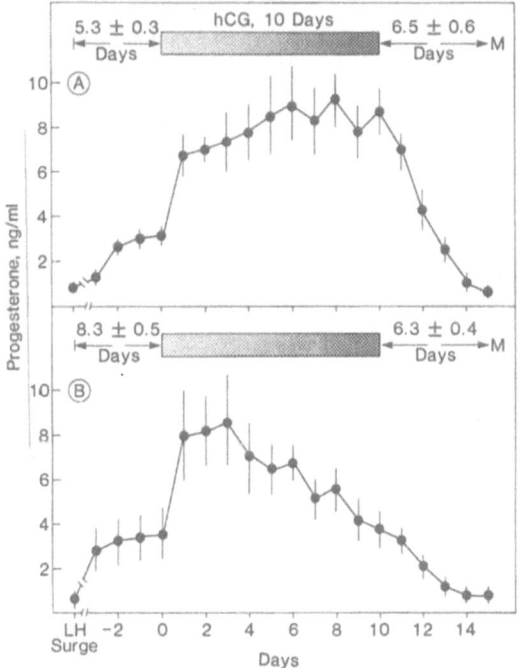

Fig. 5. Response of the macaque corpus luteum to pregnancy-like patterns of circulating hCG initiated during the early luteal phase of the menstrual cycle (A) versus around the typical time of implantation in the fertile cycle (B). Peripheral levels of progesterone are standardized to the onset of hCG treatment (day 0). Lengths of intervals from the LH surge to onset of treatment and from cessation of treatment to menses (M) are given at the top of each panel. CG treatment begun early in the luteal phase resulted in a persistent, rather than transient, stimulation of luteal progesterone production. Data adapted from reference 16.

the pattern of progesterone secretion. Circulating levels of estradiol (16) remained elevated and relaxin-like activity (17) increased at the time when progesterone concentrations declined. Considering that the gonadotropin-responsive adenylate cyclase system in the corpus luteum was desensitized by this stage, the direct role of CG or at least CG-dependent cAMP-mediated events in promoting these secretory activities is unclear. CG stimulated estrogen production in vitro by macaque luteal cells obtained during the menstrual cycle (51), but the intracellular pathways mediating the response were not investigated. Investigations of cAMP-independent pathways, such as the phosphoinositide-Ca^{++}-C kinase system (52,53), may elucidate other important mediators of gonadotropin action in the primate corpus luteum. Alternatively, the change from a gonadotropin-responsive to a CG-desensitized state may be important for the shift in luteal activity from predominantly progesterone secretion to other functions, such as relaxin secretion.

SUMMARY AND FUTURE DIRECTIONS

Recent advances confirm a vital luteotropic role for the placental gonadotropin, CG, during early pregnancy in primates. However, the precise actions of CG leading to the extension of the life span of the

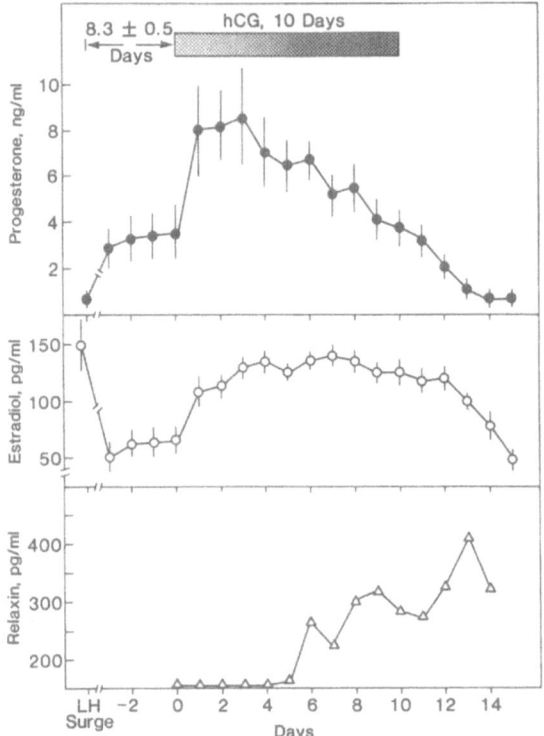

Fig. 6. Multiple divergent responses of the macaque corpus luteum to pregnancy-like patterns of circulating hCG initiated around the typical time of implantation. Serum levels of progesterone, estradiol, and relaxin are standardized to the onset of hCG treatment (day 0). See text for discussion. Data adapted from references 16,17.

216

corpus luteum, the transient stimulation of progesterone production, and the delayed expression of relaxin synthesis are not known. The corpus luteum of early pregnancy adapts to the rising gonadotropin milieu by desensitizing an important effector pathway for CG—the adenylate cyclase system and cAMP production. The membrane events leading to a CG-insensitive adenylate cyclase and the relationship of this phenomenon to the changes in luteal secretory activity in early pregnancy await investigation. Pioneering work from the laboratories of Niswender (36), Hansel (54) and others indicated that corpora lutea of domestic animals contain at least 2 populations of luteal cells which (a) differ in morphologic, functional, and regulatory properties, and (b) change dramatically in response to pregnancy or gonadotropin treatment. Discerning the characteristics of primate luteal cells, including their response to CG, could lead to major advances in our understanding of the corpus luteum and its rescue in early pregnancy. Many of the changes described in this chapter result from further differentiation or deregulation of one or more luteal cell types.

As a final enigma, the primate corpus luteum of early pregnancy is different from that of the menstrual cycle in that its initial regression is not final. In the rhesus monkey (see review by diZerega and Hodgen, 55), the corpus luteum of pregnancy involutes, remains "quiescent" at midpregnancy, and then rejuvenates to form a functional gland at term pregnancy, as judged by morphologic and hormonal criteria. The regulatory processes and cellular changes responsible for restoring gonadotropin-responsive, steroidogenic luteal tissue are unknown. Perhaps, as Schwall and Niswender suggested recently (56), there is a stem cell or "undifferentiated" cell type within the corpus luteum that can serve as the progenitor for functional luteal tissue. The nonhuman primate corpus luteum of early-to-mid pregnancy may be an appropriate model for investigating this issue.

ACKNOWLEDGMENTS

The authors would like to thank our laboratory associates and collaborators in the Department of Physiology at the University of Arizona and in the Division of Reproductive Biology and Behavior at the Oregon Regional Primate Research Center for their assistance in this research project. We gratefully acknowledge hormone donations from CPR-NICHHD, the National Hormone and Pituitary Program—NIADDK, and Ayerst Laboratories. This work was supported by NIH Grants HD-20869, HD-18185, and RR-00163. A special thanks to Mrs. Pat Kosharek for preparing this manuscript. This is paper No. 1516 from the Oregon Regional Primate Research Center.

REFERENCES

1. Knobil E. On the regulation of the primate corpus luteum. Biol Reprod 1973; 8:246-58.
2. Tullner WW. Comparative aspects of primate chorionic gonadotropins. In: Kuhn H, ed. Contributions to Primatology vol 3. Basel, Switzerland: S Karger, 1984:235-57.
3. Goodman AL, Hodgen GD. Corpus luteum-conceptus-follicle relationships during the fertile cycle in rhesus monkeys: pregnancy maintenance despite early luteal removal. J Clin Endocrinol Metab 1979; 49:469-71.
4. Hodgen GD, Niemann WH, Tullner WW. Duration of chorionic gonadotropin production by the placenta of the rhesus monkey. Endocrinology 1975; 96:789-91.
5. Hearn JP. The embryo-maternal dialogue during early pregnancy in

primates. J Reprod Fertil 1986; 76:809-19.

6. Meyer RK. Chorionic gonadotropin, corpus luteum function and embryo implantation in the rhesus monkey. Acta Endocrinol [suppl] 1972; 166:214-7.

7. Prahalada S, Venkatramaiah M, Rao AJ, Moudgal NR. Termination of pregnancy in macaques (Macaca radiata) using monkey antiserum to ovine LH. Contraception 1975; 12:137-47.

8. Talwar GP, Sharma NC, Dubey SK, et al. Isoimmunization against hCG with conjugates of processed β-subunit of the hormone and tetanus toxoid. Proc Natl Acad Sci USA 1976; 73:218-22.

9. Stevens VC. Immunization of female baboons with hapten-coupled gonadotropins. J Obstet Gynecol 1973; 42:496-506.

10. Thau RB, Sundaram K. The mechanisms of action of an antifertility vaccine in the rhesus monkey: reversal of the effects of antisera to β-oLH by medroxyprogesterone acetate. Fertil Steril 1980; 33:317-20.

11. Strott CA, Yoshimi T, Ross GT, Lipsett MB. Ovarian physiology: relationship between plasma LH and steroidogenesis by the follicle and corpus luteum; effect of hCG. J Clin Endocrinol Metab 1969; 29:1157-67.

12. Hanson FW, Powell JE, Stevens VC. Effects of hCG and human pituitary LH on steroid secretion and functional life of the human corpus luteum. J Clin Endocrinol Metab 1971; 32:211-5.

13. Neill JD, Knobil E. On the nature of the initial luteotropic stimulus of pregnancy in the rhesus monkey. Endocrinology 1972; 90:34-8.

14. Surve AH, Harrington FE, Elton RL. Effect of chorionic gonadotropin on corpus luteum of the monkey. Proc Soc Exp Biol Med 1973; 144:963-8.

15. Wilks JW, Noble AS. Steroidogenic responsiveness of the monkey corpus luteum to exogenous chorionic gonadotropin. Endocrinology 1983; 112:1256-66.

16. Ottobre JS, Stouffer RL. Persistent vs. transient stimulation of the macaque corpus luteum during prolonged exposure to hCG: a function of age of the menstrual cycle. Endocrinology 1984; 114:2175-82.

17. Ottobre JS, Nixon WE, Stouffer RL. Induction of relaxin secretion in rhesus monkeys by hCG: dependence on the age of the corpus luteum of the menstrual cycle. Biol Reprod 1984; 31:1000-6.

18. Ellendorff F, Koch E, eds. Early pregnancy factors. Proceedings of an International Workshop April 17-19, 1985, Mariensee, West Germany. New York: Perinatology Press, 1985.

19. Aschheim S, Zondek B. Hypophysenvorderlappenhormon and ovarial hormon im harn von schwangeren. Klin Wochenschr 1927; 6:1322-30.

20. Tyrey L. Human chorionic gonadotropin: structural, biologic and immunologic aspects. Semin Oncol 1982; 9:163-73.

21. Schwartz M, Jewelewicz R, Dyrenfurth I, Tropper P, VandeWeile RL. The use of human menopausal and chorionic gonadotropins for induction of ovulation: sixteen years' experience at the Sloane Hospital for Women. Am J Obstet Gynecol 1980; 138:801-7.

22. Bavister BD, Boatman DE, Collins K, Dierschke DJ, Eisele SG. Birth of rhesus monkey infant after in vitro fertilization and nonsurgical embryo transfer. Proc Natl Acad Sci USA 1984; 81:2218-22.

23. Cameron JL, Stouffer RL. Comparisons of the species specificity of gonadotropin binding to primate and non primate corpora lutea. Biol Reprod 1981; 25:568-72.

24. Cameron JL, Stouffer RL. Gonadotropin receptors of the primate corpus luteum: I. Characterization of ^{125}I-labeled hLH and hCG binding to luteal membranes from the rhesus monkey. Endocrinology 1982; 110:2059-67.

25. Cameron JL, Stouffer RL. Gonadotropin receptors of the primate corpus luteum: II. Changes in available LH and CG binding sites in macaque luteal membranes during the nonfertile menstrual cycle. Endocrinology 1982; 110:2068-73.

26. Ottobre JS, Ottobre AC, Stouffer RL. Changes in available gonadotropin receptors in the corpus luteum of the rhesus monkey during simulated early pregnancy. Endocrinology 1984; 115:198-204.

27. Eyster KM, Stouffer RL. Characterization of the adenylate cyclase system in the nonhuman primate (Macaca mulatta) corpus luteum. II. Sensitivity to gonadotropins, other hormones and nonhormonal activators. Endocrinology 1985; 116:1552-8.

28. Stouffer RL, Gulyas BJ, Nixon WE, Hodgen GD. Gonadotropin-sensitive progesterone production by rhesus monkey luteal cells in vitro: a function of age of the corpus luteum during the menstrual cycle. Endocrinology 1977; 100:506-12.

29. Rao CH V, Griffin LP, Carman FR Jr. Gonadotropin receptors in human corpora luteal of the menstrual cycle and pregnancy. Am J Obstet Gynecol 1976; 128:146-53.

30. Marsh JM, LeMaire WJ. Cyclic AMP accumulation and steroidogenesis in the human corpus luteum: effect of gonadotropins and prostaglandins. J Clin Endocrinol Metab 1974; 38:99-106.

31. Crowley WF Jr, Filicori M, Spratt DI, Santoro NF. The physiology of GnRH secretion in men and women. Recent Prog Horm Res 1985; 41:473-532.

32. Ellinwood WE, Norman RL, Spies HG. Changing frequency of pulsatile luteinizing hormone and progesterone secretion during the luteal phase of the menstrual cycle of rhesus monkeys. Biol Reprod 1984; 31:714-22.

33. Hutchison JS, Nelson PB, Zeleznik AJ. Effects of different gonadotropin pulse frequencies on corpus luteum function during the menstrual cycle of rhesus monkeys. Endocrinology 1986; 119:1964-71.

34. Hutchison JS, Zeleznik AJ. The corpus luteum of the primate menstrual cycle is capable of recovering from a transient withdrawal of pituitary gonadotropin support. Endocrinology 1985; 117:1043-49.

35. Soules MR, Steiner RA, Clifton DK, Bremner WJ. The effects of inducing a follicular phase gonadotropin secretory pattern in normal women during the luteal phase. Fertil Steril 1986; 47:45-53.

36. Niswender GD, Schwall RH, Fitz TA, Farin CE, Sawyer HR. Regulation of luteal function in domestic ruminants: new concepts. Recent Prog Horm Res 1985; 41:101-51.

37. Bazer FW, Vallet JV, Roberts RM, Sharp DC, Thatcher WW. Role of conceptus secretory products in establishment of pregnancy. J Reprod Fertil 1986; 76:841-50.

38. Tulchinsky D, Hobel CJ. Plasma hCG, estrone, estradiol, estriol, progesterone and 17α-hydroxyprogesterone in human pregnancy III. Early normal pregnancy. Am J Obstet Gynecol 1973; 117:884-93.

39. Stouffer RL, Nixon WE, Hodgen GD. The refractory state of luteal cells isolated from rhesus monkeys after prolonged exposure to CG during early pregnancy. Biol Reprod 1978; 18:858-64.

40. Gwynne JT, Strauss JF III. The role of lipoproteins in steroidogenesis and cholesterol metabolism in steroidogenic glands. Endocr Rev 1982; 3:299-329.

41. Carr BR, MacDonald PC, Simpson ER. The role of lipoproteins in the regulation of progesterone secretion by the human corpus luteum. Fertil Steril 1982; 38:303-11.

42. Golos TG, August AM, Strauss JF III. Expression of low density lipoprotein receptor in cultured human granulosa cells: regulation by hCG, cyclic AMP and sterol. J Lipid Res 27:1089-96.

43. Booher C, Enders AC, Hendrickx AG, Hess DL. Structural characteristics of the corpus luteum during implantation in the rhesus monkey (Macaca mulatta). Am J Anat 1981; 160:17-36.

44. Ellinwood WE, Resko JA. Effect of inhibition of estrogen synthesis during the luteal phase on function of the corpus luteum in rhesus monkeys. Biol Reprod 1983; 28:636-44.

45. Schoonmaker JN, Bergman KS, Steiner RA, Karsch FJ. Estradiol-

induced luteal regression in the rhesus monkey: evidence for an extraovarian site of action. Endocrinology 1982; 110:1708-15.

46. Auletta FJ, Kamps DL, Pories S, Bissett J, Gibson M. An intracorpus luteum site for the luteolytic action of $PGF_{2\alpha}$ in the rhesus monkey. Prostaglandins 1984; 27:285-98.

47. Auletta FJ, Paradis DK, Wesley M, Duby RT. Oxytocin is luteolytic in the rhesus monkey (Macaca mulatta). J Reprod Fertil 1984; 72:401-6.

48. Birnbaumer L, Kirchick HJ. Regulation of gonadotropic action: the molecular mechanisms of gonadotropin-induced activation of ovarian adenylyl cyclases. In: Greenwald G, Terranova P, eds. Factors regulating ovarian function. New York: Raven Press, 1983:287-310.

49. Ottobre JS, Stouffer RL. Receptors for chorionic gonadotropin in the corpus luteum of the rhesus monkey during simulated early pregnancy: lack of down-regulation. Endocrinology 1986; 1594-1602.

50. VandeVoort C, Molskness T, Stouffer R. Adenylate cyclase in the primate corpus luteum during CG treatment simulating early pregnancy: homologous (gonadotropin) versus heterologous (prostaglandin) desensitization [Abstract]. Abstract 4 at the Sixth Ovarian Workshop. Ithaca, NY July 14-15, 1986.

51. Stouffer RL, Bennett LA, Hodgen GD. Estrogen production by luteal cells isolated from rhesus monkeys during the menstrual cycle: correlation with spontaneous luteolysis. Endocrinology 1980; 106:519-25.

52. Clark MR, Kawai Y, Davis JS, LeMaire WJ. Ovarian protein kinases. In: Toft DO, Ryan RJ, eds. Proceedings of the Fifth Ovarian Workshop. Champaign: Ovarian Workshops, 1985:383-401.

53. Davis JS, West LA, Weakland LL, Farese RV. hCG activates the inositol 1,4,5-triphosphate-Ca^{+2} intracellular signalling system in bovine luteal cells. FEBS Lett 1986; 208:287-91.

54. Hansel W, Dowd JP. New concepts of the control of corpus luteum function. J Reprod Fertil 1986; 78:755-68.

55. diZerega GS, Hodgen GD. Changing functional status of the monkey corpus luteum. Biol Reprod 1980; 23:253-63.

56. Schwall RH, Gamboni F, Mayan MH, Niswender GD. Changes in the distribution of sizes of ovine luteal cells during the estrous cycle. Biol Reprod 1986; 34:911-19.

IV. CORPUS LUTEUM FUNCTION (CONTINUED)

THE PRODUCTION AND FUNCTION OF OVARIAN RELAXIN

Gerson Weiss, M.D.

UMDNJ-New Jersey Medical School
185 South Orange Avenue
Newark, New Jersey 07103

INTRODUCTION

Available evidence suggests that the source of circulating relaxin in primates is the corpus luteum. Since the sources and secretion patterns of relaxin is rather variable among different mammalian species, this manuscript will be limited, whenever possible, to primates.

HISTORY

Over six decades ago, Hisaw described three major ovarian hormones, estrogen, progesterone and relaxin (1). Relaxin was defined as the luteal principle which caused relaxation of the pelvic ligaments in estrogen-primed guinea pigs. During the course of isolation and purification of the steroid hormones, relaxin activity was lost. In the fourth decade of this century, detailed radiographic studies revealed that slight relaxation of the pelvic joints is a normal physiological occurrence in human pregnancy, and this relaxation occurred as early as pregnancy could be detected (2,3). This led to the hypothesis that relaxin was present in early human pregnancy. Abramson et al. (4) concentrated serum from early pregnant women and demonstrated relaxin-like activity on the pubic symphysis of the guinea pig. They were unable to make this observation using sera obtained later in pregnancy. They concluded that relaxin was present in the serum of women from earliest pregnancy. They, in fact, suggested that relaxin could be used as a pregnancy test but that this would be impractical. Pommerenke (5) reported a drop in the level of serum relaxin in midpregnancy and an absence by the eighth month. In sharp contrast, Zarrow et al. (6) in 1955 reported relaxin bioactivity in the serum of pregnant women, which increased from a low point at 7 to 10 weeks to a maximum at 38 to 42 weeks. Thus, the secretion pattern of relaxin during pregnancy was unclear. In the 1950s, there was brief excitement over the use of porcine relaxin in women to ripen the cervix or prevent premature labor. Many preparations became available, all of them quite impure and some of them totally devoid of relaxin activity. After initial excitement based on poorly controlled experimentation, there was confusion and a general disenchantment with the use of relaxin. In an evaluation of the subject in 1958, Stone et al. (7) opined that there was little doubt of the existence of biologically-active relaxin, but beyond this point, its physiology or uses in the human were unknown.

Studies on relaxin physiology in the human were stymied until the 1970s, when observations made during the purification of porcine relaxin provided the tools for study of human relaxin function and secretion. Porcine relaxin was purified and its structure elucidated (8,9). The molecule could not be iodinated since it contained no tyrosine or histidine. However, Sherwood (10) developed a method for iodinating relaxin by first tyrosylating the relaxin molecule. This allowed for development of specific relaxin radioimmunoassays (RIAs). Although Bryant had reported an RIA which detected human relaxin both in pregnancy and nonpregnancy (11), these studies were later proven to be invalid, since they were based on direct iodination of the porcine relaxin molecule. O'Byrne and Steinetz (12) developed an anti-porcine relaxin antibody capable of detecting relaxin immunoactivity in human serum. This development provided the tools for the resumption of study of relaxin in primates.

STRUCTURE OF HUMAN RELAXIN

Relaxin is a peptide of approximately 6,000 molecular weight. It consists of dissimilar A and B chains linked by two disulfide linkages. There is an additional intrachain disulfide link in the A chain. There is remarkable structural similarity to that of insulin. However, there is less than 25% amino acid homology. The structural similarity between relaxin and insulin is such that a molecular model of porcine relaxin fits on the coordinates of porcine insulin without strain (13).

Hudson et al. (14) have determined the putative structure of human relaxin by isolation of cDNA clones obtained from human ovaries. There are two non-allelic genes for human relaxin, both located on the ninth chromosome (15). One of these genes is expressed by the human ovary. It is not clear whether the second gene is expressed in other tissues or is a pseudogene. Both sequences have been synthesized and both are biologically active. Utilizing a yeast vector, the Genentech Corporation has produced analogs of human ovarian relaxin and the native molecule for experimental use.

Since there are limited biological sources of human relaxin and since it is a small lipophilic peptide with an isoelectric point of 10.4, it has never been purified to homogeneity from a human source. Assuming a 10% yield, purification of 1 mg of human luteal relaxin would require 20,000 corpora lutea of term pregnancy. O'Byrne et al. (16) have reported studies on the extraction and isolation of immunoreactive relaxin from human corpora lutea.

Relaxin is present in human seminal plasma at a concentration of approximately 50 ng/ml. This may be the most appropriate source for complete purification of human relaxin. Weiss et al. (17) have reported on a partial purification of relaxin from human seminal plasma to a level of purity which allows production of monoclonal antibodies. Completion of these studies should allow complete purification of human seminal relaxin by immunoaffinity chromatography. It can then be determined if the genes expressed in the male and in the female are similar.

MEASUREMENT OF RELAXIN

The traditional bioassays for relaxin depend on the ability of relaxin to increase the length of an interpubic ligament in either guinea pigs or mice (18). These assays are qualitative and require approximately a microgram of relaxin per animal. All relaxins from varying species have

224

been active in the guinea pig pubic symphysis palpation assay. Shark relaxin, active in the guinea pig assay, is not active in the mouse pubic symphysis assay.

Relaxin has been shown to decrease the amplitude of myometrial contractions in vitro. This has been also used as a basis for a bioassay. This assay is not as specific as the guinea pig pubic symphysis assay but is more sensitive. As little as 10 ng/ml can be detected by this method. Estrogen pretreatment is necessary in all bioassays of relaxin. Relaxin synergizes with progesterone to decrease the amplitude of myometrial contractions. Progesterone has been utilized to increase the sensitivity of relaxin assays (19).

Most studies that described relaxin secretion in the human utilized antibody R6 developed by O'Byrne and Steinetz (12). This antibody, raised in a rabbit against purified porcine relaxin, detects relaxin immunoactivity in many species. Because of differences in amino acid sequence in different relaxin molecules, most other anti-porcine relaxin antisera do not cross-react with relaxin from other species. Purified porcine relaxin and extracts of human pregnancy corpora lutea were assayed in both guinea pig pubic symphysis palpation assay and in the R6 RIA. The ratio of bioactivity to immunoactivity in the porcine system was set at one. The bioactivity to immunoactivity ratio in humans approached unity as well, suggesting that most of the human relaxin is detected by the R6 RIA (20). Several studies have demonstrated the specificity of this assay. Recently Eddie et al. (21) have described the radioimmunoassay of relaxin based on an antibody raised to an analog of human relaxin. It is anticipated that additional homologous human radioimmunoassays will be developed in the near future.

SECRETION PATTERNS OF RELAXIN

Nonpregnant Women

While relaxin is a hormone of pregnancy, it is rarely detected in serum of nonpregnant women. It is found in the corpora lutea of nonpregnant women at 100 times lower concentration than in the corpora lutea of pregnancy (20). While Thomas et al. (22) were unable to detect immunoreactive relaxin in nonpregnant women during the normal menstrual cycle, they did note small concentrations detected during the preovulatory phase in women whose ovulation was stimulated with human menopausal gonadotropins (hMG). Loumaye et al. (23) observed immunoreactive relaxin in peritoneal fluid from women with normal ovulatory cycles. It was rarely detected before day 20 of the cycle. However, it was invariably detected from days 21 to 24 in the peritoneal fluid. Since this is the period of nidation, they postulate a role for relaxin during this phase.

Pregnancy

Evidence from many directions indicates that the corpus luteum is the source of circulating relaxin in pregnancy. At the time of term cesarean section, simultaneous peripheral blood samples and ovarian vein blood samples were obtained for relaxin assay. Relaxin concentrations were similar in peripheral blood and in the blood draining the ovary not containing the corpus luteum of pregnancy. Relaxin concentrations were substantively higher in the ovarian vein draining the ovary containing the corpus luteum of pregnancy (24). Mathieu et al. (25) immunohistochemically localized relaxin to the corpus luteum during pregnancy. These investigators were not able to demonstrate relaxin in adjacent ovarian tissue or in corpora lutea during the early luteal phase of a nonfertile menstrual cycle. Luteectomy at term pregnancy results in a prompt fall in levels of circulating relaxin (26). The half-life of relaxin appears to be less then one h. In contrast, in the absence of luteectomy after delivery there is a gradual fall of relaxin secretion over 72 h.

Quagliarello et al. (27) were unable to detect peripheral relaxin in 51 nonpregnant women. Relaxin was found in peripheral blood in conception cycles by the time of the missed menses (27). Relaxin concentrations rapidly rise and peak by the middle of the first trimester of pregnancy. Serum levels then fall by approximately 20% and remain stable throughout pregnancy (28) (Fig. 1). This secretion pattern has been confirmed by other groups using the R6 RIA (29,30). Recently, Bell et al. (31) have observed a very similar pattern using a homologous RIA as described (21) based on an analog to human relaxin (Fig. 2). However, MacLennan et al., using the R6 RIA, did not show changes in relaxin secretion during pregnancy. We have been unable to find a diurnal variation in serum relaxin concentration. No significant changes were noted between antepartum and intrapartum relaxin concentrations in 10 patients sampled serially (33). However using nonserially collected samples, MacLennan observed higher relaxin levels in labor then in the third trimester (23). To detect prelabor relaxin surges, serum samples were obtained from 74 women at the end of their gestations. These women went into spontaneous labor and samples were again obtained. There were no significant differences between antepartum and intrapartum concentrations of serum relaxin (34). This suggests there is no significant prelabor elevation in relaxin secretion in women as there is in rodents and pigs. Since samples were only obtained daily, transient short-lived prelabor elevations may not have been detectable.

Relaxin was detectable in only 10% of amniotic fluid samples. Relaxin was undetectable in umbilical cord blood at term (35). Relaxin concentrations in serum of patients harboring hydatidiform moles were similar to those in normal women at corresponding weeks of gestation even though hCG levels were substantively higher (36). Relaxin concentrations in toxemic pregnancies were similar to those of normal pregnancy in the third trimester. In contrast, relaxin concentrations in pregnancies beyond 43 weeks' gestation and in women with premature labor were significantly lower then levels in normal women during the third trimester of pregnancy (29). Serum relaxin concentrations were similar in normal patients and patients treated with human menopausal gonadotropins (hMG) who conceived singleton pregnancies. However, women given hMG with multiple fetuses had significantly higher concentrations of relaxin (37). Since this latter group demonstrates a high incidence of premature birth, this may represent a human syndrome of hyperrelaxinemia which may result in cervical incompetence early in pregnancy.

Utilizing relaxin as an indicator of luteal activity and chorionic gonadotropin as an indicator of placental function, women were prospectively studied in early pregnancy. Some of these women had spontaneous abortions. In these women destined to abort, hCG levels fell before relaxin levels fell. In fact, relaxin levels were normal while chorionic gonadotropin levels were low for that stage of gestation in some patients. This indicates that, at least in the pregnancies studied, the loss of the pregnancy was due to an initial loss of placental function rather than a loss of luteal function which resulted in pregnancy wastage (38).

NONHUMAN PRIMATES

No relaxin immunoactivity was detected in serum from 5 intact male rhesus monkeys or from 6 cycling female rhesus monkeys sampled every 2 to

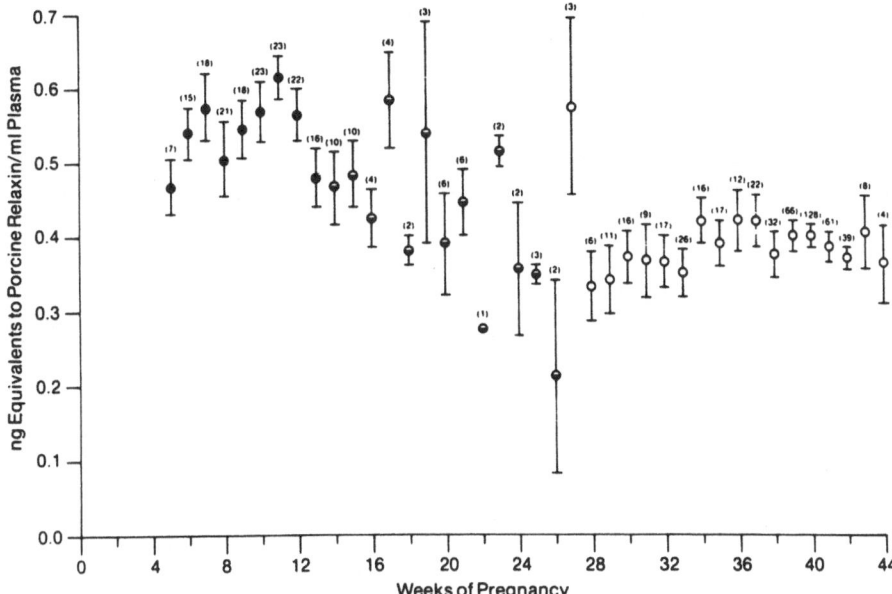

Fig. 1. Immunoreactive relaxin in plasma of women throughout the course of gestation. Numbers in parenthesis indicate the numbers of women sampled at each time interval. Vertical bars indicate ± SEM. ●, first trimester; ◕, second trimester; ○, third trimester. Assay used was based on R6 antisera, raised against porcine relaxin (28). Reproduced with permission of Williams and Wilkins.

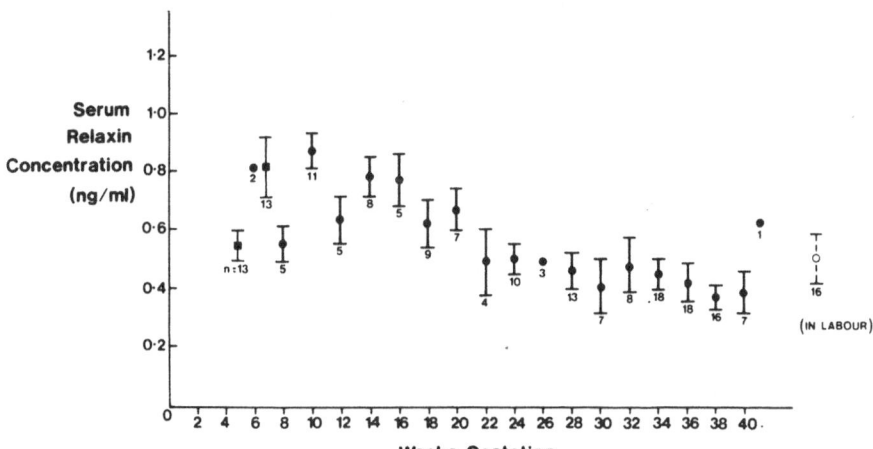

Fig. 2. Relaxin levels at 2-week intervals from 6 weeks' gestation until term in 19 normal antenatal patients studied serially (closed circles); n = number of measurements at each gestation. Also shown are relaxin levels in 13 pregnant patients measured on two occasions only (closed squares) and relaxin levels in a group of patients in labor at term (open circle). Assay used was a homologous human RIA based on an antibody raised to a human relaxin antibody (31). Reprinted with permission from The American College of Obstetricians and Gynecologists. (Obstetrics and Gynecology, 1987; 69:587.)

227

3 days during the entire menstrual cycle. Relaxin was detected in serum from pregnant monkeys after the third week of gestation to the end of pregnancy. Relaxin was undetectable in the serum of 3 ovariectomized pregnant monkeys, indicating the ovary is the source of circulating relaxin in rhesus monkeys. Luteal relaxin is detectable in monkeys at a time when the ovary is secreting little progesterone (39). In contrast to the rhesus monkey, relaxin is present in serum of pregnant women from the time of the missed menses. Thus, there are major differences in luteal function in early pregnancy between rhesus monkeys and women with regard to secretion profiles of relaxin and progesterone.

Low concentrations of relaxin are detectable in the late luteal phase of the menstrual cycle in the baboon. A significant increase in plasma relaxin concentrations occurs in pregnant baboons by day 12 postovulation. Plasma relaxin levels increase rapidly during early pregnancy and remain elevated throughout pregnancy. Removal of the corpus luteum bearing ovary during pregnancy results in a rapid fall in relaxin concentration to below the limits of detection. The concentration of circulating relaxin in the baboon is similar to the circulating concentration in women. Progesterone concentration rises in early pregnancy similar to those changes seen in women. It would appear that the baboon is a reasonable nonhuman primate model for further studies of the regulation and action of relaxin (40).

CONTROL OF LUTEAL RELAXIN SECRETION

In Vivo Studies

HCG. Relaxin is detectable in pregnancy serum from the time of the missed menses. We have hypothesized that an early signal from the blastocyst induces luteal relaxin secretion. To test this hypothesis, we gave hCG injections every other day starting on day 8 of the luteal phase. This resulted in a prompt rescue of the corpus luteum and an abrupt rise in progesterone secretion (Fig. 3). Relaxin became detectable only after 2 to 6 days. In fact, relaxin concentrations were still rising while progesterone concentrations in the serum were already falling for several days. Thus, hCG can induce relaxin secretion in nonpregnant women (41). There may be different control mechanisms for relaxin and progesterone secretion, even though the same exogenous hormone, hCG, is the stimulus for both.

The timing of the hCG stimulus is critical to relaxin secretion. When an identical experimental paradigm was used, starting hCG injections on day 2 to 3 of the luteal phase, no relaxin was detectable (Fig. 3). This suggests that the corpus luteum is a dynamic structure and must be in the appropriate condition to respond to hCG with relaxin secretion. Ottobre et al. (42), studying the rhesus monkey, noted that the induction of relaxin secretion by hCG was also a function of the age of the corpus luteum of the menstrual cycle. These authors also noted a dissociation in the secretion pattern of progesterone and relaxin. Castracane et al. (40) showed a similar response in the baboon. When hCG was administered on days 9 through 11 postovulation, there was a rapid increase in plasma progesterone which declined in a few days. Increases in relaxin were seen only 4 to 6 days following the first hCG administration. Progesterone levels were declining while relaxin levels increased.

While relaxin is present throughout pregnancy in women, administration of hCG is incapable of maintaining relaxin secretion for more than two weeks, when administered starting in the late luteal phase in nonpregnant women. Thus, other factors must also contribute to relaxin secretion in pregnant women.

228

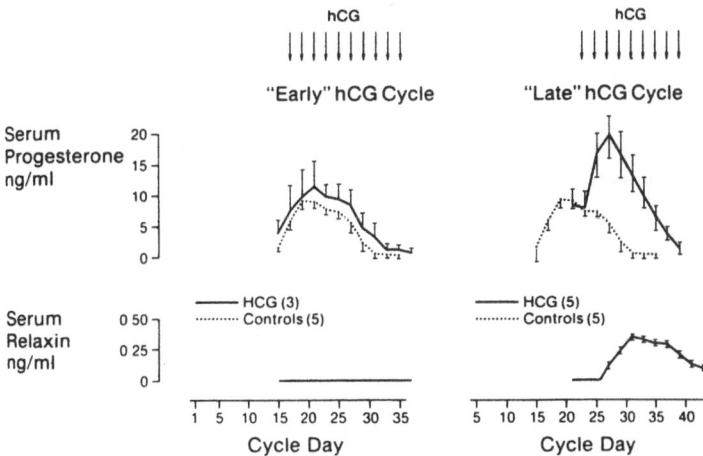

Fig. 3. Induction of relaxin secretion in nonpregnant women using hCG. Ovulation has been standardized as day 14 in a composite of all 5 patients. Serum progesterone and serum relaxin concentrations are shown on the y-axis, and cycle days are given on the x-axis. HCG injections (2500 IU im, every 2 days) are shown as arrows. ···, Control cycle values; ——— hCG-treated cycles. Relaxin is noted in late hCG-treated cycles only in association with statistically significant (P<0.05) increases in mean serum progesterone determinators (41). Reproduced with permission of Williams and Wilkins.

Lactogenic hormones. Prolactin (PRL) and placental lactogen (PL) are luteotropic in rodents and some other species (43). PRL is capable of binding to human corpora lutea (44). To determine if endogenous prolactin is luteotropic, daily serum samples were obtained from 13 lactating and 15 nonlactating women for 3 days postpartum. None of these women were treated with neuroleptics, narcotics, hormones or dopamine agonists. The pattern of decline of circulating relaxin in the lactating and nonlactating women patients were similar, suggesting that the higher prolactin concentrations seen in nursing mothers are not luteotropic. We were unable to obtain binding of radiolabeled hPL to corpora lutea of late pregnancy. Thus, the above data suggests that the lactogenic hormones may not have a role in the maintenance of the human corpus luteum of term pregnancy (45).

GnRH. In two cycles of hMG treatment, patients developed rapid ovarian hyperstimulation. Thomas (22) observed small concentrations of detectable relaxin in these patients. When GnRH was given in an attempt to induce ovulation, progesterone levels increased and there was an increase of relaxin secretion as well. However, relaxin concentrations were always in a very low range. In unpublished studies, we have been unable to induce relaxin secretion with GnRH in normal women either during the menstrual cycle or during pregnancy.

Prostaglandins. Although prostaglandin (PG) F2α causes a rapid and significant increase in serum relaxin concentration in pigs at term, we have noted that PGF2α in doses capable of inducing labor in women at term does not result in an alteration in relaxin secretion (46). Thus, PGF2α is not either acutely luteolytic or luteotropic in women at term pregnancy. Similar observations were made utilizing PGE2 to induce midtrimester abortion. Concentrations of PGE2 which were effective in inducing uterine emptying had no effect on circulating levels of relaxin (47).

Oxytocin. Oxytocin is also produced by the human corpus luteum. Infusions of oxytocin which were capable of inducing labor did not significantly alter serum relaxin concentration (46).

IN VITRO STUDIES

To study the control mechanisms of the human corpus luteum, Goldsmith et al. (48) established a monolayer culture system for human luteal cells. Human corpora lutea from term pregnancy and the menstrual cycle were dispersed by enzymatic digestion aided by mechanical disruption. Cells were maintained as monolayer cultures for at least 26 days. Progesterone and relaxin in the culture medium were measured by radioimmunoassay. Luteal cells from both the menstrual cycle and pregnancy secreted progesterone throughout the culture period. Chorionic gonadotropin increased progesterone secretion by menstrual cycle luteal cells but not by pregnancy luteal cells. Relaxin was not detected in the media of menstrual cycle cells nor in media of these cells incubated with hCG. Relaxin was detected in media of luteal cells of pregnancy for only 6 days. Treatment with hCG caused a significant increase in media relaxin levels only on the second day of culture. Similar observations were noted by Schmidt et al. (49), who reported that smooth-surfaced endoplasmic reticulum was increased in the hCG-treated cells compared with controls. Gap junctions were also increased in the treated cells. These studies show that morphologic and functional aspects of luteal cell activity can be investigated by these long-term culture techniques. It appears that either hCG is not a direct stimulus to relaxin secretion or other factors are also necessary for hCG to directly induce relaxin secretion.

Nixon (50) detected relaxin in media of monolayer cell cultures from rhesus monkey corpora lutea of early gestation and term pregnancy for 4 and 6 days respectively after initiation of the cultures. Incubation with hCG extended the time of relaxin secretion for an additional 2 days. Prolactin and hPL extended relaxin secretion from luteal cells of pregnancy for 2 days whereas a combination of prolactin and hCG extended the secretion for 4 days.

EXTRALUTEAL RELAXIN

It is clear that the corpus luteum is necessary for pregnancy maintenance in primates for only a portion of the first trimester of pregnancy. After this point, pregnancies can progress normally after luteectomy without any evidence of circulating relaxin. These data would suggest a trivial role for relaxin in pregnancy if the corpus luteum were its only source. There have been conflicting reports of the presence of relaxin in nonluteal tissues during pregnancy. Bigazzi et al. (51) found no placental relaxin, but high concentrations of relaxin in human term decidua. He estimated that the concentration of relaxin in decidua is as high as 11 micrograms per gram wet weight of tissue. Fields and Larkin (52) reported relaxin of low biopotency isolated from 3 of 5 human term placentae. They estimated that one gram of fresh placenta contains 6 micrograms of relaxin. This is roughly four times the concentration of relaxin found in human corpora lutea of pregnancy. Yamamoto et al. (53) found 7.7 ng of immunoreactive relaxin per gram of tissue from the basal plate of human placenta obtained by cesarean section. These results were higher than those obtained from placentas after labor. The authors found a thousandfold greater level of bioactivity then immunoactivity in their specimens. Schmidt et al. (54), utilizing an R6 RIA, the guinea pig pubic symphysis palpation assay, the mouse pubic ligament assay and a sensitive rat uterine inhibition assay, demonstrated only small quantities of relaxin in decidua and placenta. Highest levels were seen in decidua from first trimester pregnancies. Concentrations were in the picogram to nanogram range. There is general agreement that relaxin is present in nonluteal tissues but the concentrations appear to be somewhat disputed.

A more significant question is whether either decidual or placental relaxin is made locally in these tissues or is sequestered there. In an attempt to answer this question, Castracane et al. (55) removed the corpus luteum-bearing ovary from 5 baboons in early pregnancy. Intact pregnant baboons served as controls. Peripheral, uterine and ovarian venous blood samples were collected before hysterotomy, which was performed in late pregnancy. After hysterotomy, samples of placenta, decidua, myometrium, fetal membranes and omentum were obtained. Relaxin concentrations were determined in all samples utilizing R6. Peripheral plasma levels of relaxin were undetectable for 100 days following ovarian removal, while the levels in control pregnant animals were greater than 1 ng/ml. Relaxin levels in uterine venous plasma were comparable to peripheral plasma levels in both groups suggesting that there is no uterine contribution to circulating relaxin. Relaxin was found in decidua, placenta and myometrium in pregnant baboons whose corpus luteum bearing ovary had been removed 100 days earlier. In fact, concentrations of relaxin in the decidua of the ovariectomized baboons were significantly higher then in the intact controls, suggesting that there may be a feedback mechanism between decidual and circulating relaxin. Thus, available evidence suggests that there are uterine sources as well as ovarian sources of relaxin. This is currently a subject of active investigation.

FUNCTION OF RELAXIN IN PREGNANCY

Endometrial Effects

Hisaw and Hisaw (56) demonstrated that relaxin, in conjunction with estrogen and progesterone, produces a much greater hypertrophy of monkey endometrium then steroid treatment alone. Recently, Tseng and Mazella (57) demonstrated that relaxin induces endometrial aromatase activity.

Myometrium

Szlachter et al. (58) demonstrated that human relaxin can decrease the amplitude of spontaneous contractions in human myometrial strips obtained from nonpregnant premenopausal women. The mechanism of this action is unknown. However, relaxin increases the secretion of prostacyclin by human myometrial cells in vitro (59). Prostacyclins also decrease myometrial contractility. In the rat, uterine cAMP is increased by relaxin (60). Nishikori et al. (61) have suggested a mechanism of action of relaxin on myometrial activity, demonstrating myosin light chain kinase activity, myosin light chain phosphorylation and calcium-activated ATPase activity are decreased by relaxin.

Cervix

Several groups have clearly demonstrated that exogenous porcine relaxin can ripen the human cervix at term, thereby inducing labor or allowing an easier induction of labor by oxytocin (62,63). Wiqvist et al. (64) have demonstrated that relaxin significantly influences tritiated hydroxyproline incorporation by cervical tissues in vitro. The role of endogenous relaxin on cervical ripening and dilatation is unknown. It is clear, however, that endogenous relaxin is necessary for cervical dilatation in the rat and the cow.

Pubic Symphysis

As previously noted, there is clear radiographic evidence that there are changes in the pubic symphysis during early pregnancy. It is likely that these are due to a relaxin effect. The significance of this finding in human pregnancy is probably minimal since there is a rather minor change in pelvic diameter during human pregnancy.

Glucose Metabolism

Relaxin increases the affinity of insulin for its own receptor in human adipocytes isolated from women at term gestation, in vitro (65). Thus, it is possible that circulating relaxin may have a protective effect from the diabetogenetic effects of pregnancy.

Mammary Glands

In several species relaxin is clearly a growth stimulator for the mammary gland (8). Relaxin may subserve this function in humans as well.

Intraovarian Effects

There are few data as to when relaxin becomes detectable in human ovaries during the menstrual cycle. We have not detected relaxin in follicular fluid (unpublished study). There is at present no direct evidence that relaxin has any intraovarian effects in primates. In pigs, relaxin can be produced by the graafian follicle in vitro (66) as well as by LH treated granulosa cells from large follicles (67). Too et al. (68) demonstrated that relaxin stimulated plasminogen activator secretion by rat granulosa cells in vitro. Collagenase and proteoglycanase were also increased. However, the dosage of relaxin used (5 μg/ml) was several orders of magnitude higher than the preovulatory endogenous levels. Plasminogen activator catalyses the conversion of plasminogen to plasmin which activates latent collagenases and degrades follicular fluid proteoglycans. It is, thus, tempting to speculate that relaxin may be one of the substances involved in the process of ovulation in primates. As yet, however, there are little data in support of this hypothesis.

CONCLUSION

While significant strides have been made in understanding the secretion and control of relaxin in human pregnancy, there are still many unanswered questions. It is likewise clear that relaxin is involved in a variety of ways in the remodeling of the reproductive tract during pregnancy and in the control of labor. It is certain that relaxin does not function alone but in association with many other hormones and paracrine substances. The challenge of the next decade is to unravel these interrelationships to achieve a better understanding of the control of ovarian function, pregnancy and parturition.

ACKNOWLEDGMENT

Supported by NIH grant HD 22338.

232

REFERENCES

1. Fevold H, Hisaw FL, Leonard SL. Hormones of the corpus luteum. The separation and purification of three active substances. J Am Chem Soc 1932; 54:254.
2. Abramson D, Roberts SM, Wilson P. Relaxation of pelvic joints in pregnancy. Surg Gynecol Obstet 1934; 58:595.
3. Barnes JM. Concerning x-ray and clinical studies of pelvic joints in pregnancy humans. Roentogenol 1934; 32:333.
4. Abramson D, Hurwitt E, Lesnick G. Relaxin in human serum as a test of pregnancy. Surg Gynecol Obstet 1937; 65:335.
5. Pommerenke WJ. Experimental ligamentous relaxation in the guinea pig pelvis. Am J Obstet Gynecol 1934; 27:708.
6. Zarrow MX, Holmstrom EG, Salhanick HA. The concentration of relaxin in the blood serum and other tissues of women during pregnancy. J Clin Endocrinol Metab 1955; 15:22.
7. Stone ML, Sedlis A, Zuckerman M. Relaxin--a critical evaluation. Ann NY Acad Sci 1958; 76:544.
8. Schwabe C, Steinetz BG, Weiss G, et al. Relaxin. Recent Prog Horm Res 1978; 34:123.
9. James R, Niall H, Kwok S, Bryant-Greenwood G. Primary structure of porcine relaxin: homology with insulin and related growth factors. Nature 1977; 267:544.
10. Sherwood OD, Rosentreter KR, Birkhimer ML. Development of a radioimmunoassay for porcine relaxin using ^{125}I labeled polytyrosyl-relaxin. Endocrinology 1975; 96:1106.
11. Bryant GD, Panter M, Stelmasiuk T. Immunoreactive relaxin in human serum during the menstrual cycle. J Clin Endocrinol Metab 1975; 41:1065.
12. O'Byrne EM, Steinetz BG. RIA of relaxin in sera of various species using an antiserum to porcine relaxin. Proc Soc Exp Biol Med 1976; 152:272.
13. Bedarkar S, Blundell T, Gowan LK, McDonald JK, Schwabe C. On the three-dimensional structure of relaxin. Ann NY Acad Sci 1982; 380:22.
14. Hudson P, Haley J, John M, et al. Structure of a genomic clone encoding biologically active human relaxin. Nature 1983; 301:628.
15. Crawford RJ, Hudson P, Shine J, Niall HD, Eddy RL, Shows TB. Two human relaxin genes on chromosome 9. EMBO J 1984; 3:2341.
16. O'Byrne EM, Weiss G, Steinetz BG. The isolation of human relaxin from the corpus luteum. In: Bigazzi M, Greenwood FC, Gasparri F, eds. Biology of relaxin and its role in the human. Excerpta Medica International Congress Series 610, 1983:370.
17. Weiss G, Goldsmith LT, Schoenfeld C, D'Eletto R. Partial purification of relaxin from human seminal plasma. Am J Obstet Gynecol 1986; 154:749.
18. Steinetz BG, O'Byrne EM, Sarosi P, Weiss G. Bioassay of relaxin: present status and future prospects. In: Bigazzi M, Greenwood FC, Gasparri F, eds. Biology of relaxin and its role in the human. Excerpta Medica International Congress Series 610, 1983;140.
19. Brenner SH, Lessing JB, Weiss G. The effect of in vivo progesterone administration on relaxin-inhibited rat uterine contractions. Am J Obstet Gynecol 1984; 148:946.
20. O'Byrne EM, Flitcraft JF, Sawyer WI, Hochman J, Weiss G, Steinetz BG. Relaxin bioactivity and immunoactivity in the human corpus luteum. Endocrinology 1978; 102:1641.
21. Eddie LW, Bell RJ, Lester A, et al. Radioimmunoassay of relaxin in pregnancy with an analog of human relaxin. Lancet 1986; 1:1344.
22. Thomas K, Loumaye E, Ferin J. Relaxin in non-pregnant women during ovarian stimulation. Gynecol Obstet Invest 1980; 11:75.
23. Loumaye E, Donnez J, Thomas K. Immunoreactive relaxin in the human

menstrual cycle. In: Bigazzi M, Greenwood FC, Gasparri F, eds. Biology of relaxin and its role in the human. Excerpta Medica International Congress Series 610, 1983;337.

24. Weiss G, O'Byrne EM, Steinetz BG. Relaxin: a product of the human corpus luteum of pregnancy. Science 1976; 194:948.

25. Mathieu PH, Rahier J, Thomas K. Localization of relaxin in human gestational corpus luteum. Cell Tissue Res 1981; 219:213.

26. Weiss G, O'Byrne EM, Hochman JA, Goldsmith LT, Rifkin I, Steinetz BG. Secretion of progesterone and relaxin by the human corpus luteum of midpregnancy and at term. Obstet Gynecol 1977; 50:679.

27. Quagliarello J, Steinetz BG, Weiss G. Relaxin secretion in early pregnancy. Obstet Gynecol 1979; 53:62.

28. O'Byrne EM, Carriere BT, Sorensen L, Segaloff A, Schwabe C, Steinetz BG. Plasma immunoreactive relaxin levels in pregnant and non-pregnant women. J Clin Endocrinol Metab 1978; 47:1106.

29. Szlachter BN, Quagliarello J, Jewelewicz R, Osathanondh R, Spellacy WN, Weiss G. Relaxin in normal and pathogenic pregnancies. Obstet Gynecol 1982; 59:167.

30. Loumaye E, Teuwissen B, Thomas K. Characterization of relaxin RIA using Bolton-Hunter reagent. First results in plasma during pregnancy and in placenta, corpora lutea and ovarian cysts in women. Gynecol Obstet Invest 1978; 9:262.

31. Bell RJ, Eddie LW, Lester AR, Wood EC, Johnston PD, Niall HD. Relaxin in human pregnancy serum measured with an homologous radioimmunoassay. Obstet Gynecol 1987; 69:585.

32. MacLennan AH, Nicolson R, Green RC. Serum relaxin in pregnancy. Lancet 1986; 2:241.

33. Quagliarello J, Nachtigall R, Goldsmith LT, et al. Serum immunoreactive relaxin concentrations in human pregnancy, labor and the puerperium. In: Channing CP, Marsh JM, Sadler WA, eds. Ovarian follicular and corpus luteum function. New York: Plenum Publishing, 1979:743.

34. Quagliarello J, Lustig DS, Steinetz BG, Weiss G. Absence of a prelabor relaxin surge in women. Biol Reprod 1980; 22:202.

35. Weiss G, O'Byrne EM, Hochman J, Steinetz BG, Goldsmith L, Flitcraft JG. Distribution of relaxin in women during pregnancy. Obstet Gynecol 1978; 52:569.

36. Seki K, Vesato T, Tabei T, Kato K. Serum relaxin in patients with hydatidiform mole. Obstet Gynecol 1986; 67:381.

37. Haning RV, Steinetz B, Weiss G. Elevated serum relaxin levels in multiple pregnancy after mexotropin treatment. Obstet Gynecol 1985; 66:42.

38. Quagliarello J, Szlachter W, Nisselbaum JS, Schwartz MK, Steinetz B, Weiss G. Serum relaxin and human chorionic gonadotropin concentrations in spontaneous abortions. Fertil Steril 1981; 36:399.

39. Weiss G, Steinetz BG, Dierschke DJ, Fritz G. Relaxin secretion in the rhesus monkey. Biol Reprod 1981; 24:565.

40. Castracane VD, D'Eletto R, Weiss G. Relaxin secretion in the baboon (Papio Cynocephalus). In: Greenwood GS, Terranova PI, eds. Factors regulating ovarian function. New York: Raven Press, 1983:415.

41. Quagliarello J, Goldsmith L, Steinetz B, Lesstig DS, Weiss G. Induction of relaxin secretion in non-pregnant women by human chorionic gonadotropin. J Clin Endocrinol Metab 1980; 51:74.

42. Ottobre JS, Nixon WE, Stouffer RL. Induction of relaxin secretion in rhesus monkeys by human chorionic gonadotropin: dependence of the age of the corpus luteum of the menstrual cycle. Biol Reprod 1984; 31:1000.

43. Astwood EB. The regulation of corpus luteum function by hypophysial luteotrophin. Endocrinology 1941; 28:209.

44. Saito S, Saxena B. Specific receptors for prolactin in the ovary. Acta Endocrinol (Copenh) 1975; 80:126.

45. Quagliarello J, Goldsmith L, Szlachter N, Hochman J, Weiss G. Absence of a luteotropic effect of prolactin and human placental lactogen on the human corpus luteum of pregnancy. In: Goldstein M, ed. Ergot compounds and brain function: neuroendocrine and neuropsychiatric aspects. New York: Raven Press, 1980:229.

46. Hochman J, Weiss G, Steinetz BG, O'Byrne EM. Serum relaxin concentrations in prostaglin and oxytocin-induced labor in women. Am J Obstet Gynecol 1978; 130:473.

47. Quagliarello J, Cederqvist L, Steinetz BG, Weiss G. Serum relaxin levels in prostaglandin E_2 induced abortions. Prostaglandins 1978; 16:1003.

48. Goldsmith LT, Essig M, Sarosi P, Beck P, Weiss G. Hormone secretion by monolayer cultures of human luteal cells. J Clin Endocrinol Metab 1981; 53:890.

49. Schmidt CL, Black VH, Sarosi P, Weiss G. Progesterone and relaxin secretion in relation to the ultrastructure of human luteal cells in culture: effects of human chorionic gonadotropin. Am J Obstet Gynecol 1986; 155:1209.

50. Nixon WE. In vitro relaxin and progesterone secretion by nonhuman primate (macaca mulatta) luteal cells [Abstract 778]. Endocrine Society Annual Meeting, 1982.

51. Bigazzi M, Nardi E, Bruni P, Petrucci F. Relaxin in human decidua. J Clin Endocrinol Metab 1980; 51:939.

52. Fields PA, Larkin LH. Purification and immunohistochemical localization of relaxin in the human term placenta. J Clin Endocrinol Metab 1981; 52:79.

53. Yamamoto S, Kwok SCM, Greenwood FC, Bryant-Greenwood GD. Relaxin purification from human placental basal plates. J Clin Endocrinol. Metab 1981; 52:601.

54. Schmidt CL, Sarosi P, Steinetz BG, et al. Relaxin in human decidua and term placenta. Eur J Obstet Gynecol Reprod Biol 1984; 17:171.

55. Castracane VD, Lessing J, Brenner S, Weiss G. Relaxin in the pregnant baboon: evidence for local production in reproductive tissues. J Clin Endocrinol Metab 1985; 60:133.

56. Hisaw FL Jr, Hisaw FL. Effect of relaxin in the uterus of monkeys (macaca mulatta) with observations on the cervix and symphysis pubis. Am J Obstet Gynecol 1964; 89:141.

57. Tseng L, Maxella J. Effects of relaxin on human endometrium. Regulation of estrogen synthesis and metabolism in primary cell culture [Abstract 285]. Society for Gynecologic Investigation, 1986.

58. Szlachter N, O'Byrne EM, Goldsmith L, Steinetz BG, Weiss G. Myometrial-inhibiting activity of relaxin containing extracts of human corpora lutea of pregnancy. Am J Obstet Gynecol 1980; 136:584.

59. Richardson M, Mitchell MD, MacDonald PC, Casey ML. Effect of relaxin on prostacyclin production by human myometrial cells in monolayer culture. Society for Gynecologic Investigation Annual Program, 1983.

60. Sanborn BM, Kuo HS, Weisbrodt NW, Sherwood OD. The interaction of relaxin with the rat uterus I. Effect on cyclic nucleotide levels and spontaneous contractile activity. Endocrinology 1980; 106:1210.

61. Nishikori K, Weisbrodt NW, Sherwood OD, Sanborn BM. Relaxin alters rat uterine myosin light chain phosphorylation and related enzymatic activities. Endocrinology 1982; 111:1743.

62. MacLennan AH, Green RC, Bryant-Greenwood GD, Greenwood FC. Ripening of the human cervix and induction of labour with purified porcine relaxin. Lancet 1980; 1:220.

63. Evans MI, Dougan MB, Moawad AH, Evans WJ, Bryant-Greenwood G, Greenwood FC. Ripening of the human cervix with porcine ovarian relaxin. Am J Obstet Gynecol 1983; 147:410.

64. Wiqvist I, Norstrom A, O'Byrne EM, Wiquist N. Regulatory influence of relaxin on human cervical and uterine connective tissue. Acta Endocrinol (Copenh) 1984; 106:127.

65. Jarrett JC, Ballejo G, Saleem TH, Tsibris JCM, Spellacy WN. The effect of prolactin and relaxin on insulin binding by adipocytes from pregnant women. Am J Obstet Gynecol 1984; 149:250.

66. Bryant-Greenwood GD, Jeffrey R, Ralph MM, Seamark RF. Relaxin production by the porcine ovarian graafian follicle in vitro. Biol Reprod 1980; 23:792.

67. Loeken MR, Channing CP, D'Eletto R, Weiss G. Stimulatory effect of luteinizing hormone upon relaxin secretion by cultured porcine preovulatory granulosa cells. Endocrinology 1983; 112:769.

68. Too CKL, Bryant-Greenwood GD, Greenwood FC. Relaxin increases the release of plasminogen activator, collagenase and proteoglycanase from rat granulosa cells in vitro. Endocrinology 1984; 115:1043.

RECEPTOR-MEDIATED DIFFERENCES IN THE ACTIONS OF OVINE

LUTEINIZING HORMONE VS. HUMAN CHORIONIC GONADOTROPIN

G. D. Niswender, D. A. Roess, and B. G. Barisas

Departments of Physiology and Chemistry
Colorado State University
Fort Collins, Colorado 80523

INTRODUCTION

In primates, as in most other species, continued secretion of progesterone from the corpus luteum is a requirement for maintenance of early
pregnancy. Luteinizing hormone (LH) plays the key role in stimulating
ovulation and formation of the corpus luteum (1). If pregnancy occurs,
concentrations of human chorionic gonadotropin (hCG) in serum begin to
rise as early as 8 days after ovulation or 1 day after implantation (2).
The secretion of hCG by the developing conceptus is apparently the only
hormonal signal required for maternal recognition and maintenance of
pregnancy.

There has been evidence available for a number of years that LH and
hCG have similar biological and immunological activities. However, it has
also been clear that some of the biological effects of LH and hCG are
different, particularly as related to the duration of the response following a single injection of these hormones. For example, in 1969 Vande-
Wiele and Turskoy (3) reported that induction of ovulation in anovulatory
women with a single injection of hCG resulted in a corpus luteum with a
normal life span, while induction with LH (1) was followed by a dramatically shortened luteal phase of the menstrual cycle. At the time these
experiments were performed, the different responses were attributed to the
fact that LH was cleared from blood much more rapidly than was hCG (4).

Human LH (hLH) and hCG are composed of two nonidentical subunits.
They have a common α-subunit which contains 92 amino acids with 2 branched
chain carbohydrates attached at the asparaginyl residues at positions 52
and 78. The β-subunit of hCG contains 145 amino acids with branched chain
carbohydrates linked through asparaginyl residues at the 13 and 30 positions and short linear sugars linked via serines at positions 121, 127,
132 and 138 (5). The β-subunit of hLH, on the other hand, has only 121
amino acids with a single carbohydrate moiety at the asparaginyl residue
at position 30. Although there is considerable homology in the amino acid
composition of the β-subunits of hLH and hCG, 24 amino acids differ
between the two molecules and hCG has an additional 24 amino acids (6).
Based on their chemical composition, it appears that differences in the
chemical compositions of the β-subunits of the two hormones are responsible for the differences observed in the rates of clearance from blood

and are likely responsible for the different actions at the level of the receptor for LH to be discussed below.

Ovine LH (oLH) rather than hLH has been used for most of the experiments to be discussed since sheep luteal tissue was used for these studies. The α-subunit of oLH contains 96 amino acids of which 71 are homologous with those in the α-subunit of hLH. Thirty-nine of the 119 amino acids in the β-subunit of oLH are different from those in the β-subunit of hLH which has 121 total (6). The α-subunit of oLH has carbohydrates linked at asparaginyl residues at the 56 and 82 positions while the β-subunit of oLH has carbohydrate linked at the 13 asparaginyl position.

The ovine corpus luteum has been used for the studies described below because in ewes and in women, the luteal phase of the estrous cycle lasts 14 days (7). In both species, the corpus luteum is composed of two types of steroidogenic luteal cells (8,9), and LH and hCG bind to the same luteal receptor in both species (10,11).

DIFFERENTIAL EFFECTS OF LH AND HCG ON THE LUTEAL CELL

Effects on Secretion of Progesterone

When ovine luteal cells were exposed to a maximally stimulating dose (10 or 100 ng) of oLH for 15 min, there was an eightfold increase in progesterone secretion within 1 h after initiation of treatment (12). By 3-4 h progesterone secretion had returned to pretreatment levels. Progesterone secretion was also maximal within 1 h when luteal cells were exposed to 2 or 20 ng hCG; however, following stimulation with hCG, the secretion of progesterone remained elevated for the 6-h duration of the experiment. Thus, the steroidogenic response to hCG is dramatically prolonged over that observed following treatment with oLH. In addition, the steroidogenic response obtained with a 15-min pulse of a maximally stimulatory dose of hCG was not different from that observed with continuous (6 h) exposure to the same levels of hormone.

Segaloff et al. (13) had previously demonstrated a prolonged steroidogenic response when Leydig cells (both normal and tumor cells) were treated with a maximal stimulatory dose of hCG compared to oLH. Thus, this difference in the effects of oLH vs. hCG does not appear to be species specific. However, these studies need to be conducted with primate luteal tissue and primate gonadotropins to determine whether the differences that we observed in the steroidogenic responses to oLH and hCG also occur in primates.

Rate of Internalization of Hormone

One possible explanation for the prolonged steroidogenic effect of hCG vs. oLH was that the hCG receptor complex was internalized more slowly than was the oLH receptor complex. When this hypothesis was tested directly (14), it was found that the time required for internalization of one-half ($t_{\frac{1}{2}}$) of ^{125}I-hCG bound to ovine luteal receptors for LH was 22.8 ± 2.3 h. The $t_{\frac{1}{2}}$ for internalization of ^{125}I-oLH was 0.4 ± 0.2 h, which was similar to that (0.3 ± 0.1 h) observed for ^{125}I-mouse epidermal growth factor (mEGF). Thus, oLH was internalized approximately 50 times more rapidly than was hCG. The fact that the rates of internalization of oLH and mEGF were similar to each other and to the rates observed for EGF and insulin in other cell types (15,16) suggested that hCG had some unique property which prevented rapid internalization of the hCG-occupied receptor. Since there was an inverse relationship between the rate of internalization and the duration of the steroidogenic response following treatment of luteal cells with oLH and hCG, it was suggested that internalization of the hormone-receptor complex is a primary mechanism for termination of the gonadotropin-mediated steroidogenic response.

Mock et al. (14) also studied the rate of internalization of hLH and found a $t_{\frac{1}{2}}$ of 15.1 ± 1.4 h. This value was intermediate between those observed for oLH and hCG and indicated that hLH had properties more similar to those of hCG than to oLH when the rate of internalization of the receptor for LH was determined.

In a second series of experiments, all possible recombinants were made with the α- and β-subunits of oLH and hCG (17). When the radioiodinated β-subunit of hCG was recombined with the α-subunit of hCG, the $t_{\frac{1}{2}}$ for internalization was 22.8 ± 3.8 h while recombination with the α-subunit of oLH resulted in a $t_{\frac{1}{2}}$ for internalization of 8.9 ± 4.5 h. When the radioiodinated β-subunit of oLH was recombined with the α-subunit of oLH, the $t_{\frac{1}{2}}$ for internalization was 0.7 ± 0.2 h while recombination with the α-subunit of hCG resulted in a $t_{\frac{1}{2}}$ of 0.5 ± 0.1 h. It was obvious from these data that the α-subunit played little, if any, role in modulating the rate of internalization of the tropic hormone. On the other hand, the β-subunit of hCG appeared to be the primary determinant of the slow rate of internalization of hCG. This was not surprising since most of the chemical differences in the composition of oLH and hCG reside in the β-subunits of the two hormones.

Finally, the rate of internalization of hCG-occupied LH receptors ($t_{\frac{1}{2}}$ = 22.8 h) is very similar to the rate of internalization of radioiodinated membrane proteins ($t_{\frac{1}{2}}$ = 25 h). This suggests that hCG immobilizes the receptor within the plasma membrane and that internalization occurs only as a consequence of generalized membrane recycling (18).

Differences in Mobility of the LH Receptor

The prolonged residency of hCG-occupied receptors on the plasma membrane, compared to oLH-occupied receptors, suggested that differences exist in the physical behavior of these complexes in the membrane. To investigate this possibility, initial studies were performed to determine if the slow rate of internalization of hCG relative to oLH was due to differences in the lateral mobilities of the LH receptor in the plasma membrane when occupied by the two hormones (19). Tetramethylrhodamine isothiocyanate (TRITC)-labeled oLH and hCG, which retained biological activity and demonstrated receptor specificity, were bound to LH receptors on small ovine luteal cells obtained by enzymatic dispersion. Diffusion coefficients of hormone-occupied receptors were measured using fluorescence photobleaching recovery techniques (19). The oLH receptor complex had a diffusion coefficient of $1.9 \pm 1.0 \times 10^{-10}$ cm^{2}sec^{-1}, which was comparable to that of membrane proteins on ovine luteal cells labeled nonspecifically with TRITC-succinyl concanavalin A (S Con A) and to other membrane proteins on lymphocytes, fibroblasts, and other cell types (20). In contrast, hCG receptor complexes had a diffusion coefficient of $<1 \times 10^{-11}$ cm^{2}sec^{-1}, suggesting that most hCG-occupied receptors were immobile.

In subsequent studies the lateral dynamics of the mobile hCG-occupied receptors were measured by performing three complete photobleaching experiments at a single site on the luteal cell membrane. In the first photobleaching experiment, exposure of TRITC-labeled molecules to intense laser light for 500 msec irreversibly bleached fluorophores in the beam path. Subsequent fluorescence photobleaching recovery experiments at the same spot then measured fluorescence from unbleached, mobile fluorophores.

Although fluorescence was reduced dramatically in the second and third experiments, the recovery after photobleaching was between 60 and 80%. The fraction of mobile TRITC-hCG-labeled receptors was obtained from the first experiment. The rate of lateral diffusion of the mobile fluorophores was obtained on the second or third experiment. The diffusion coefficients agree well with the values obtained from the initial photobleaching experiments but are considerably more precise. The mobile hCG receptor complexes had a mean diffusion coefficient of 3.3×10^{-10} $cm^2 sec^{-1}$ (Table 1). The fraction of mobile fluorophores, estimated from mean values for fluorescence recovery after photobleaching obtained on the first bleach was 10.3%.

The immobilization of the LH receptor by hCG is probably not due to TRITC-induced hCG degradation or structural alterations in the hCG molecule for several reasons. (1) TRITC-hCG can compete for ^{125}I-hCG binding sites on luteal cell membranes (19). (2) TRITC-hCG binds specifically to small luteal cells and this binding can be blocked in cells pretreated with a one-hundred- to five-hundredfold excess of unlabeled hCG (19). If there were appreciable amounts of nonspecific hormone binding, it seems likely that values obtained for fluorophore lateral diffusion would increase rather than decrease since virtually every protein we have studied on the luteal cell membrane, with the exception of hCG-occupied receptors, has a diffusion coefficient of $1-2 \times 10^{-10}$ $cm^2 sec^{-1}$. (3) As is shown below, the binding of unlabeled hCG to small luteal cells causes an identical reduction in the lateral diffusion of the LH receptor.

The next question to be addressed was whether occupancy of the LH receptor by oLH influenced the lateral mobility of the receptor. Diffusion of unoccupied and occupied receptors was measured with a monoclonal antibody directed against the LH receptor. This antibody was produced following immunization of mice with a cell membrane fraction obtained from purified small ovine luteal cells. Hybridomas were screened for the ability to secrete antibody which could be used to immunoprecipitate detergent-solubilized hCG-occupied LH receptors.

Monovalent Fab fragments of this monoclonal antibody were used to probe the lateral diffusion of the LH receptor in the presence and absence of LH and hCG (Table 1). When studied by fluorescence photobleaching recovery, TRITC-derivatized Fab fragments of antibody bound to the LH receptor had a diffusion coefficient of 1.5×10^{-10} $cm^2 sec^{-1}$ with fluorescence recovery after photobleaching of 53.2%. After cells were incubated with oLH (1 nM), the diffusion coefficient for TRITC-Fab was

Table 1. Lateral diffusion of occupied and unoccupied LH receptors.

Ligand	Treatment	Diffusion Coefficient (10^{-10} $cm^2 sec^{-1}$)		Mean % Recovery
Anti-LHR (Fab)	none	1.5 ± 0.8^{a}	(10)*	53.2
oLH	none	1.9 ± 1.0^{a}	(27)	34.0
hLH	none	1.4 ± 0.1^{a}	(12)	59.0
anti-LHR (Fab)	1 nM oLH	2.0 ± 0.7^{a}	(8)	39.2
hCG	none	0.33 ± 0.1^{b}	(7)	10.3
anti-LHR (Fab),	1 nM hCG	0.42 ± 0.1^{b}	(8)	<20
deglyco hCG	none	1.1 ± 0.1^{a}	(9)	61.0

*Numbers in parentheses represent the number of FPR experiments.
[a,b] Numbers followed by different superscripts are different (P<0.05).

$2.0\text{x}10^{-10}\text{cm}^2\text{sec}^{-1}$ with 39.2% fluorescence recovery after photobleaching. The diffusion coefficient was similar to that of the unoccupied LH receptor and to that obtained using TRITC-oLH as a probe for LH receptor lateral diffusion. However, when cells were incubated with hCG (1 nM), the diffusion coefficient was reduced to approximately $0.4\text{x}10^{-10}\text{cm}^2\text{sec}^{-1}$ with fluorescence recovery of less than 20%. Thus, the antibody is an effective probe for monitoring molecular motions and distribution of receptors for LH on viable cell membranes. Using the antibody as a probe, the fluorescence recovery after photobleaching was still less than 40% for oLH-occupied receptors and less than 20% for hCG-labeled LH receptors which was quite low. Fluorescence recovery for other membrane proteins is typically 50-60% (21,22), suggesting that the lateral diffusion of an appreciable fraction of oLH receptor complexes might also be physically constrained.

Another question is what chemical component of hCG is involved in the actions of this hormone to immobilize the receptor for LH. Ryan et al. (23) has proposed a model for the biological activity of hCG in which hCG binding to LH receptor is accompanied by a secondary association between the carbohydrates of hCG and membrane proteins. Both receptor binding and secondary protein associations are needed for the biological function of hCG. If there are additional interactions between hCG and proteins adjacent to the receptor, it would not be unreasonable to expect that lateral motions of the hCG molecule would be reduced compared to LH-occupied receptors. From fluorescence photobleaching recovery experiments it appears that the carbohydrate portion of the hCG molecule plays a role in decreasing the mobility of the receptor for LH. Deglycosylated hCG-TRITC bound to LH receptor had a diffusion coefficient, $1.1\pm0.1\text{x}10^{-10}\text{cm}^2\text{sec}^{-1}$, similar to that of receptors occupied by oLH (Table 1). It is known that deglycosylation reduces the biological activity of hCG and uncouples cAMP production (24,25). Thus, further studies of the interactions of possible receptor-associated proteins with the unique components of the β-subunit of hCG are merited.

Involvement of the Cytoskeleton in Receptor Immobilization

Interactions of the hormone-LH receptor complex with cell structural components such as the cytoskeleton or an intra-membrane protein network, may restrict receptor motions. Microfilaments and microtubules have been implicated in other aspects of luteal cell function (26). Therefore, the next question to be answered was whether components of the cytoskeleton were involved in the reduced lateral mobility of the hCG-occupied receptor. In cells treated with cytoskeletal disrupters, the rate of lateral diffusion and the fractional recovery of hCG-labeled receptor increased, suggesting that some cytoskeletal modulation of receptor complex mobility occurs (Table 2). Colchicine and cytochalasin D treatment resulted in the largest increase (about sevenfold) in lateral diffusion while cytochalasin B caused a smaller threefold increase.

As shown in Table 3, cytoskeletal disrupters had no major effect on the lateral diffusion of S Con A labeled glycoproteins in luteal cell membranes. A diffusion coefficient of $1.24\text{x}10^{-10}\text{cm}^2\text{sec}^{-1}$ was measured in untreated luteal cells. In cells exposed to cytoskeletal disrupters, diffusion coefficients for S Con A labeled glycoproteins ranged from 1.0 to $1.8\text{x}10^{-10}\text{cm}^2\text{sec}^{-1}$. The average recovery after photobleaching for these proteins was low compared to rates of lateral diffusion of glycoproteins in other cells. Fluorescence recovery on the first bleach was no more than 47% for the S Con A-labeled molecules.

A treatment which induced vesiculation of the luteal cell membrane was used as a second approach to evaluate the role of the cytoskeleton in

Table 2. Effects of cytoskeletal disruptors on the lateral diffusion and fluorescence recovery of hCG-occupied receptors.*

Ligand	Treatment	Diffusion Coefficient (10^{-10} cm^2 sec^{-1})		% Recovery After Photobleaching
hCG	none	0.33 ± 0.08^a	(9)	10.3 ± 2.5^a
hCG	cytochalasin B	0.90 ± 0.01^b	(17)	26.4 ± 3.7^b
hCG	cytochalasin D	2.20 ± 0.42^c	(18)	24.9 ± 3.8^b
hCG	colchicine	2.25 ± 0.34^c	(16)	33.3 ± 3.6^b

*Small luteal cells were pretreated for 1 h with cytochalasin B (20 µg/ml), cytochalasin D (20 µg/ml) or colchicine (40 µg/ml) and then labeled with 0.5 µg/ml TRITC-hCG. Results are the mean and SEM of the number of individual experiments shown in parentheses.

[a,b,c] Diffusion coefficients or values for percent recovery having different superscripts are different at the 95% confidence level by Student's t test.

limiting the lateral mobility of the hCG-occupied receptor. Luteal cells were exposed to 25 mM formaldehyde and 2 mM dithiothreitol in phosphate-buffered saline (VES) which produced membrane protrusions of varying diameters that were uniformly labeled with TRITC-hCG. The viability of cells with membrane blebs was >90% as measured by fluorescein diacetate staining (27). NBD-phallacidin labeling of F-actin in conjunction with image processing techniques indicated that these membrane blebs on ovine luteal cells were free of underlying actin filaments. On the membrane vesicle the fraction of mobile membrane proteins, including the hCG-occupied receptors was increased (Table 4). However, unlike proteins examined on membrane blebs of lymphocyte and muscle cell membranes (28,29), luteal cell membrane proteins and lipids labeled with the lipid probe DiI never become fully mobile and hCG-occupied receptor diffusion coefficients are at least tenfold less than reported for lymphocyte and muscle cell surface proteins.

Table 3. Effects of cytoskeletal disruptors on the lateral diffusion and fluorescence recovery after photobleaching of TRITC-succinyl concanavalin A labeled membrane proteins.*

Ligand	Treatment	Diffusion Coefficient (10^{-10} cm^2 sec^{-1})		% Recovery After Photobleaching
S Con A	none	1.24 ± 0.12	(26)	26.8 ± 3.1
S Con A	cytochalasin B (20 µg/ml)	1.01 ± 0.36	(19)	37.8 ± 6.2
S Con A	cytochalasin D (20 µg/ml)	1.49 ± 0.08	(12)	46.8 ± 7.4
S Con A	colchicine (40 µg/ml)	1.83 ± 0.15	(12)	27.4 ± 4.3

*Luteal cells were preincubated with the indicated concentration of cytocytoskeletal disruptors and then labeled with 10 µg/ml TRITC-S Con A. Results are the mean and SEM of the number of experiments shown in parentheses.

Ligand	Treatment	Diffusion Coefficient $(10^{-10} cm^2 sec^{-1})$		% Recovery After Photobleaching
DiI	none	13.9 ± 1.7	(17)	80.8 ± 2.4
DiI	VES	28.3 ± 2.8	(11)	88.6 ± 5.0
TRITC-S Con A	none	1.2 ± 0.1	(26)	26.8 ± 3.1
TRITC-S Con A	VES	4.2 ± 0.4	(8)	61.6 ± 6.1
TRITC-hCG	none	0.3 ± 0.2	(8)	10.3 ± 2.5
TRITC-hCG	VES	1.7 ± 0.2	(16)	52.3 ± 3.5

*Membrane blebs formed on small luteal cells treated with a vesiculent (VES) consisting of 25 mM formaldehyde and 2 mM dithiothreitol in phosphate-buffered saline containing 0.9 mM Ca^{2+} and 0.5 mM Mg^{2+}. Cells were incubated 30 min with VES at room temperature, washed two times in balanced salt solution (BSS), and resuspended in 1 ml of BSS. VES-treated small luteal cells and untreated small luteal cells were labeled with 0.5 µg DiI, 10 µg TRITC-S Con A or 0.1 µg TRITC-hCG. Results are the mean and SEM of the number of experiments shown in parentheses.

That a comparatively small molecule such as hCG can immobilize its receptor is not unique to luteal cells. Yahara and Edelman (30) were the first to propose that binding of a protein, in their case the plant lectin Concanavalin A (Con A), could globally restrict the mobility of cell surface receptors through anchorage of receptors to cytoskeletal components. Binding of Con A to membrane glycoproteins on fibroblast membranes (31) and lymphocytes (32) immobilizes its receptor. Even limiting Con A binding to localized regions of the fibroblast membrane using Con A-coated platelets caused a global immobilization of unoccupied Con A-binding proteins at distant sites (32). This may occur through the rapid association of transmembrane glycoproteins and cytoskeletal components (33,34). Global restriction of Con A receptors and surface immunoglobulin receptors on murine B cells by Con A-coated platelets can be fully reversed, but only by simultaneous treatment with both colchicine and cytochalasin B (32). Treatment of luteal cells with either microfilament or microtubule disrupters also increases the rate of hCG-occupied LH receptor lateral diffusion (Table 2).

To determine whether hCG occupancy of the LH receptor by cytoskeletal components might, in some way, restrict the lateral diffusion of other proteins, we examined the lateral diffusion of the EGF receptor following binding of hCG to its receptor. TRITC-EGF bound to EGF receptors on luteal cells has a diffusion coefficient of $1.97 \times 10^{-10} cm^2 sec^{-1}$ (Table 5). When LH receptors were occupied by hCG, the lateral motions of EGF-occupied receptors were not perturbed. These results suggest that an obligatory reduction in the diffusion of all membrane proteins did not occur in response to hCG binding to the LH receptor. Henis (35) has shown that while Con A-coated platelets inhibit the movement of surface Ig and Con A receptors on lymphocytes, there is no reduction in the lateral diffusion coefficients measured for the H-2K antigens. Axelrod et al. (36) have shown that acetylcholine receptors located in discrete patches on the membrane of embryonic rat muscle cells are immobile. However, TRITC-S Con A had unconstrained lateral motions within these patches of immobile acetylcholine receptors (37).

Table 5. The effect of hCG on the lateral mobility and
fluorescence recovery of EGF-occupied receptors.*

Ligand	Treatment	Diffusion Coefficient $(10^{-11} cm^2 sec^{-1})$		% Recovery After Photobleaching
TRITC-EGF	none	1.97 ± 0.28	(13)	26.4 ± 2.0
TRITC-EGF	hCG	2.07 ± 0.26	(15)	35.5 ± 3.2

*Luteal cells were incubated with 0.1% sodium azide in BSS for 30 min
prior and then incubated for 30 min with 0.1 µg/ml hCG. After a 30-min
incubation, cells were washed three times and labeled with TRITC-EGF.
Results are the mean and SEM of the number experiments shown in
parentheses.

Rotational Movements of Receptors for LH

There have been indications that receptor aggregation might be
necessary for biological action of the hormone, internalization of the
hormone-receptor complex, receptor recycling, or desensitization to the
hormone (38,39). The size of receptor-hormone aggregates increases on
cells exposed to LH concentrations up to and beyond the LH concentration
which results in maximum progesterone secretion (40). In other cell
systems, receptor aggregation is a prerequisite for biological response.
About 10% of cyanogen bromide-treated EGF can bind EGF receptors but
remains biologically inactive until cross-linked with divalent anti-EGF
antibody (41). Studies of insulin receptor function have shown that anti-
body-induced cross-linking of monovalent fragments of anti-receptor antibody can produce insulin-like effects in target cells (42). In pituitary
cells, aggregation of receptors for gonadotropin-releasing hormone (GnRH)
may play a role in the secretion of LH (43). A GnRH antagonist has
agonist activity if GnRH receptors are brought into close proximity (<150
A°). An enhancement of agonist action can also be obtained using antibody
cross-linking of GnRH agonist dimers. Conn (44) suggests receptors must
lie within a critical distance for GnRH agonist activity. These results
suggest that, in general, aggregation of the protein hormone-occupied
receptor may be a prerequisite for target cell response.

One consequence of LH receptor aggregation on the luteal cell surface
would be an increase in the physical size of aggregates. Molecular
rotational relaxation times depend strongly on molecular size and asymmetry (45). Rotational motion measurements thus have the potential to
probe subtle changes in the aggregation state of proteins. Measurement of
protein rotation also can provide a means of choosing between factors
which might restrict the lateral motions of the LH receptor, such as
cytoskeletal interactions, receptor-protein interactions, receptor-
receptor interactions (46) or "caging" of receptors within a membrane
protein network. Zidovetzki et al. (47) have used phosphorescence emission anisotropy to measure the rotational motions of EGF-occupied EGF
receptors on human epidermoid carcinoma cells. When EGF-labeled cells
were warmed from 4 to 37°C, there was a rapid decrease in the rate of
rotational movement. They have estimated from these data that EGF receptors are aggregated in small clusters containing about 2-3 receptors prior
to binding EGF. Upon warming, the aggregate size increases until it
contains a maximum of about 50 receptors.

We have used time-resolved phosphorescence anisotropy (TPA)
techniques in the laboratory of T. M. Jovin at Goettingen, Federal Repub-

lic of Germany, to measure rotational diffusion of LH receptors on ovine luteal cells using erythrosin (ErITC) conjugates of hCG and a monoclonal antibody against LH receptor as probes (48). ErITC is a long-lived triplet probe. An orientationally asymmetric population of triplet labels is produced by a polarized pulse of laser light in a microscope optical system. The remaining ground state fluorophores have a corresponding orientationally asymmetric depletion. Fluorescence from ground state fluorophores, which can be elicited by a low powered laser beam, is polarized. This fluorescence polarization decays over 10–200 µsec due to rotation of fluorophore-bearing proteins. Effects of triplet decay, being much slower, are easily separated. In the absence of hCG, antibody-labeled LH receptor exhibits rotational correlation times (ϕ) of 48 µsec at 4°C and 52 µsec at 37°C. With 10^{-8} M hCG, ϕ is 80 µsec at 4°C and 46 µsec at 37°C. Anisotropies (r) of LH receptor-bound antibody fall over 0–200 µsec at 37°C and rise at 4°C, although r falls at both temperatures for the antibody in glycerol. This suggests a temperature-induced change in the orientation of LH receptor-bound antibody. Small values of the ratio $(r_0-r_\infty)/r_0$ indicates that most LH receptor-bound antibody is rotationally immobile. Binding of hCG further reduces rotational mobility of the LH receptor at 4°C. ErITC-hCG bound to the LH-receptor is completely immobile in these experiments. Thus, LH receptors may undergo aggregation which is both thermotropic and ligand (hCG)-linked.

SUMMARY

The results of the experiments described in this communication have demonstrated that hCG occupancy of ovine luteal receptors for LH results in a number of different responses when compared to occupancy of the same receptor with oLH. The steroidogenic response to hCG is prolonged as compared to the response following treatment with oLH. This prolonged steroidogenic response appears to result from a dramatically reduced rate of internalization of the LH receptor when occupied by hCG vs. oLH. The reduced rate of internalization of the hCG-LH receptor complex is likely the result of immobilization of the LH receptor in the plasma membrane due to binding of hCG. Immobilization of the receptor appears to involve interactions between the β-subunit of hCG and, more specifically, the unique carbohydrate moieties associated with this portion of the molecule, and the cytoskeleton of the luteal cell.

These results have very interesting implications for the maintenance of pregnancy in primates. It appears that the unique chemical composition of hCG has at least two major actions to insure continued secretion of progesterone and maintenance of pregnancy. First, hCG has a dramatically reduced rate of clearance from circulation compared to LH. Second, hCG produces a more prolonged steroidogenic response by preventing rapid internalization of the hormone-LH receptor complex. In fact, the data suggest that hCG receptor complexes are only internalized as a result of recycling of the components of the plasma membrane. However, these results should be interpreted with caution since the results were obtained with hCG, oLH and ovine luteal cells. It remains to be demonstrated that hLH and hCG will have similar actions on human luteal cells.

REFERENCES

1. VandeWiele RL, Bogumil J, Dryenfurth I, et al. Mechanisms regulating the menstrual cycle in women. Recent Prog Horm Res 1971; 26:63-90.
2. Jaffe RB, Lee PA, Midgley AR Jr. Serum gonadotropins before, at the inception of, and following human pregnancy. J Clin Endocrinol 1969; 1281-3.

3. VandeWiele RL, Turksoy RN. Treatment of amenorrhea and of anovulation with human menopausal and chorionic gonadotropins. J Clin Endocrinol 1965; 25:369-84.

4. Midgley AR Jr, Jaffee RB. Regulation of human gonadotropins: II. Disappearance of human chorionic gonadotropins following delivery. J Clin Endocrinol 1968; 28:1712-8.

5. Birken S, Canfield RE. Structural and immunochemical properties of human choriogonadotropin. In: McKerns KW, ed. Structure and function of the gonadotropins. New York: Plenum Press, 1978:47-80.

6. Ward, Darrel. Personal communication. Spring 1987.

7. Niswender GD, Nett TM, Akbar AM. The hormones of reproduction. In: Hafez ESE, ed. Reproduction in farm animals. Philadelphia: Lee & Febiger, 1975:57-88.

8. Guraya SS. Morphology, histochemistry and biochemistry of human ovarian compartments and steroid hormone synthesis. Physiol Rev 1971; 785-897.

9. Fitz TA, Mayan MH, Sawyer HR, Niswender GD. Characterization of two steroidogenic cell types in the ovine corpus luteum. Biol Reprod 1982; 27:703-11.

10. Diekman MA, O'Callahan P, Nett TM, Niswender GD. Validation of methods and quantification of luteal receptors for LH throughout the estrous cycle and early pregnancy in ewes. Biol Reprod 1978; 19:999-1009.

11. Wardlaw S, Lauersen NH, Saxena BB. The LH-hCG receptor of human ovary at various stages of the menstrual cycle. Acta Endocrinol (Copenh) 1975; 79:568-76.

12. Bourdage RJ, Fitz TA, Niswender GD. Differential steroidogenic response of ovine luteinizing hormone and human chorionic gonadotropin. Proc Soc Exp Biol Med 1984; 175:483-6.

13. Segaloff DL, Puett D, Ascoli M. The dynamics of the steroidogenic response of perifused Leydig tumor cells to human chorionic gonadotropin, ovine luteinizing hormone, cholera toxin and adenosine 3',5'-cyclic monophosphate. Endocrinology 1981; 108:632-8.

14. Mock EJ, Niswender GD. Differences in the rates of internalization of ^{125}I-human chorionic gonadotropin, luteinizing hormone and epidermal growth factor by ovine luteal cells. Endocrinology 1983; 113:259-64.

15. Carpenter G, Cohen S. ^{125}I-labeled human epidermal growth factor: binding, internalization and degradation in human fibroblasts. J Cell Biol 1976; 71:159-71.

16. Haigler HT, Maxfield FR, Willingham MC, Pastan I. Dansylcadaverine inhibits internalization of ^{125}I-epidermal growth factor in BALB 3T3 cells. J Biol Chem 1980; 255:1239-41.

17. Mock EJ, Papkoff H, Niswender GD. Internalization of ovine luteinizing hormone/human chorionic gonadotropin recombinants: differential effects of the alpha and beta subunits. Endocrinology 1983; 113:265-9.

18. Ahmed CE, Sawyer HR, Niswender GD. Internalization and degradation of human chorionic gonadotropin in ovine luteal cells: kinetic studies. Endocrinology 1981; 109:1380-7.

19. Niswender GD, Roess DA, Sawyer HR, Silvia WJ, Barisas BG. Differences in the lateral mobility of receptors of luteinizing hormone (LH) in the luteal cell membrane when occupied by ovine LH vs. human chorionic gonadotropin. Endocrinology 1985; 116:164-9.

20. Almers W, Stirling C. Distribution of transport proteins over animal cell membranes. J Membr Biol 1984; 77:169-86.

21. Dragsten P, Henkart P, Blumenthal R, Weinstein J, Schlessinger J. Lateral diffusion f surface immunoglobulin, Thy-1 antigen, and a lipid probe in lymphocyte plasma membranes. Proc Natl Acad Sci USA 1979; 76:5163-7.

22. Peters R. Translational diffusion in the plasma membrane of single

cells as studied by fluorescence microphotolysis. Naturwissenschaften 1983; 70:294–302.

23. Keutmann HT, McIlroy PJ, Bergert P, Ryan R. Chemically deglycosylated human chorionic gonadotropin subunits: characterization and biochemical properties. Biochemistry 1983; 22:3067–72.

24. Manjunath P, Sairam MR. Biochemical, biological, and immunological properties of chemically deglycosylated human choriogonadotropin. J Biol Chem 1982; 257:7109–15.

25. Chen HC, Shimohigashi Y, Dufau ML, Catt KJ. Characterization and biological properties of chemically deglycosylated human chorionic gonadotropin. J Biol Chem 1982; 257:14446–52.

26. Silavin SL, Moss GE, Niswender GD. Regulation of steroidogenesis in the corpus luteum. Steroids 1980; 36:229–41.

27. Rotman B, Papermaster BW. Membrane properties of living mammalian cells as studied by enzymatic hydrolysis of fluorogenic esters. Proc Natl Acad Sci USA 1966; 55:134–41.

28. Tank DW, Wu E-S, Webb WW. Enhanced molecular diffusion in muscle membrane blebs: release of lateral constraints. J Cell Biol 1982; 92:207–12.

29. Wu E-S, Tank DW, Webb WW. Unconstrained lateral diffusion of concanavalin A receptors on bulbous lymphocytes. Proc Natl Acad Sci USA 1982; 76:4962–6.

30. Yahara I, Edelman GM. Restriction of the mobility of lymphocyte immunoglobulin receptors by concanavalin A. Proc Natl Acad Sci USA 1972; 69:608–12.

31. Yahara I, Edelman GM. Modulation of lymphocyte receptor mobility by locally bound concanavalin A. Proc Natl Acad Sci USA 1975; 72:1579–83.

32. Schlessinger J, Elson EL, Webb WW, Yahara I, Ruthishauser O, Edelman GM. Receptor diffusion on cell surfaces by locally bound concanavalin A. Proc Natl Acad Sci USA 1977; 74:1110–4.

33. Painter RG, Gerrard W, Ginsberg MH. Direct evidence for the interaction of platelet surface membrane proteins GDIIb and III with cytoskeletal components: protein crosslinking studies. J Cell Biochem 1985; 27:277–90.

34. Wheeler ME, Gerrard JM, Carrol RC. Reciprocal transmembranous receptor-cytoskeleton interactions in concanavalin A-activated platelets. J Cell Biol 1985; 101:993–1000.

35. Henis YI. Mobility modulation by local concanavalin A binding: selectivity toward different membrane proteins. J Biol Chem 1984; 259:1515–9.

36. Axelrod D, Ravdin P, Koppel DE, et al. Lateral motion of fluorescently labeled acetylcholine receptors in membranes of developing muscle fibers. Proc Natl Acad Sci USA 1976; 73:4594–8.

37. Axelrod D, Randin PM, Podleski TR. Control of acetylcholine receptor mobility and distribution in cultured muscle membranes: a fluorescence study. Biochim Biophys Acta 1978; 511:23–38.

38. Niswender GD, Sawyer HR, Chen TT, Endres DB. Action of luteinizing hormone at the luteal cell level. In: Thomas JA, Singhal RL, eds. Advances in sex hormone research; vol 4. Baltimore: Urban & Schwarzenberg, 1979:153–86.

39. Amsterdam A, Berkowitz A, Nimrod A, Kohen F. Aggregation of luteinizing hormone receptors in granulosa cells: a possible mechanism for desensitization to the hormone. Proc Natl Acad Sci USA 1980; 77:3440–4.

40. Luborsky JL, Slater WT, Behrman HR. Luteinizing hormone (LH) receptor aggregation: modification of ferritin-LH binding and aggregation by prostaglandin $F_{2\alpha}$ and ferritin-LH. Endocrinology 1984; 115:2217–25.

41. Schechter Y, Hernaez L, Schlessinger J, Cuatrecasas P. Local aggregation of hormone-receptor complexes is required for activation

by epidermal growth factor. Nature 1979; 278:835-8.

42. Kahn CR, Baird KL, Jarrett DB, Flier JS. Direct demonstration that receptor crosslinking or aggregation is important in insulin action. Proc Natl Acad Sci USA 1978; 75:4209-13.

43. Conn PM, Rogers DC, Stewart JM, Niedel J, Sheffield T. Conversion of a gonadotropin-releasing hormone antagonist to an agonist. Nature 1982; 296:653-5.

44. Conn PM, Rogers DC, McNeil R. Potency enhancement of a GnRH-agonist: GnRH-receptor microaggregation stimulates gonadotropin release. Endocrinology 1982; 111:335-7.

45. Saffman PG, Delbruck M. Brownian motion in biological membranes. Proc Natl Acad Sci USA 1975; 72:3111-6.

46. Koppel DE, Sheetz MP, Schindler M. Matrix control of protein diffusion in biological membranes. Proc Natl Acad Sci USA 1981; 78:3576-80.

47. Zidovetzki R, Yarden Y, Schlessinger J, Jovin T. Rotation diffusion of epidermal growth factor complexed to cell surface receptors reflects rapid microaggregation and endocytosis of occupied receptors. Proc Natl Acad Sci USA 1981; 78:6981-5.

48. Roess DA, Niswender GD, Jovin TM, Barisas BG. Rotational diffusion of luteal cell LH receptors studied by time-resolved phosphorescence anisotropy. Biophys J 1987; 51:419a.

THE PRIMATE OVARY:

CRITIQUE AND PERSPECTIVES

David T. Baird

Department of Obstetrics and Gynecology
Center for Reproductive Biology
37 Chalmers Street, Edinburgh EH3 9EW

INTRODUCTION

The primate belongs to a small group of mammals in which only a single follicle is selected for ovulation each month. It is of considerable biological importance for each species that the number of ovulations matches the number of offspring which can be reared successfully (1,2). The deleterious consequences of multiple births in man is well illustrated by the fact that the perinatal mortality rate of twins is tenfold higher than that of singleton births (3).

This conference has illustrated the complex strategies devised to ensure that a single oocyte in optimal condition is ovulated each month. The fact that the primate has only a single dominant preovulatory follicle has certain advantages for studying its function and control. By day 7 of the cycle, the dominant follicle is easily recognizable by its size and vascularity and it has already acquired unique biochemical characteristics (e.g., high concentration of estradiol in follicular fluid, LH receptors on the granulosa cells, etc.) which distinguish it from other follicles (1). Its secretory activity in vivo can be studied by comparing the concentration of hormones in the ovarian venous effluent on the side containing the preovulatory follicle with that of the contralateral side (4). By following the changes in hormone levels following enucleation of the preovulatory follicle or corpus luteum, it is possible to investigate the regulatory roles of these dominant structures (5).

The ovary has proved to be a particularly favorable organ for study of the different compartments and their cellular components in vitro. Corpora lutea and large graafian follicles are easily identifiable and can be enucleated free from contamination of the rest of the ovary. These structures can be perfused or incubated in whole or in part in vitro. Pure preparations of dispersed granulosa cells can be prepared from the follicle by simple mechanical dispersion and techniques for their culture and incubation are well established (6). The cultured granulosa cell is a powerful experimental model for studying the mechanism of hormone action and cell differentiation and growth. Similar preparations of dispersed cells from the theca and corpus luteum have been much more difficult to develop. Dispersion of the cells with enzyme inevitably leads to a variable loss of cell surface receptors. Although luteal cells have been separated on the basis of their physical characteristics (such as density, size, etc.), no satisfactory techniques have yet been developed to obtain undamaged preparations of "pure" theca lutein and granulosa lutein cells. It has been demonstrated that small and large luteal cells differ in their biochemical properties as tested in vitro, but we still do not know whether these reflect different cell types or whether they are the same cell at different stages of development.

The graafian follicle has proved to be a biological Pandora's box with a new hormone or factor being isolated from follicular fluid each month (7). Follicular fluid provides a readily accessible source of hormones produced by the granulosa cells and apparently in many instances retained in high concentrations. Porcine follicular fluid was the source from which estradiol 17β was first identified. Some 50 years later it is still providing material for the isolation of new hormones, such as inhibin and related peptides, GnRH-like peptides, etc. (8-11).

The follicular cavity provides a very special environment in which the germ cell develops, and we now know that the somatic (granulosa) cells play a key role in the orderly maturation of the oocyte prior to ovulation (12). The oocyte is the largest cell in the body and its special metabolic requirement can be studied in vitro after aspiration from the follicle.

We have heard much about the wide galaxy of paracrine and autocrine factors influencing ovarian function. While these factors are important in regulating the response of the individual cell types to trophic stimuli, we should not forget the overriding importance of the hypothalamo-pituitary system (13,14). Without gonadotropins there is minimal ovarian function, and both the preovulatory follicle and corpus luteum are dependent throughout their life span on gonadotropins.

In the rhesus monkey and women, there is good evidence which indicates that ovulation occurs at random in successive cycles without preference for the presence or absence of the site of the corpus luteum from the previous cycle (15,16). This fact alone indicates that local paracrine factors are unlikely to play a major role in determining the selection of the preovulatory follicle. Moreover, the fact that once established the preovulatory follicle dominates the other follicles including those in the contralateral ovary makes it likely that it does so via the systemic circulation.

Among the many questions posed during this meeting, perhaps five are of central importance.

WHY DOES THE FOLLICULAR PHASE LAST 14 DAYS?

A remarkable feature of the primate ovarian cycle is that the follicular phase lasts for 14 days. Evidence from hypogonadotropic women and monkeys suggests that treatment with gonadotropins must be maintained for at least 10 days to stimulate the development of a small antral follicle to the preovulatory stage (14,17). In women, all antral follicles of >4 mm are atretic during the luteal phase of the cycle. Hence, when follicular selection commences at luteal regression, there are no large healthy antral follicles available for further development. We have previously suggested that the length of the follicular phase is related to the secretory products of the corpus luteum (18). In primates, the corpus luteum secretes steroids and other factors which suppress FSH secretion drastically, and follicular development is inhibited. In other species, like the sheep and the cow, the levels of FSH do not fall during the luteal phase of the cycle and follicular development continues until

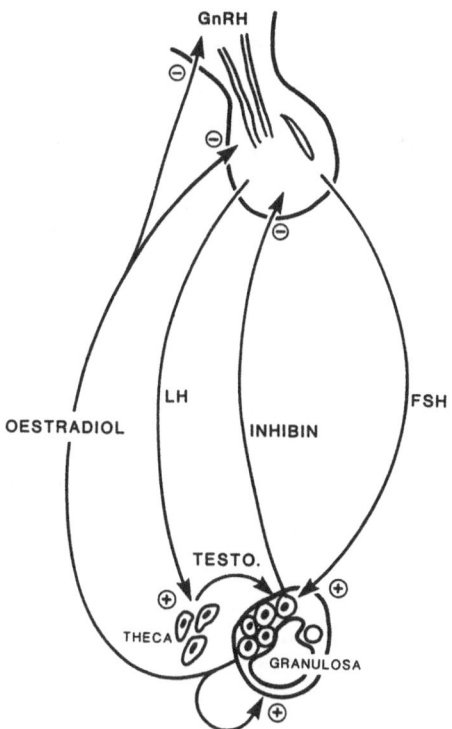

Fig. 1. Model of the feedback system operating between the hypothalamic-pituitary unit and ovarian hormones in the follicular phase. The theca cells of the follicle are stimulated by LH to produce testosterone and androstenedione which is converted into estradiol by the aromatase enzyme system in the granulosa cells. FSH stimulates aromatase and production of inhibin by the granulosa cells which feeds back to suppress the secretion of FSH by the anterior pituitary.

within a few days of ovulation. In these species, final maturation of the follicle during the luteal phase is only prevented by the fact that the frequency of LH pulses is markedly slowed due to the high level of progesterone secreted by the corpus luteum (19). When this structure is removed, the concentration of progesterone falls strikingly, the frequency of LH pulse increases, and the preovulatory rise in estradiol secretion by the large antral follicle(s) is stimulated. We originally suggested that the almost unique capacity of the primate corpus luteum to secrete estradiol was responsible for the marked suppression of FSH during the luteal phase. While estrogen is undoubtedly important, recent preliminary evidence suggests that the corpus luteum may also be a major source of inhibin, a polypeptide which selectively suppresses FSH (20,21).

The Role of Inhibin

Inhibin has been identified in high concentrations in follicular fluid of all species examined (22). Its production by granulosa cells

cultured in vitro is stimulated by FSH and testosterone and its secretion
in vivo is stimulated by the administration of hMG or FSH (23-25).
Inhibin bioactivity has been measured in ovarian venous plasma of the rat,
nonhuman primate and women (26-28). Recent data in sheep confirm that
inhibin is secreted by the ovary but, surprisingly, the secretion of
inhibin is relatively high on day 12 of the luteal phase and falls during
the follicular phase after luteal regression (20). Preliminary data in
this species suggests that the concentration of inhibin in ovarian venous
plasma is higher on the side bearing the corpus luteum. These data
suggest that inhibin is secreted by the sheep corpus luteum (C. G. Tsonis,
B. Campbell, D. T. Baird, and R. J. Scaramuzzi, unpublished observation).

The evidence that the primate corpus luteum secretes inhibin is
indirect. In women hyperstimulated with gonadotropins, the levels of
inhibin rise in parallel to those of estradiol during the follicular
phase, fall sharply at mid-cycle and then rise again in the early luteal
phase of the cycle (24). Luteinized granulosa cells secrete inhibin into
the culture medium when stimulated with LH (29). These findings suggest
that the secretion of inhibin by the corpus luteum may contribute to the
suppression of FSH secretion and, hence, the inhibition of the later
stages of follicular development in the luteal phase of the cycle in
women.

The biological advantage of a prolonged follicular phase is difficult
to determine. It may be that at least 14 days is required for repair and
subsequent growth of the endometrium following its disposal at menstruation. Estradiol is known to stimulate the synthesis of progesterone
receptors, and unless the uterus has been exposed to unopposed estrogen
for at least 7 days, it may be unable to form a secretory endometrium
adequate to sustain implantation of the developing blastocyst. With the
development of techniques of ovum transplantation to agonadal females, it
should be possible to test experimentally the minimum period of estrogen
replacement.

HOW IS A SINGLE PREOVULATORY FOLLICLE SELECTED?

Current evidence suggests that the follicle which will eventually
ovulate is selected from a group of small antral follicles (in women,
2-4 mm diameter) present in the ovaries at the end of the luteal phase of
the cycle (1,30). The rise in the concentration of FSH occurring at this
time is crucial and "activates" the future ovulating follicle by inducing
a series of maturational changes in the function of its granulosa cells,
including stimulation of aromatase activity. This activity is important
for the synthesis of estradiol and permits the chosen follicle to secrete
large quantities of estradiol both within the follicle and into the
ovarian venous effluent.

This process has been termed recruitment or activation (5). I prefer
the latter term because recruitment from the pool of primordial oocytes
occurs continuously uninfluenced by fluctuations in levels of gonadotropins or steroids. We still do not know what special properties are
possessed by the single favored small antral follicle which distinguishes
it from other apparently identical small antral follicles. It may be
simply at the correct stage in its development to benefit from the optimal
gonadotropic environment present in the early follicular phase of the
cycle.

The most plausible mechanism to explain the dominance of the
preovulatory follicle involves the suppression of FSH. Secretion of
estradiol by the dominant follicle suppresses the concentration of FSH

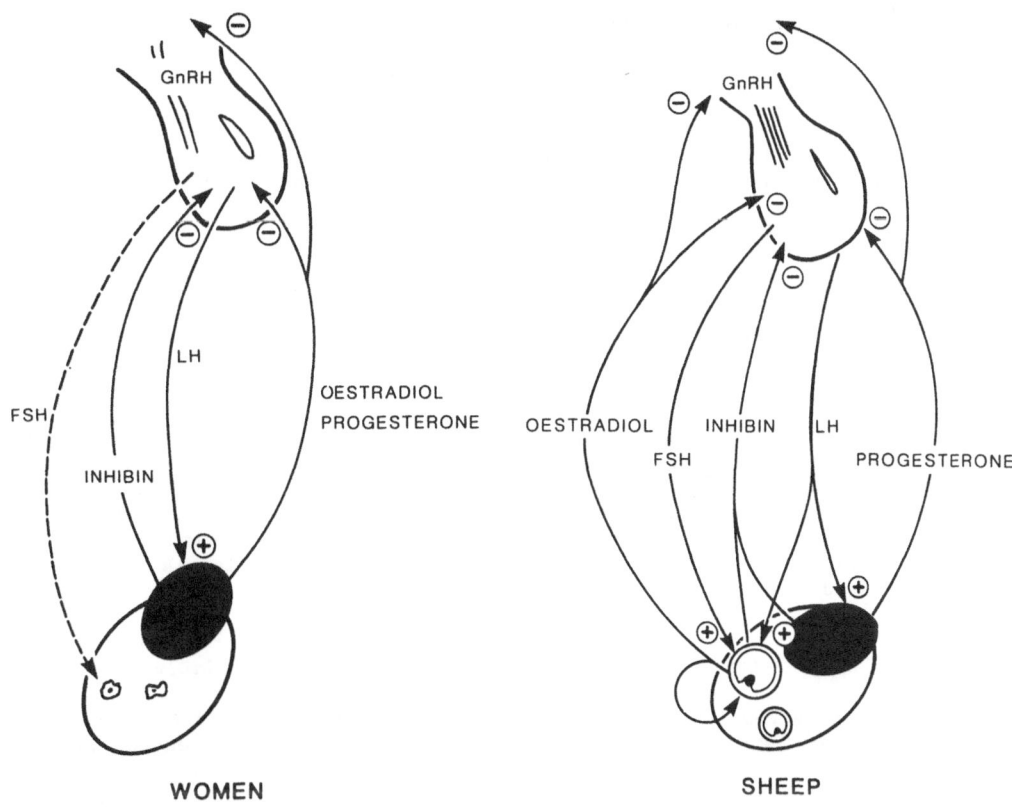

WOMEN   SHEEP

Fig. 2. Model of the hypothalamo-pituitary-ovarian axis in the
luteal phase of (a) women and (b) sheep. In women, the corpus
luteum secretes estradiol, progesterone and inhibin and, hence,
the levels of FSH are very low. In sheep, inhibin is secreted
by both the corpus luteum and the large antral follicles. In
contrast to women, estradiol is not secreted by the corpus
luteum but by the large antral follicles which continue to
develop throughout the luteal phase.

below a threshold level so that other small antral follicles can no longer
be activated. Infusion of FSH to maintain the concentration above the
threshold level throughout the follicular phase results in the development
of several preovulatory follicles (17). This hypothesis does not preclude
the existence of other factors such as Follicle Regulatory Protein which
inhibit the development of other follicles and reduce their responsiveness
to FSH (31).

The chosen follicle then exerts dominance over other antral follicles
by suppression of FSH due to its secretion of estradiol. As the levels of
FSH fall below the threshold necessary to activate small antral follicles,
only the dominant follicle can continue to grow. Zeleznik et al. (32)
have recently provided direct evidence that the follicle can continue to
develop in the presence of subthreshold levels of FSH. In monkeys ren-
dered hypogonadotropic by administration of an antagonist of GnRH, follicular development continued even when the amount of exogenous FSH was
reduced below the threshold level. We have recently found similar results
in hypogonadotropic women in whom follicular development was induced with
hMG and FSH administered by a subcutaneous pulse every 90 min. Devel-

opment of the dominant follicle as measured by serial ultrasound continued even when the dose of FSH was reduced during the 5 days prior to ovulation to a value below that found necessary to activate follicular growth (A. F. Glasier, J. Wickings, S. G. Hillier and D. T. Baird, unpublished observation). These data confirm that the dominant follicle becomes increasingly sensitive to FSH and, hence, can continue to develop in the mid- and late-follicular phase of the cycle when the secretion of FSH is falling.

We still do not know the relative importance of estradiol and inhibin in the regulation of FSH under physiological conditions. Infusion of estradiol or inhibin preparations suppresses the concentration of FSH in the rhesus monkey, sheep and many other species (33,34). The levels of FSH rise into the castrate range in sheep immunized against estradiol (35), whereas the rise is modest in those immunized against a semipurified inhibin prepared from follicular fluid (36).

Although the levels of inhibin rise in women whose ovaries are stimulated with gonadotropins, the levels remain constant or fall in the mid- to late-follicular phase of spontaneous cycles (C. G. Tsonis, A. F. Glasier, A. S. McNeilly, S. G. Hillier, and D. T. Baird, unpublished observation). When follicular development is stimulated with clomiphene, the negative feedback mechanism still operates and the levels of FSH are suppressed by the rising levels of estradiol.

The concentration of inhibin remains low until the mid-cycle surge. Thus, while estradiol secretion by the preovulatory follicle is mainly dependent on LH and the supply of androgen precursor, the production of inhibin is directly related to the level of FSH. These findings suggest that either estradiol is more important in the feedback control of FSH and/or that the inhibin operates through an estrogen-dependent mechanism. Further work is necessary to define the relative importance of these two factors in the control of FSH in different physiological circumstances.

DOES THE OOCYTE INFLUENCE GRANULOSA CELL FUNCTION?

Although it is well established that the granulosa cells of the cumulus play an important role in the nourishing of the oocyte and regulating its cytoplasmic maturation, the evidence for a reciprocal arrangement is much more fragmentary (37). An ovary devoid of oocytes is unable to initiate the differentiation of the somatic cells into granulosa and theca cells, so clearly the oocyte must be involved in the initial stages of folliculogenesis. As the function of ovulation is to ensure that a mature oocyte is delivered from the ruptured follicle, it would make sense if the oocyte had some way of ensuring that the preovulatory LH surge was only provoked by a follicle containing a mature egg. Attempts to study the function of the follicle after removal of the oocyte have been fraught with technical problems associated with damage to the follicular wall (38). Although removal of the oocyte in the rabbit is followed by luteinization of the granulosa cells, this may be due to hemorrhage and vascularization of the granulosa cell layer associated with puncture of the follicle wall. Further studies with in vitro systems are needed to investigate this problem further.

DOES THE PRIMATE CORPUS LUTEUM REQUIRE CONTINUOUS
PITUITARY LUTEOTROPIC SUPPORT?

This question has been the source of considerable controversy over the last decade (39). It is virtually certain that pituitary LH is an

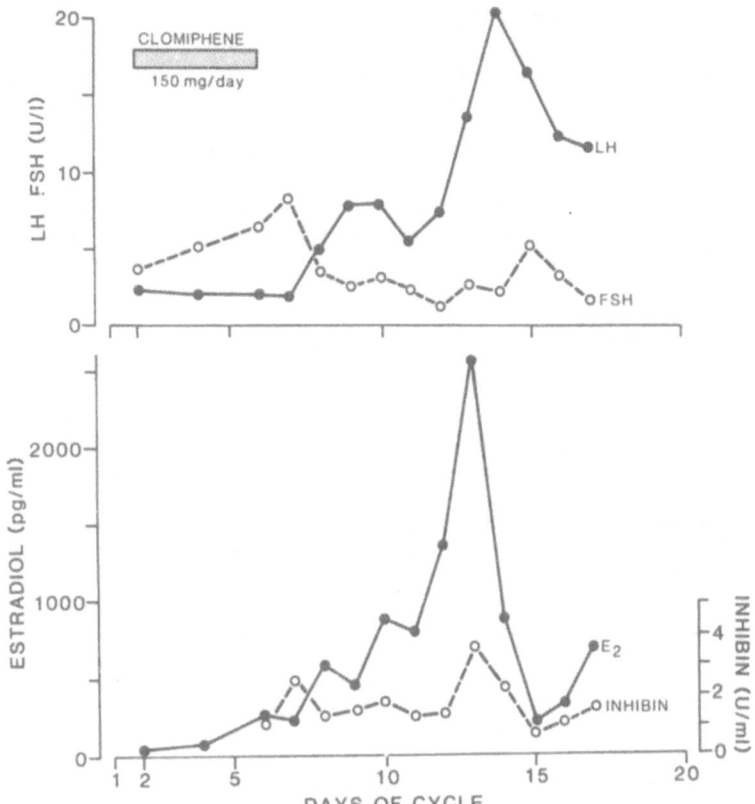

Fig. 3. Concentration of estradiol, LH, FSH and inhibin in a woman treated with the antiestrogen-clomiphene 150 mgm per day as indicated. Note that as the concentration of estradiol rises, the levels of FSH are suppressed while those of inhibin remain constant until the mid-cycle surge of LH. (Data from reference 24.)

important (perhaps the sole) component of the pituitary luteotropic complex. Receptors for LH reach their maximum levels by the mid-luteal phase and endogenous and exogenous LH stimulate the production of progesterone and estradiol by luteal tissue in vivo and in vitro (40). Recent data using LHRH antagonists to suppress pituitary LH secretion have helped clarify the luteal requirement for LH support (41). In the stump-tailed macaque, suppression of LH results in reduced secretion of progesterone and premature luteal regression at any stage of the luteal phase. Similar preliminary results have been reported in women (42). Earlier reports of normal luteal function in rhesus monkeys following hypophysectomy in the luteal phase were probably due to residual amounts of LH (43). However, as in other species, the recently formed corpus luteum is relatively resistant to withdrawal of LH, presumably because of the presence of LH on the receptors following the mid-cycle surge. In the mid- and late-luteal phases, the frequency of LH pulses slows drastically and each pulse of LH is followed by a marked increase in progesterone concentration (44). It is at this stage that the corpus luteum becomes increasingly sensitive to a variety of potentially luteolytic agents.

WHAT IS THE MECHANISM OF LUTEAL REGRESSION?

In many animal species (e.g., sheep, guinea pig, cow), luteal regression is induced by release of prostaglandin F2α (PGF2α) from the uterus (45). Hysterectomy in these species results in maintenance of the corpus luteum. Recent evidence suggests that progesterone and estradiol prime the endometrium to synthesize PGF2α which is then released from the uterus in response to oxytocin secreted by the corpus luteum (46,47). In turn, PGF2α stimulates the release of luteal oxytocin so that a positive feedback loop between the uterus and the corpus luteum is established.

In primates, hysterectomy has no effect on ovarian cyclicity, and the mechanism of luteal regression is still unknown. Under certain conditions estradiol, PGF2α, oxytocin and LHRH—like peptides can all suppress the production of progesterone (46). These hormones and/or their receptors are found in the corpus luteum, and it seems possible, therefore, that they are involved in luteal regression. These potentially luteolytic factors are all more effective in the mid— to late—luteal phase of the cycle when the pituitary LH support is at a minimum (48). It seems unlikely, however, that luteolysis in the primate is solely due to withdrawal of pituitary luteotropic support. In the late luteal phase of the cycle, the LH pulse frequency increases again and yet the corpus luteum can no longer respond to LH. Unless hCG is secreted by the blastocyst by day 10 of the luteal phase, rescue of the corpus luteum does not take place. It seems likely, therefore, that the maintenance of the corpus luteum depends on a very fine balance between luteotropic factors (LH, hCG and possibly prolactin) and a variety of local luteolytic agents (PGF2α, estradiol, LHRH—like peptides, oxytocin) (48).

The mechanism by which hCG rescues the corpus luteum at pregnancy is not fully understood. While hCG and LH bind to the same receptor, the stimulation of progesterone secretion by the luteal cell is prolonged following hCG. Recent evidence suggests that internalization of the hCG/receptor complex is 50 times slower than that of LH and may explain why in contrast to the state existing in the cycle, over 90% of the receptors on the corpus luteum at pregnancy are occupied (49).

SUMMARY AND CONCLUSIONS

The papers presented at this meeting have highlighted the complexities of the regulation of the dynamics of ovarian function. The structures within the ovary are continually in a state of flux involving growth and differentiation of a range of cell types. At the same time, the oocytes probably require a very carefully controlled environment in which to develop properly. An exciting development has been the recognition of the role of intragonadal peptides and growth factors as regulators of the action of gonadotropins. Somatomedin, insulin, GnRH, inhibin-related peptides apparently enhance or suppress the response of the cell to FSH or LH. By this mechanism the individual cellular compartments can respond selectively to circulating levels of gonadotropins. For example, the increased sensitivity of the preovulatory follicle to both FSH and LH may be achieved by the actions of gonadal peptides on the granulosa and theca cells respectively. One cellular compartment may even influence the other in a paracrine fashion. For example, inhibin of granulosa cell origin may enhance the LH stimulated production of androgens by the theca cells.

A better understanding of the means by which ovarian function is controlled should enable the development of better means to enhance or suppress ovarian function.

ACKNOWLEDGMENTS

I am grateful to my colleagues, Drs. H. M. Fraser, A. F. Glasier, S. G. Hillier, A. S. McNeilly and C. G. Tsonis, for helpful discussion; to Tom McFetters and Ted Pinner for preparation of figures; and to Margaret Harper for typing the manuscript. This work was supported by a grant from the Medical Research Council (G 426375).

REFERENCES

1. Baird DT. Factors regulating the growth of the preovulatory follicle in the sheep and human. J Reprod Fertil 1983; 69:343-52.
2. Baird DT. A model for follicular selection and ovulation: lesson from superovulation. J Steroid Biochem 1987 (in press).
3. Macgillivary I. Twins and other multiple deliveries. Clin Obstet Gynecol 1980; 7:581-600.
4. Baird DT, Fraser IS. Concentration of oestrone and oestradiol in follicular fluid and ovarian venous blood of women. Clin Endocrinol 1975; 4:259-66.
5. Hodgen GD. The dominant ovarian follicle. Fertil Steril 1982; 38:281-300.
6. Channing CP, Anderson LD, Hoover DJ, et al. The role of non steroidal regulators in control of oocyte and follicular maturation. Recent Prog Horm Res 1982; 38:331-400.
7. McNatty KP. Follicular fluid. In: The vertebrate ovary. New York: Plenum Press, 1978:215-59.
8. de Jong FH, Sharpe RM. Evidence for inhibin-like activity in bovine follicular fluid. Nature 1976; 263:71-2.
9. Mason AJ, Hayflick JS, Ling N, et al. Complementary DNA sequences of ovarian follicular fluid inhibin show precursor structure and homology with transforming growth factor. Nature 1985; 318:659-63.
10. Robertson DM, Foulds LM, Leversha L, et al. Isolation of inhibin from bovine follicular fluid. Biochem Biophys Res Commun 1985; 126:220-6.
11. Li CH, Ramasharma K, Yamashiro D, Chung D. Gonadotropin-releasing peptide from human follicular fluid: isolation, characterization and chemical synthesis. Proc Natl Acad Sci USA 1987; 84:959-62.
12. Moor RM, Osborn JC. Somatic control of protein synthesis in mammalian oocytes during maturation. In: Molecular biology of egg maturation (Ciba Found Symp No. 98). London: Pitman; Newark, NJ: Ciba Pharmaceutical Co., 1983:178-96.
13. Yen SSC, Lasley BL, Wang CF, Leblanc H, Siler TM. The operating characteristics of the hypothalamic-pituitary system during the menstrual cycle and observations of biological action of Somatostatin. Recent Prog Horm Res 1975; 31:321-57.
14. Knobil E. The neuroendocrine control of the menstrual cycle. Recent Prog Horm Res 1980; 36:53-88.
15. Clark JR, Dierschke DJ, Wolf RC. Hormonal regulation of ovarian folliculogenesis in rhesus monkeys. 1. Concentration of serum luteinizing hormone and progesterone during laparoscopy and patterns of follicle development during successive menstrual cycles. Biol Reprod 1978; 18:779-83.
16. Sallam HN, Whitehead MI, Collins WP. The incidence of mature follicles in spontaneous and induced ovarian cycles. Lancet 1983; i:357.
17. Brown JB. Pituitary control of ovarian function—concepts derived from gonadotrophin therapy. Aust NZ J Obstet Gynaecol 1978; 18:47-54.
18. Baird DT, Baker TG, McNatty KP, Neal P. Relationship between the secretion of the corpus luteum and the length of the follicular phase

of the ovarian cycle. J Reprod Fertil 1975; 45:611-9.

19. Baird DT, McNeilly AS. Gonadotrophic control of follicular development and function during the oestrous cycle of the ewe. J Reprod Fertil (suppl) 1981; 30:119-33.

20. Tsonis CG, McNeilly AS, Baird DT. Inhibin secretion by the sheep ovary during the luteal and follicular phases of the oestrous cycle and following stimulation with FSH. 1987 (in preparation).

21. Tsonis CG, McNeilly AS, Baird DT. Production and secretion of ovarian inhibin. Proceedings of Ares-Serono Symposium. Tokyo: 1987 (in press).

22. Tsonis CG, Sharpe RM. Dual gonadal control of follicle-stimulating hormone. Nature (London) 1986; 321:724-5.

23. Henderson KM, Franchimont P. Regulation of inhibin production by bovine ovarian cells in vitro. J Reprod Fertil 1981; 63:431-42.

24. Tsonis CG, Messinis IE, Templeton AA, McNeilly AS, Baird DT. Gonadotropic stimulation of inhibin secretion into peripheral blood by the human ovary during the follicular and early luteal phase of the cycle. J Clin Endocrinol Metab 1987 (in press).

25. McLachlan RI, Robertson DM, Healy DL, de Kretser DM, Burger HG. Plasma inhibin levels during gonadotropin-induced ovarian hyperstimulation for IVF: a new index of follicular function. Lancet 1986; i:1233-4.

26. de Paolo LV, Shander P, Wise PM, Barraclough CA, Channing CP. Identification of inhibin-like activity in ovarian venous plasma of rats during the estrous cycle. Endocrinology 1979; 105:647-54.

27. Hoover DJ, Tanabe K, Channing CP. Inhibin secretion by the primate ovary. Seminars in Reprod Endocrinol 1983; 1:279-94.

28. Channing CP, Gagliano P, Tanabe K, Fortuny A, Cortes-Prieto J. Demonstration of a gradient in inhibin activity, estrogen progesterone and Δ^4-androstenedione in follicular fluid, ovarian vein blood, and peripheral blood of normal women. Fertil Steril 1985; 43:142-5.

29. Tsonis CG, Hillier SG, Baird DT. Production of inhibin bioactivity by human granulosa-lutein cells: stimulation by LH and testosterone in vitro. J Endocrinol 1987; 112:R11-4.

30. McNatty KP. Ovarian follicular development from the onset of luteal regression in humans and sheep. In: Follicular maturation and ovulation. Amsterdam: Excerpta Medica, 1982:1-18.

31. diZerega GS, Goebelsmann U, Nakamura RM. Identification of protein(s) secreted by the preovulatory ovary which suppress the follicle response to gonadotrophins. J Clin Endocrinol Metab 1982; 54:1091-6.

32. Zeleznik AJ, Kubik CJ. Ovarian responses in macaques to pulsatile infusion of follicle-stimulating hormone (FSH) and luteinizing hormone: increased sensitivity of the maturing follicle to FSH. Endocrinology 1986; 119:2025-32.

33. Zeleznik AJ. Premature elevation of systemic estradiol reduces serum levels of follicle stimulating hormone and lengthens the follicular phase of the menstrual cycle in rhesus monkeys. Endocrinology 1981; 109:352-5.

34. Salamonsen LA, Jonas HA, Burger HG, et al. A heterologous radioimmunoassay in follicle-stimulating hormone: application to measurement of FSH in the ovine estrous cycle and several other species including man. Endocrinology 1973; 93:610-8.

35. Scaramuzzi RJ, Martenz ND, Van Look PFA. Ovarian morphology and the concentration of steroids, and of gonadotrophins during the breeding season in ewes actively immunized against oestradiol 17 or oestrone. J Reprod Fertil 1980; 59:303-10.

36. Henderson KM, Franchimont P, Lecomte-Yerna MJ, Hudson N, Ball K. Increase in ovulation rate after active immunisation of sheep with inhibin partially purified from bovine follicular fluid. J

Endocrinol 1984; 102:305–9.

37. Hillensjo T, Magnusson C, Ekholm C, Billig H, Hedin L. Role of cumulus cells in oocyte maturation. In: Intraovarian control mechanisms. New York: Plenum Press, 1982:175–88.

38. El-Folly MA, Cook B, Nekola M, Nalbandov AV. The role of the ovum in follicular luteinization. Endocrinology 1970; 87:288–93.

39. Rothchild I. The regulation of the mammalian corpus luteum. Recent Prog Horm Res 1981; 37:183–298.

40. McNeilly AS, Kerin J, Swanston IA, Bramley TA, Baird DT. Changes in the binding of human chorionic gonadotrophin/luteinizing hormone, follicle stimulating hormone and prolactin to human corpora lutea during the menstrual cycle and pregnancy. J Endocrinol 1980; 87:315–25.

41. Fraser HM, Baird DT, McRae GI, Nestor TJ, Vickery BH. Suppression of luteal progesterone secretion in the stump tailed macaque by an antagonist analogue of luteinizing hormone-releasing hormone. J Endocrinol 1985; 104:R1–4.

42. Mais V, Kazer RR, Cetel NS, Rivier J, Vale W, Yen SSC. The dependency of folliculogenesis and corpus luteum function on pulsatile gonadotropin secretion in cycling women using a gonadotropin-releasing hormone antagonist as a pulse. J Clin Endocrinol Metab 1986; 62:1250–5.

43. Asch RH, Abou-Samra M, Braunstein GD, Pauerstein CJ. Luteal function in hypophysectomized rhesus monkeys. J Clin Endocrinol Metab 1982; 55:154–61.

44. Healy DL, Schenken RS, Lynch A, Williams RF, Hodgen GD. Pulsatile progesterone secretion: its relevance to clinical evaluation of corpus luteum function. Fertil Steril 1984; 41:114–21.

45. Horton EW, Poyser NL. Uterine luteolytic hormone: a physiological role for prostaglandin F2. Physiol Rev 1976; 56:595–651.

46. Baird DT. Control of luteolysis. In: Jeffcoate SL, ed. The luteal phase. New York: Wiley, 1985:25–42.

47. Flint APF, Sheldrick EL. Evidence for a systemic role for ovarian oxytocin in luteal regression in sheep. J Reprod Fertil 1983; 67:215–22.

48. Richardson MC. Hormonal control of ovarian luteal cells. Oxf Rev Reprod Biol 1986; 8:321–78.

49. Bramley TA, Stirling D, Swanston IA, Menzies GS, McNeilly AS, Baird DT. Specific binding sites for gonadotrophin-releasing hormone LH/chorionic gonadotrophin, low-density lipoprotein, prolactin and FSH in homogenates of human corpus luteum. II: Concentrations throughout the luteal phase of the menstrual cycle and early pregnancy. J Endocrinol 1987; 113:317–27.

Editor's Note: On Saturday evening, May 16, 1987, after the traditional Symposium banquet, Dr. Luigi Mastroianni presented a thoughtful discussion on a number of ethical concerns important to researchers in the field of reproductive biology. Dr. Mastroianni has provided us with a manuscript of the address, and we include it here as a part of the proceedings.

SCIENTIFIC, LEGAL AND ETHICAL ISSUES

IN REPRODUCTIVE RESEARCH

Luigi Mastroianni, Jr., M.D.

Department of Obstetrics and Gynecology
University of Pennsylvania School of Medicine
3400 Spruce Street, Philadelphia, Pennsylvania 19104

The past decade has witnessed dramatic advances in reproductive technology and its clinical applications. The societal implications of research in the reproductive sciences have been the focus of attention, and investigators and clinicians in the field find themselves in the vertex of a whirlpool of ethical and legal deliberations. Huxley's 1984 is now three years behind us and possibilities of genetic manipulation and even cloning have conjured up the image projected in his "Brave New World." As attention is focused on later reproductive events, fetal experimentation becomes the issue. Most recently, a series of court-ordered obstetrical interventions, many based on dubious legal grounds, coupled with expanding physicians' liability, has compounded the ethical issues surrounding late pregnancy (1,2). The fundamental question as to how new knowledge will be used cannot be separated from the issues surrounding the initial appropriateness of the experimentation which would generate the new information. John Ziman, Chairman of the Council for Science and Society of London, put it aptly when he stated, "A society holds together by the rules that people are bound to obey. Human behavior varies surprisingly from country to country and from era to era. But however bizarre it may appear to the outsider, it must always follow the constraints of biological reality. The trouble with science is that it changes biological reality. The boundary conditions on the rules of social behavior are suddenly altered, and many people become very frightened" (3).

It is clear that almost any new technology carries with it the possibility of misuse. The mechanisms which operate in the early stages of human development undoubtedly offer a greater opportunity for misuse. Multiple and sometimes realistic concerns have fostered a climate which demands repeated and detailed evaluation of reproductive research—and this is good and appropriate. As is so often the case—and especially true when the reproductive process is the subject of scrutiny—the most conservative voices are the loudest. Some have taken the position that no experimentation involving human fertilization, the human conceptus, the embryo, or the fetus is appropriate under any circumstances. Unfortunately, the debate has been inexorably linked with that of pregnancy termination and with larger metaphysical questions as to when life begins and when the fetus is entitled to all of the rights of the First Amendment to the U.S. Constitution. Let us first review some of the concerns surrounding reproductive research on the fetus and then focus attention on research on human gametes, fertilization, and the human embryo.

For those who take the position that the fetus is not a person until the time of viability, fetal experimentation takes on a straightforward dimension. Within that mind-set, the principal issues in cases of intrauterine manipulations are related to any potential harm to the mother and also potential harm to the fetus if it is to be allowed to proceed to viability. If the fetus is to be aborted after the experimental manipulations, the potential of subsequent harm is terminated at that point. The overriding ethical dilemma centers about procedures which are life-sustaining and the consequent birth of a child for whom the quality of life is severely compromised. One could argue that any quality of life is better than no life at all, but most of us would look upon that as a rather extreme position. The fundamental difficulty is that the fetus cannot give the investigator an informed consent. Consider that providing experimental treatment might allow survival in an otherwise lethal condition and that in treating to avoid death, one may have produced or sustained irreparable physical harm. Surely the investigator might realistically be accused of "wrongful birth" by a disfigured or suffering person.

Issues surrounding experimentation on the nonviable fetus which has already been delivered are somewhat less complex. Here, the rights of the embryo and fetus before viability are at issue. The discussion centers about the determination of the point in time at which the value placed on human life applies during embryonic development. At present, federal guidelines severely curtail experiments on the living, nonviable fetus in the United States. Beyond the point of viability, the principle of protection of human life held by almost every culture would apply, and any research or manipulation which would cause harm would be considered unacceptable. These issues are blurred by our increasing ability to support extrauterine life. Keep in mind that in the united States a woman can legally abort her fetus to the point of viability. After that, she loses that right unless her health or life is in jeopardy. Thus, viable fetuses have legal rights. One such right is not to be aborted. Another such right certainly is not to be experimented on except when there is no risk or when the benefit far outweighs any risk. These rights do not extend by law to the previable fetus. The problem is the line of demarcation. The legal cutoff point for viability is currently set at 24 weeks, but new medical procedures are rapidly shifting that point to earlier and earlier dates. Predictably, there will be a continuing controversy over the legal status of the previable fetus. The issue is a philosophical one and also one of attitude. Experimentation on the fetus which is clearly previable and yet has the appearance of a formed human being is much more repugnant than manipulation of individual cells in an embryo which does not have distinct human features. The issues include projection and identification and the psychological implications are far reaching.

The use of human in vitro fertilization and embryo culture in the treatment of infertility has done more to focus attention on the ethical and legal aspects of reproductive research than any other advance. For the first time, human procreation could be separated from the heretofore inaccessible environments of the fallopian tube and uterus. It was clear from the start that it would be essential to consider some carefully thought-out guidelines for research in this important area. Yet our own United States Public Health Service, to this day, does not officially support research on human in vitro fertilization. Such research was interdicted in the early 70s when our own program at the University of Pennsylvania, designed to explore the physiology of human fertilization, was curtailed. Much later, an NIH Advisory Committee did meet to explore the issues surrounding in vitro fertilization and did present a report to the Secretary of Health and Human Services. The report was pigeonholed and no official action has been taken to this date. Thus, in the United States it was left principally to the medical profession and the wider scientific community to spearhead further efforts to consider the ethical issues surrounding human gamete manipulation.

In Great Britain, a government-sponsored commission was established which, in 1984, issued the Warnock Report entitled, "A Question of Life." Such subjects as artificial insemination, in vitro fertilization, egg donation, embryo donation, and surrogacy were reviewed in detail. The wider use of these techniques, including freezing and storage of human semen, eggs and embryos, scientific issues and possible future developments in research were considered. Guidelines for research were recommended. The majority of the committee agreed that research on human embryos should continue but that the handling of such embryos should be permitted only under license and that, furthermore, any unauthorized use of an in vitro embryo should constitute a criminal offense. They would restrict research on the human embryo only to those questions which could not be answered appropriately in other species. Having decided that research on the human in vitro-produced embryo was acceptable, they set a time limit beyond which the embryo would not be kept alive in vitro, beyond which it would no longer be appropriate to use it as a research subject. That limit was set at 14 days, the reference point being the development of the primitive streak on day 15. It was reasoned that that event marked the beginning of individual development of the embryo. Clearly, then, the potential for differentiation into an increasingly unique human form was pivotal. Particularly forceful was their recommendation that the placing of the human embryo in the uterus of another species for gestation should be a criminal offense.

Shortly after the Warnock Report was published, the American Fertility Society established a Committee on Ethics which was charged with exploring in vitro fertilization (surrogacy, gamete donation, cryopreservation, genetic manipulation, cloning, etc.) and donor insemination including cryopreservation. The committee included representatives from a wide variety of disciplines. Their recommendations on research also embraced the concept that somehow the first 14 days were different from the days which follow. They endorsed the term "pre-embryo" which is considered to last until 14 days after fertilization. They were quick to point out, however, that "this definition is not intended to imply a moral evaluation of the pre-embryo." Nevertheless, they endorsed the concept that although a pre-embryo is not a person, it should be treated with special respect because it is a genetically unique living human entity that might become a person. They subscribed to the 14-day limit beyond which research would be inappropriate but acknowledged that the limitation was somewhat arbitrary.

Such arbitrary definitions, including the designation of the term pre-embryo, are a source of comfort to those who look upon the newly formed conceptus and embryo as something much more than simple biological material. The embryo's rights somehow increase as the primitive streak is being laid down, although it is quite clear that, even if transferred, there is no guarantee of normal implantation and, therefore, of continued existence. There is seeming consensus, then, that research beyond the fourteenth day is unacceptable. Under the British system, the guidelines of the Warnock Report, in practical terms, represent standards from which there will likely be little or no deviation. In the United States, acceptance of a definition as to when meaningful life begins, be it at 14 days or actually at some point during the course of conception, would certainly have far-reaching implications in our pluralistic society. The importance of the fundamental issue as to when meaningful human life begins was highlighted by an effort to put the matter into legislation. I refer to Bill S158, introduced by Mr. Jesse Helms, in the Senate of the United States. This was a bill "to provide that human life should be deemed to exist from conception." If such a bill had been enacted, no form of fetal experimentation, except that which would absolutely insure the continued existence of the products of conception, would be legally sanctioned.

The bill stated that "Congress finds that present day scientific evidence indicates a significant likelihood that actual human life exists from conception. Congress further finds that the fourteenth amendment to the Constitution of the United States was intended to protect all human beings." This, then, was an effort to move that protection into the uterus—indeed, into the fallopian tube.

"Upon the basis of these findings, and in the exercise of the powers of Congress, including its power under Section 5 of the fourteenth amendment to the Constitution of the United States, that Congress hereby declares that for purpose of enforcing the obligation of the States under the fourteenth amendment not to deprive persons of life without due process of law, human life shall be deemed to exist from conception without regard to race, sex, age, health, defect, or condition of dependency; and for this purpose 'person' shall include all human life as defined herein."

This bill went on to propose, and here is the heart of the matter, that States shall have the responsibility of issuing a restraining order which would protect the rights of human persons between conception and birth and prohibit the performance of abortions. Again, the abortion issue and the issue of the ethics of fetal experimentation and, for that matter, any treatment which involves manipulation of embryos or fetuses are inexorably entwined.

Not surprisingly, S158 engendered substantial public debate. Scientists and physicians were being asked by Congress essentially to define the onset of human life. Congress was about to put into law a judgment with which theologians and philosophers had grappled over the centuries and on which there is no clear consensus. To be sure, the present view of the Roman Catholic Church is that meaningful human life begins at conception, specifically at the time of fusion of the male and female pronuclei. There are those of other persuasions who do not accept this concept. On the matter of scientific definition as to when life begins, we are asking the impossible. We are dealing with a metaphysical issue and not a scientific one. It was my view and that of many of my colleagues that in the pluralistic society of the United States, it was inappropriate to define in law a position which would have to be embraced by all of our citizens, the violation of which would put those whose beliefs are contrary to those expressed in the law in jeopardy. Furthermore, those who wish to have enacted into law their own religious position would surely run the risk that at some point others might wish to impose their views on them.

Moral and litigious issues aside, let us consider the scientific information pertinent to any discussion of when life begins. Early on, at a time when the process of fertilization and early development was not understood, the position was held that life began with the movement of the fetus or "quickening." When it was appreciated that pregnancy occurred as the result of union of sperm and egg, many then defined the beginning of life as representing that event. As the physiology of fertilization is scrutinized in greater detail, however, it becomes evident that at the scientific level the issue is not quite so straightforward.

Spermatozoa are living cells. They are unique. They are equipped with a very effective mechanism for movement in the form of a tail which beats under the control of cytoplasmic droplets within the head. This living cell which has been manufactured in the testes, is released into the environment provided by the male reproductive tract. It cannot move efficiently and it is not yet capable of fertilization. It must first come under the influence of the male reproductive tract where it acquires an additional ability to function in fertilization. Even after ejaculation, it is still incapable of penetrating the egg until it is modified further by exposure to the female reproductive tract. I don't believe there is any theologian who would deny that the spermatozoan is human from the very point when it is manufactured and that it is living. The decision then must be made as to whether the spermatozoan itself, being living and human and having the <u>potential</u> for continued life as part of the new conceptus once fertilization has occurred, is entitled to the right of protection as a person. Those who would deny this right to the spermatozoan might argue that it is not a complete human cell chromosomally. It contains only the haploid number of chromosomes. Paradoxically, those who would take that position would undoubtedly insist that an individual born with fewer or more chromosomes than normal is human and entitled to all the rights of "personhood." The decision to base the definition of "human life" solely on the number of chromosomes in a given cell has far-reaching implications. This admittedly whimsical example of an effort to apply scientific fact to a metaphysical definition can be highlighted as we take the argument further.

This living human structure, the spermatozoan, possibly not completely human because it does not have a complete complement of chromosomes, becomes more human as it takes on the ability to fertilize under the influence of the female reproductive tract. It undergoes certain biochemical and morphological changes which condition it further so that it can finally begin to enter the egg. Thereafter, fertilization involves not only the egg itself, but the various vestments which surround the egg at the time it is released from the follicle in the ovary. The sequence of events which occurs during penetration is still not completely understood, although the process has been studied extensively in experimental animals, including the subhuman. Suffice it to say that the spermatozoan must penetrate a cellular coat which surrounds the egg and must find its way to and attach to the zone pellucida, a protein layer which immediately surrounds the egg cytoplasm. The penetrating spermatozoan must have been conditioned further such that it can traverse the zona pellucida, must attach itself to the egg membrane and finally penetrate into the egg cytoplasm. It is then modified further to form a pronucleus. Thereafter, the male pronucleus and the female pronucleus, formed at about the same time, join. At some point thereafter, there is division of this egg to the 2-cell stage. This clearly represents a continuum of events. If we take the scientific position that it is the completion of the fertilization process which is important, there are those who could equally take the position that it is the <u>potential</u> for completion of the fertilization process which is important. The latter position, vis-a-vis fertilization, would be similar to the position of those who state that the recently fertilized egg represents the beginning of human personhood because it has the <u>potential</u> of proceeding on through further development in the oviduct and uterus. The fallacy here is that a high percentage of oocytes which have been penetrated never proceed on to further development in nature, and that many fertilized oocytes which do are thwarted so early in their development that their presence is not even recognized in the form of a skipped menstrual period.

Can we then, as scientists, give to our legislators, based on our knowledge of fertilization, a clear-cut definition on the beginning of life? I doubt seriously that any scientist with genuine expertise in this field would be able to label one event or another in this complicated chain of events as the pivotal one on which to base a decision on exactly when "meaningful human life" begins. This is not to imply that theological and philosophical opinions on this issue should be taken lightly. Rather, they should be regarded as religious positions and, as such, accorded all due respect.

Modern reproductive technology has raised many ethical issues. Observations on gametes offer unparalleled opportunities to gain insight into the processes of human fertilization and early development and to treat human infertility. Embryo freezing, embryo transfer, and use of surrogate uteri are but a few of the systems stemming from this work which has sparked the interest of ethicists. The ethical aspects of this work will continue to occupy the minds of those physicians and scientists who have chosen to work in these areas. De facto, all of us will be called upon to consider such ethical issues in the foreseeable future.

REFERENCES

1. Kolder VEB, Gallagher J, Parsons MT. Court ordered obstetrical interventions. N Engl J Med 1987; 316:1192.
2. Annas GJ. Protecting the liberty of pregnant patients. N Engl J Med 1987; 316:1213.
3. Ziman J. Human procreation: ethical aspects of the new techniques. Council for Science and Society. Oxford University Press, 1984.
4. Warnock M. A question of life. Oxford: Blackwell Ltd., 1985.
5. Ethical considerations of new reproductive technology. Report of the Ethics Committee of the American Fertility Society. Fertil Steril 1986; 46(suppl 1).
6. Ratzinger J, Bovone A. Instruction on respect for human life in its origin and on the dignity of procreation: replies to certain questions of the day. Vatican Polyglot Press, 1987.

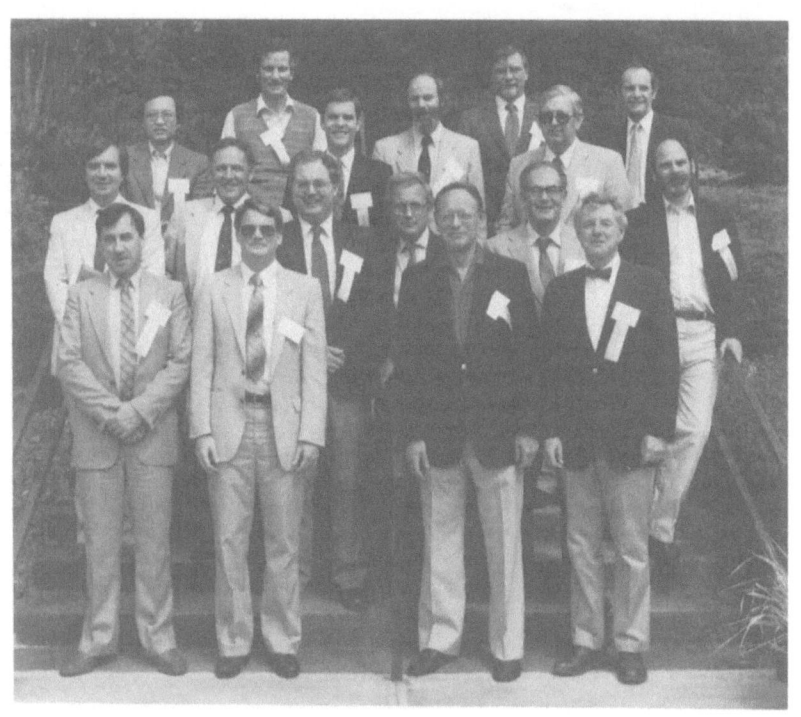

SPEAKERS AND CHAIRMEN

The Primate Ovary
Oregon Regional Primate Research Center
Beaverton, Oregon
May 16-17, 1987

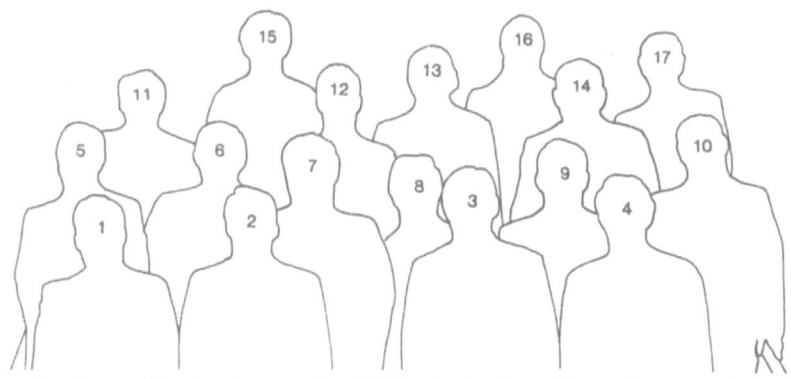

1, Barry D. Bavister; 2, Richard L. Stouffer; 3, Kenneth J. Ryan; 4, Luigi Mastroianni, Jr.; 5, Stephen G. Hillier; 6, David W. Schomberg; 7, Gary D. Hodgen; 8, William J. LeMaire; 9, Robert M. Brenner; 10, Anthony J. Zeleznik; 11, Aaron J. W. Hsueh; 12, Gere S. diZerega; 13, John J. Eppig; 14, Gordon D. Niswender; 15, David T. Baird; 16, Harold R. Behrman; 17, Charles H. Phoenix. Not pictured: Vaughn Critchlow, Lars Hamberger, Marilyn J. Koering, and Gerson Weis.

AUTHOR INDEX

A
Aten, R.F., 175

B
Baird, D.T., 249
Barisas, B.G., 237
Bavister, B.D., 119
Behrman, H.R., 175
Bicsak, T.A., 35
Brannstrom, M., 91

C
Clark, M.R., 91
Curry, T.E.,Jr., 91

D
Dixson, A.F., 61
diZerega, G.S., 49

E
Eppig, J.J., 77

F
Fay, J., 49
Fujimori, K., 49

H
Hahlin, M., 191
Hamberger, L., 191
Harlow, C.R., 61
Hillier, S.G., 61
Hodgen, G.D., 139
Hodges, J.K., 61
Hsueh, A.J.W., 35
Hutchison, J., 163

I
Ireland, J., 49
Ireland, J.J., 175

K
Koering, M.J., 3
Koos, R.D., 91

L
LeMaire, W.J., 91
Lindblom, B., 191

M
Makris, A., 113
Mastroianni, L.,Jr., 261
Morioka, N., 91
Musicki, B., 175

N
Niswender, G.D., 237

O
Ottobre, J.S., 207

P
Pepperell, J.R., 175

R
Roess, D.A., 237
Ryan, K.J., 113

S
Schomberg, D.W., 25
Shaw, H.J., 61
Soodak, L.K., 175
Stouffer, R.L., 207

T
Tonetta, S.A., 49

V
VandeVoort, C.A., 207

W
Weiss, G., 223
Westhof, G., 49
Westhof, K., 49
Wickings, E.J., 61
Woessner, J.F., 91

Z
Zeleznik, A.J., 163

SUBJECT INDEX

Abortion
  legality, 264
  spontaneous, 207
Acetylcholine receptor, 243
Activin, 26, 29, 41
  see Heteroactivin, Homoactivin
Adenosine, 81–84
Adenosine monophosphate, cyclic,
        38, 40, 65, 80, 85, 86,
        93, 94, 122, 123, 178,
        179, 192–199, 201, 209,
        212, 213, 216, 217
Adenosine triphosphate, 84,
        183, 184
Adenylate cyclase, 55, 80, 84, 93,
        178, 180, 181, 209, 212–21∢
  desensitization, 212, 216, 217
Adrenaline, 196
American Fertility Society, 263
p-Aminophenylmercuric acetate, 98,
        100, 103
Androgen, 40–43, 50, 51, 61, 68,
        70, 149
Androitin, see Testosterone
Androstenedione, 6, 27, 38, 95,
        149, 251
Angiogenesis, 30, 113–118
  assay, 114–115
  factors of, 115–116
  and tumor, 114
Angiogenin, 116
Anovulation, 55–56
Antrum, 4, 5, 8
Aromatase, 28, 42, 49–52, 54–56,
        63–64, 68–71, 251
Arrest, meiotic, 80–84, 122
Aspirin, 96
Atresia, 50, 56, 113, 142, 145
  and follicle maturation, 3–23
Axis, hypothalamic-pituitary,
        3, 11, 161
Azocoll, 101, 102

Bredinin, 83
Blastocyst, 256

Calcium, 178–180
  ionophore A23187, 179
Callithrix jacchus, see Marmoset
        monkey
Capillary, 114–115
Catecholamine, 194–205
Cell
  "castration" cell, 35
  endothelial, 114–115
    growth factor, 116
  –effector combination, 25
  follicular, 25, 49
  granulosa, see Granulosa cell
  hypertrophy, 35
  Leydig, 35, 42, 43, 238
  luteal, 30, 210–212, 216, 217,
        230, 238–245
  and angiogenesis, 30
  pituitary, 26, 35, 37
  Sertoli, 35
  testicular, 35
  thecal, 42, 52, 53, 149, 251
Cholera toxin, 40, 80
Cholesterol, 212
Chromatography, 36
CI-1 (collagenase inhibitor),
        102, 103
Clomiphene citrate, 55, 141, 151
Cohort follicle, 144, 145
Colchicine, 241, 242
Collagen, 99, 100, 102, 105
Collagenase, 97–102
  inhibitor, 102, 103
Concanavalin A, 242, 243
Corona cell, 122, 123, 127
Corpus luteum, 3–7, 10, 14, 18, 51,
        113–117, 176, 177, 250, 253
  aberrant, 4
  clock, "luteal," 166
  function, 163–248
  and gonadotropin, see
        Gonadotropin
  human, 181, 191–205
    and catecholamine, 194–205
    clinical application, 200–203
    and prostaglandins, 191–205

Corpus luteum (continued)
  life span, 164–168, 207–208
    rescue of, 207–208, 228, 256
  and pregnancy, early, 207–220
  of primate, 207–220
  rescue of life span, 207, 208,
    228, 256
  response to gonadotropin, 208–216
  of rhesus monkey, 163–174
  see Luteinizing hormone
Creatine phosphate, 184
Creatine phosphokinase, 184
Cumulus cell, 80–86, 125–127,
  130–133
Cycle, menstrual
  conceptualization, 141
  luteinizing hormone surge,
    147–149
    blockage of, 147–149
  natural, ovarian, 140–143
    stimulation, gonadotropic,
      147–157
  stimulation, gonadotropic,
    147–157
  terminology, 143–146
  see Cohort, Dominance, Follic-
    ulogenesis, Hormonogensis,
    Recruitment
Cynomolgus monkey, 5, 11–15, 18,
  20, 41
Cytokeratin, 27
Cytoskeleton, 241–243

1,2-Diacylglycerol, 84, 180, 184
Diethylstilbestrol (DES), 11, 13,
  14, 170
Diglyceride, 180
20α-Dihydroprogesterone, 176
5α-Dihydrotestosterone, 70
Dominance, follicular, 146

Embryo
  culture, 120, 262
  development, 120
    after transfer, 128
  fertilization in vitro, 49
  loss during pregnancy, 119, 127
  pre-embryo concept, 263
  transfer therapy, 49, 139
  two-cell theory, 149–156
  wastage, 119, 127
Endometrium, 256
Epidermal growth factor, 26, 29,
  30, 38, 116, 238
Epostane, 94
17β-Estradiol, 6, 7, 14–20, 29, 38,
  40, 49–52, 55, 62, 68, 70,
  79, 95, 96, 121, 122,
  129–133, 147, 149–151, 154,
  171, 172, 216, 251–256

Estrogen, 10, 11, 17, 27, 42,
  50–52, 56, 68, 79, 95, 147,
  153, 170–171, 212, 216,
  252
  effects, 11–16
  and follicle-stimulating
    hormone treatment, 14–15
  and regression, luteal, 170–171
Estrone, 212

Fertility of female, 140, 200
Fertilization
  assessment, 125
  description of human, 265
  in vitro, 49, 119–159, 262
    embryo transfer therapy, 49,
      139–159
  polyspermy, 125
Fetus
  a person?, 262
  viability, limit of, 262
  viable has legal rights, 262
  and wrongful birth, 262
Fibroblast growth factor, 25, 26,
  30, 39, 116, 117
Fluid, follicular, see Separate
  steroids
Fluorescence photobleaching
  recovery, 239–244
Follicle, 140, 142
  activation, 252
  antral, 4, 5, 9–15, 54, 63, 65,
    77, 79, 250, 252
  cavity, 250
  cohort, 144
  cyclic, 113–114
  development, 3, 7, 25–33
    and gonadotropin, 25–33
    and growth factors, 25–33
    and regulation, hormonal, 25–33
  dominant, 3, 6–10, 114, 146
  factors, 250
  feature, morphological, 3–11
  fluid, 5, 49, 250, see separate
    hormones
  graafian, 77, 78, 99, 250
  human, preovulatory, 64
  maturation, 3–23
    and atresia, 3–23
    induced, 143
    and stimulation, hormonal,
      11–15
  phase, 250
  preovulatory, 54–55, 64
  primordial, 6
  protein, regulatory, 49–60
  purine in, 81
  recruitment, 144–145, 252
  response to gonadotropin, 49–60
  rupture, 97, 99, 104, 105
  selection by ovary, 3, 252–254

Follicle (continued)
  size distribution, 63
  stimulation, 4
Follicle regulatory protein, 253
Follicle stimulating hormone (FSH),
      6, 11, 14-20, 28, 37-39,
      42, 49, 51, 61, 65-69, 79,
      80, 84-86, 91, 92, 95-97,
      103-105, 122, 143, 147,
      149, 153-156, 208, 251-255
    see Inhibin
  releasing protein, 26, 41
Folliculogenesis, 3-7, 61, 62, 140,
      143, 144
Forskolin, 37-40, 80, 93, 213

GLOH, see Hormone, ovarian,
      gonadotropin-like
Glycoprotein, 241, 243
Gonadotropin, 6, 7, 10, 40, 78-80,
      85, 175, 177, 182, 191-203
  antibody against, 208
  bioassay, 143
  and catecholamine, 196-197
  and cell, luteal, 238-245
  chorionic, 208-216
    action, mechanism of, 208-210
    and corpus luteum response,
        208-216
    human, see human chorionic
    in rhesus monkey, 207
    in woman, 207
  composition, 237-238
  and corpus luteum response,
      208-216
  and cycle, ovarian, 145-157
  discovery (1927), 208
  and follicle development, 25-33
  growth factor interaction, 25-33
  human
    chorionic, 38-41, 67, 69, 92,
        95-104, 119, 123, 125,
        128-131, 163-166, 169, 171,
        172, 207-216, 228-230,
        237-248
    menopausal, 49-52, 141-145
  menopausal, human, 49-52, 141-145
  and prostaglandin, 197-198
  radioimmunoassay (RIA), 35
  and relaxin, 228-229
  stimulation, 49-60
  theory, 149-157
  therapy, 150-155
Gonadotropin releasing hormone,
      38, 39
  ovarian (GLOH), 91-93, 183
Granulosa cell, ovarian, 6, 8, 9,
      11, 12, 14, 27-30, 43,
      49-54, 78, 80, 99, 101-103,
      113, 117, 122, 149, 177,
      180, 197, 212, 251-254

Granulosa cell, ovarian
      (continued)
  and angiogenic factor, 30
  culture, 65-71
  differentiation, 61-73
  and estrogen, 42
  and fibroblast growth factor, 26
  and follicle stimulating hormone,
      65
    responsiveness, 65-71
  and inhibin biosynthesis, 38-42
  and luteinizing hormone, 65-68
  number of, 63-64
  and steroidogenesis, 50-52
Growth factor
  and follicle, 25-33
  -gonadotropin interaction, 25-33
  groups, listed, 25
    epidermal, 25, 26
    fibroblast, 25, 26
    insulin-like, 25, 26
    platelet-derived, 26
    transforming, 25, 26
  production, 29-30
  responsiveness, 26-28
Guanosine, 83
Guanine nucleotide, 213
Guanosine triphosphate, 84
GVB, see Vesicle, germinal

Heparin, 115, 117
Heteroactivin, 41, 43
Homoactivin, 41, 43
Hormone
  internalization, 238-239, 244
  ovarian, 182, 183
    see separate hormones
Hormonogenesis, 144
17α-Hydroxylase/C17, 20-1yase, 52
3β-Hydroxysteroid dehydrogenase,
      50-52, 55
Hypophysectomy, 153
Hyperprolactinemia, 148
Hypothalamus, 163
Hypoxanthine, 81-85, 122
Hysterectomy, 176, 181, 256

Implantation and prostaglandin I_2,
      193
Indomethacin, 96-99, 182
Inhibin, 6, 26, 35-47, 50, 251-255
  A, 36
  adenosine monophosphate, 38
  antibody, monoclonal, against,
      36, 37
  B, 36
  biosynthesis in granulosa cell,
      38-42
  characterization, 36
  chromatography, 36
  cloning of subunit, 36-37

Inhibin (continued)
  effect, paracrine, 42–43
  in fluid, follicular, 36
  follicle stimulating hormone,
      pituitary, 35, 39
    suppression of, 35
  nomenclature, 35
  ovarian, 39
  protein, related to, 41–42
  purification, 36
  regulation, hormonal, 37–41
    ovarian, 37–40
    testicular, 40–41
  research advances, 35–47
  role of, 251–252
  subunit
    cloning, 36–37
    sequence, 36–37
Inosine, 82, 83
Inositol 1,4,5,-triphosphate, 84,
      179, 180, 184
Insect egg development
  inhibition of, 182
Insulin, 39, 238
  receptor, 244
Insulin-like growth factor (IGF),
      25–29, 39, 50
Internalization of hormone,
      238–239, 244
Ionomycin, 179
3-Isobutyl-1-methylxanthine, 80,
      93, 95
Isoproterenol, 197, 198

Lactogen, placental, 229
Leydig cell, 35, 42, 43, 238
Life
  and spermatozoon, 265
  when does it begin?, 264
Lipoprotein, low density, 28, 29
Luteinization, 10
Luteinizing hormone (LH), 38, 39,
      42, 61, 62, 67, 69, 91–98,
      102–104, 122, 147, 153–155,
      163–174, 177, 178, 181,
      183, 185
  blockade, 147–148
  and cell, luteal, 238
  composition, 237–238
  ovine, 237–248
  pituitary, 254–255
  and progesterone, 164
  receptor, see Receptor
    aggregation, 244
    interaction, 244
    mobility, 239–245
  regression, 256
  see Gonadotropin
Luteolysin, 170, 175–189
  uterine, 175, 176
  see Prostaglandin

Luteolysis, 62, 64, 68, 69, 71,
      168–170, 175–189, 194, 210,
      212
  definition, 175–176
  mechanism of, 175–189
  model
    functional, 185
    structural, 185
  in nonprimate, 176–181
  in primate, 181–182
  by prostaglandin, 62, 64, 68–71,
      194
  structural, 176, 185

Macaque, see Rhesus monkey
Marmoset monkey, 61–73
  granulosa cell culture, 64–71
  ovary, 61–73
Maturation defect, cytoplasmic,
      121, 127
Medroxyprogesterone acetate, 208
Meiosis, 77
  and gonadotropin, 77
Meiotic arrest, 80–84, 122
1-Methyladenine, 86
Mink lung, 26
Monensin, 179
Mouse, 79, 80
Mullerian inhibiting substance,
      29, 37
Mycophenolic acid, 83

Noradrenaline, 196–199
Nucleotide, cyclic, 93–94
Nucleotide, see Guanine

Oocyte, 5, 8, 124–125, 254
  arrest, see Arrest, meiotic
  denuded, 81, 82, 85, 86
  in graafian follicle, 77
  growth, 77–90
  immature, 130–134
  mammalian, 77–90
  maturation, 77–90, 119–137
    control in vitro, 86
Ouabain, 178, 179
Ovary
  angiogenesis, see Angiogenesis
  anovulation, 55–56
  artery, 191, 193
  component, 3
  cortex, 4–8, 18
  of cynomolgus monkey, see
      Cynomolgus monkey
  development, capillary, 113–118
  dysfunction, 55–56
  factor, local, 191–205
  fertilization in vitro, 139–159
    see Fertilization
  and follicle selection, 3

Ovary (continued)
  and hormone, see separate
      hormones
  of human, 51
  hyperstimulation, 123, 124,
      147-149
  and inhibin, see Inhibin
  muscle contraction, 98
  perfused, 97, 99
  phase
    follicular, 64, 250-254
    luteal, 62, 64
  of primate, 249-259, see
      separate monkeys
  of rhesus monkey, 4-12
  section, 4
  sonogram, 142
  of squirrel monkey, see
      Squirrel monkey
  stimulation, 139-159
  superstimulation, see hyper-
  terminology, 143-146
  vein, 191, 193
Ovulation, 91-111
Oxytocin, 176-177, 181, 212,
    230, 256

Paracrine system, see System
Peptide, intestinal
  vasoactive (VIP), 39
Phenanthroline, 102
Phorbol ester, 84, 94
Phosphatidylserine, 180
Phosphodiesterase inhibitor, 38-41
Phospholipase C, 84, 179
Phosphorescence anisotropy
  time-resolved, 244
Plasmin, 102-105
Plasminogen, 104
  activator, 86, 94, 102-104
Platelet-derived growth factor,
    26-28
Polyspermy, 125
Pre-embryo concept, 263
Pregnancy
  "biochemical," 120
  early, 191-194, 207-220, 223
  human
    early, 191-194
    ectopic, 200, 203
      termination, 200, 203
    loss of, 226
    termination, 208
Pregnenolone, 51
Primate, see separate monkeys
Progesterone, 6, 7, 10, 27, 28,
    49-52, 62, 65-71, 94-96,
    121, 129-133, 149, 155,
    156, 163-172 175-177, 179,
    185, 192-203, 207-209,
    211-213, 225, 228-230,

Progesterone (continued)
    238, 251-256
Progestin, 151
  synthetic, see Medroxyproges-
      terone acetate
Prolactin, 38-41, 177, 229
Propranolol, 199-202
Prostaglandin, 184
  and catecholamine, 199
  and corpus luteum, human, 191-205
  D_2, 213
  E_2, 93, 96-99, 191-194, 197,
      214, 230
  $F_{2\alpha}$, 62, 64, 68, 175-182,
      194-196, 199-202, 212,
      213, 229
  and gonadotropin, 197-198
  I_2, 193-195, 213
  and termination of pregnancy,
      200, 203
Protein, 52-55, 182-183
Proteinase, 99-104
  metalloproteinase, 101, 102
  see Collagenase
Protein kinase
  A, 39
  C, 39, 84, 94, 105, 180-181,
Purine, 81, 83

Radioimmunoassay, 35, 37, 39
Rat, 26, 35, 79, 97
Receptor of luteinizing hormone
  antibody, monoclonal, 245
  cytoskeleton, 241-243
  diffusion, lateral, 240-244
  immobilization, 240-243
  internalization, 238-239, 244
  mobility, 239-245
  movement, rotational, 244-245
Recruitment, follicular, 144-145
Relaxin, 208, 216, 217
  decidual, 230-231
  extraluteal, 230-231
  luteal secretion, 228-230
  ovarian, 223-236
    analog, 224
    antibody, 224-227
    bioassay, 224-225
    function, 223-236
    guinea pig assay, 225
    history, 223-224
    immunoreactive, 227
    and luteectomy, 226
    measurement, 224-225
    in plasma, seminal, 224
    production, 223-236
    and progesterone, 225
    purification, 224
    radioimmunoassay (RIA), 224-227
    in rhesus monkey, 226, 228
    secretion in woman, 223-226

Relaxin (continued)
  ovarian (continued)
    structure, 224
  placental, 230-231
  in pregnancy, 231-232
    early, 223-226
  uterine, 230-231
Reproduction
  experimentation, 261-266
  issues, societal, 261-266
  research, 261-266
Research, reproductive
  American attitudes, 263
  British attitudes, 263
  issues, societal, 261-266
  Warnock report, 263
Rhesus monkey, 65, 66, 119-137,
        150, 182, 207-217, 226, 228
  corpus luteum, 163-174
  oocyte maturation, 119-137
  oocyte fertilization in vitro,
    124-125

Scatchard analysis, 28
Serine protease plasmin, 100
Sertoli cell, 35, 40-43
  and inhibin production, 40, 41
Sodium, 179
Somatomedin-C, 26
Squirrel monkey
  ovary, 5, 7

Steroidogenesis, 26, 27, 30, 50-52,
        65, 70, 94, 95, 143, 168
Stimulation, ovarian, 139-159
Superovulation, 119
Surrogate primate female, 139-159
Syncytiotrophoblast, 207, 210
System, paracrine, 56

Testis and inhibin production, 40
Testosterone, 35, 50, 68-71,
        251, 252
Theca
  cell, 42, 52, 53, 149, 251
  interna, 6-9, 113
Thyroid-stimulating hormone, 208
Tranexamic acid, 103
Transforming growth factor, 25-29,
        37, 50, 116
Tumor and angiogenesis, 114
Tyrosine kinase, 39

Urokinase, 86
Uterus, 176-177
  removal, 176, 181, 256

Vesicle, germinal
  breakdown, 77-80
Vimentin, 27

Walker 256 carcinoma, 115-116